Consent To Cure

Using Holistic Options And Personal Empowerment to Reclaim Health

Judy Magalhaes, PHARMD, BCGP, CDCES

DISCLAIMER

The ideas shared in this book are meant to educate and empower you on your health journey. They are not a substitute for personalized medical advice, diagnosis, or treatment. Every person's body and health history are unique, so please consult your physician or qualified healthcare provider before making changes to your diet, lifestyle, or medications. The author shares information with the intention of inspiring informed choices, but cannot be responsible for how you apply it. Always partner with your healthcare team to determine what is right for you. The author and publisher disclaim any liability for any medical outcomes that may occur as a result of applying the methods suggested in this book.

To my family, whose love and strength have carried me; to my pastors, whose faith and wisdom have guided me; and to every patient who has trusted me on their journey. May this book remind you that we are fearfully and wonderfully made, created to heal, and that true restoration comes through God, the ultimate source of healing and HOPE.

ABOUT THE AUTHOR

Judy Magalhaes is a Doctor of Pharmacy, Board Certified Geriatric Pharmacist, Certified Diabetes Care and Education Specialist, and Lifestyle Coach, who believes true healing happens where science meets faith. As founder and CEO of Holistic Options & Personal Empowerment (HOPE, LLC), she brings over 30 years of clinical experience in diverse healthcare settings, blending functional-medicine principles with natural, holistic strategies that honor your mind, body, and spirit. In these pages, she delivers a compassionate, science-backed roadmap to break free from chronic disease, achieve and maintain long-term health, and rediscover genuine hope. Are you ready to reclaim your health—and your life?

FOREWORD

It is my honor to write this foreword for my dear colleague and friend, Dr. Judy Magalhaes. Judy has been part of my journey since the earliest days of the STORRIE Institute®, where she stood as one of the founding members of what we called the Wholistic Vitality Revolution. Her courage to reimagine her career as a pharmacist and to step into a more holistic and faith-driven approach to healing has inspired me and countless others.

In 2022, Dr. Judy became a bestselling author when she contributed her powerful story, From Pain to Purpose, in Creating the Functional Medicine Revolution. In those pages, she shared how personal health struggles, the toll of the pandemic, and decades in conventional pharmacy led her to a breaking point. That breaking point became the foundation of her purpose: to bring holistic healing, rooted in functional medicine and faith, to people who are tired of being stuck in survival mode.

What makes Dr. Judy's work extraordinary is her ability to weave together science and soul. She integrates functional lab testing, gut health, detoxification, nutrition, sleep, stress management, and lifestyle strategies with faith and spiritual grounding. Her HOPE Method - Empower, Test, Optimize - is more than a framework; it is a philosophy of healing that honors the whole person: mind, body, and spirit.

I've watched Judy evolve from student to colleague, from a pharmacist on the edge of burnout to a visionary leader creating lasting transformation for her clients. She has walked the path herself, and that authenticity is what makes her voice so trustworthy.

Consent to Cure is not just another health book. It is a movement of hope. It reminds us that true healing is possible when we seek root causes, trust the body's innate ability to heal, and anchor ourselves in faith. For anyone who feels stuck, depleted, or dismissed by conventional care, this book is a lifeline.

I am so proud of Dr. Judy for the woman she has become, the healer she has grown into, and the hope she brings to the world. May this book guide you, as it has guided so many, to reclaim your health and live with renewed vitality.

Dr. Christine Manukyan, PharmD, M.S.

Founder & CEO STORRIE Institute®, Fractional Chief Vitality Officer, Creator of NeuroBreathwork®, 6x No.1 international Bestselling Author, Wholistic Vitality® Podcast Host, Keynote Speaker

ENDORSEMENTS

Dr. Judy Magalhaes has turned her pain into purpose, and *Consent to Cure* is the powerful result. Drawing from 30+ years as a pharmacist, her own health journey, and her faith, she shows us what true healing looks like - mind, body, and spirit. With biblical wisdom, functional medicine insights, and her HOPE Method (Empower, Test, Optimize), Dr. Judy equips readers to move beyond managing disease to reclaiming vitality. This book is both a roadmap and a reminder that healing is possible when we seek the root cause, trust the body's design, and anchor ourselves in faith.

Dr. Christine Manukyan, PharmD, M.S.

Founder & CEO STORRIE Institute®, Fractional Chief Vitality Officer, Creator of NeuroBreathwork®, 6x No.1 international Bestselling Author, Wholistic Vitality® Podcast Host, Keynote Speaker

I commend Dr. Magalhaes to see beyond the confines of pharmaceutical medicine and journey through a truly holistic path to her health. I applaud her sharing that journey so that others may also find real health.

David Baltimore, MD, ND
President & CEO at Baltimore Laboratories, Inc. Monroe, Connecticut, United States

Dr. Judy Magalhaes' profound insight in *Consent to Cure*—"healing requires a combination of faith and science"—deeply resonated with me. Over two decades ago, I came to a similar realization that changed the course of my life and career. I transitioned into counseling, guided by the conviction that true healing involves more than clinical methods; it requires faith.

Through years of working with individuals facing emotional, mental, and physical challenges, I've witnessed that transformation often begins not with a treatment plan, but with a simple belief: that healing is possible. As Judy so powerfully writes, "Healing starts with a single step—and sometimes, that step is simply believing that it's possible." Her words echo the timeless truth found in Mark 9:23, "All things are possible for the one who believes."

Dr. Judy's journey of personal healing led her to a powerful discovery: that integrating science with unwavering faith can open doors conventional approaches often cannot. In *Consent to Cure*, she shares not only her story but a divine framework for healing that invites us to trust, believe, and step into wholeness.

This book is more than a resource—it's a roadmap to transformation. I wholeheartedly recommend *Consent to Cure* to anyone seeking healing, whether physical, emotional, or spiritual. It is a compelling testament to the power of faith meeting science.

Lois Flewelling, LCPC
Author, Tenacious Warrior, Author, Speaker, Coach
www.loisflewelling.com

Demystifying functional medicine page by page, chapter by chapter, this book is an intelligent, down-to-earth explanation of a powerful medical alternative that is both transformational and more accessible than most realize.

Dr. Judy has taken her decades of clinical medical training and experience, opened her mind and heart to companion or alternative treatments, and is now using all these skills to change health trajectories, prevent disease, and support an overall, holistic wellness model. If you care about preserving your good health or are frustrated with the traditional system that has failed to produce long-lasting or sustainable results, Dr. Judy is the expert, and this is the book you need NOW!

Jennifer Vaughn

Best-selling and Award Winning author of fiction
and narrative nonfiction, Award Winning TV News Anchor.

Dr. Judy Magalhaes has written a powerful and deeply needed book that brings clarity, compassion, and practical wisdom to the world of holistic health. Drawing from her decades of experience as a pharmacist and her personal journey of reversing chronic disease, she offers readers not just information but true empowerment.

What makes this work exceptional is how it weaves together science, faith, and lived experience into a framework that is both accessible and transformative. By guiding readers from "sick care" toward true health, Dr. Magalhaes provides a blueprint for reclaiming vitality—through nutrition, sleep, stress resilience, movement, detoxification, and the strength of community.

The concepts she writes about are a gift for patients and practitioners alike: one that puts root-cause healing back where it belongs—in the hands of those seeking lasting change. This book will inspire and equip anyone ready to take ownership of their health and live with purpose.

I wholeheartedly recommend this book as an essential resource for anyone seeking to bridge the gap between conventional medicine and a truly holistic model of lifelong wellness.

Dr. Dan Kalish,

Founder, Kalish Institute of Functional Medicine

TABLE OF CONTENTS

FROM PAIN TO PURPOSE

Faith shows the reality of what we hope for;
It is the evidence of things we cannot see.

— Hebrews 11:1 (NLT)

Have you ever felt as though your body is betraying you? Symptoms seem to continually creep into your life—a headache here, an ache there, a sleepless night every so often. You brush them off, thinking they're just transient annoyances. But, as time goes by, they build up, little by little, until every day feels like a struggle. Thank you for picking up this book. Maybe you've looked for an answer to your condition for a while, only to be told to take yet another drug to manage your symptoms. You take more and more medications, but you don't get better. If you're reading this, you're not alone. I've been there. For more than 30 years, I worked as a pharmacist, where I guided others in managing their chronic conditions. I thought I understood health. But nothing in my training or experience prepared me for the moment my own body began to break down.

It started with fatigue. At first, I dismissed it. Maybe I just needed more rest. Then I began having sharper headaches, some digestive issues, and *relentless* exhaustion. Slowly but surely, my health seemed to unravel on me. Traditional treatments—the same ones I had spent my career recommending to patients—offered me no relief. I became trapped in the same endless cycle I had witnessed so many patients get stuck in.

By the time I acknowledged the full extent of my symptoms, I could barely function. The realization that something had to change set me on a path of discovery—one that would redefine my entire understanding of health and healing!

You might be reading this book because you feel trapped in a similar pattern—where conventional care just hasn't worked, and nothing seems to help. As a pharmacist, I thought I had all the tools to maintain good health. Yet, despite my background in healthcare, I found myself caught in a spiral of worsening chronic conditions. My symptoms began to take over my life, and there seemed to be no relief. All of this pain and fatigue crept into my life so gradually that I failed to see all the warning signs. I dismissed the headaches and chalked up the exhaustion to age, hormones, and stress. However, by late 2020, I could no longer ignore the reality. The fatigue became crushing, making almost every normal action seem overwhelming. I had migraines, accompanied by severe back pain that robbed me of both rest and mobility.

But my situation was far from unique. The pandemic we were facing had pushed many patients to their limits. People were isolated, afraid of seeking medical care, and struggling with their physical and emotional well-being. I saw this firsthand while working in long-term and primary care settings. Their symptoms worsened in isolation—and yet I, too, was unraveling under the same pressure. Despite my expertise, I felt lost in a fog of symptoms that seemed to defy the solutions I knew of. The patients I treated expressed similar frustrations—chronic symptoms, a long list of medications, and no real recovery. Something had to change! I needed to understand *why* my body was breaking down. That moment of crisis became the turning point that set me on a journey toward true healing—a journey that would challenge and ultimately transform my entire perspective on health and wellness.

The Breaking Point

December 2020 marked a turning point. My body had reached its limit. After months of struggling with worsening symptoms—debilitating back pain, migraines, relentless fatigue and finally succumbed to COVID—I was forced to step away from my work. I could no longer manage my day-to-day responsibilities or find relief through the treatments I had so long trusted. This wasn't just regular exhaustion from stress; it was my body telling me that something was deeply wrong. Many of my patients were in a similar situation, caught in a cycle of symptoms without any answers. They would return to have their medication adjusted, but their conditions remained unchanged.

I had spent years advising them on how to manage their diseases, but now I saw how inadequate that approach could be. The pandemic made this even clearer! People were so isolated, overwhelmed by the emotional and mental stress, and unable to access proper care due to the situation. Their physical and emotional health deteriorated rapidly. Despite my clinical expertise, I found myself lost in that same desperation. Conventional medicine was failing me—just as it had for so many others. It became obvious that I couldn't continue down this path. I needed to uncover the root causes of my symptoms. This realization drove me to seek new answers and set me on a journey of healing and transformation that challenged everything I had once believed about "health care".

Functional Medicine – A New Path

It was during this search for answers that I discovered functional medicine. Unlike conventional approaches that primarily focus on suppressing symptoms, functional medicine is for the root cause(s). Why was I in so much pain? What underlying imbalances were contributing to my fatigue, migraines, back pain, and anxiety? Instead of diagnosing and treating each issue I had separately, functional medicine offered a comprehensive view—examining how different systems in the body work together and where those systems had broken down. Functional medicine changed the way I thought about health and healing. I learned how inflammation, nutrient imbalances, and hormonal dysregulation could silently undermine our well-being, just like they had for me.

This approach illuminated connections I hadn't considered before: how stress could affect our digestion, how toxic exposure might disrupt our hormones, and how deficiencies in key minerals could weaken the body's ability to recover. One of the first steps I took was undergoing functional testing to understand my own unique needs. Functional testing involves a series of specific diagnostic tools that are designed to evaluate key areas of our health, like our hormone levels, nutrient balance, gut health, inflammatory markers, and toxin exposure. These tests provide a detailed look at how the body's systems are functioning and where imbalances may lie. So, my tests revealed imbalances that had been overlooked for years. These discoveries were eye-opening! I wasn't simply dealing with isolated symptoms—my entire system was out of alignment. Functional medicine gave me the tools I needed to begin restoring balance through targeted nutrition, detoxification, and lifestyle adjustments. Bit by bit, small changes led to noticeable improvements. The debilitating pain and exhaustion began to subside, and I felt a renewed sense of hope.

This shift in mindset was transformative. Functional medicine empowered me to take control of my health in a way I never had before. It was no longer about endless prescriptions or another kind of drug. It was about creating lasting wellness by supporting my body's ability to heal itself. I realized that this approach held a lot of promise, not just for me, but for the many patients I had seen with no changes. This new path became the foundation for my healing journey and, eventually, the cornerstone of my work at HOPE.

The Role of Faith In Healing

Healing is not just a physical journey—it is deeply tied to the emotional and spiritual aspects of who we are. During the pandemic, I witnessed firsthand the heavy toll that isolation and fear took on patients. Many were trapped in their homes, scared, overwhelmed by anxiety, and unable to meet even basic self-care needs. I felt helpless as a consultant pharmacist, trying to navigate a landscape without evidence-based protocols to guide treatment. Telehealth, although available to some, was ineffective for many others who lacked the necessary technology. The emotional burden was *immense*—on both patients and providers alike. The stress of these circumstances was a big part of me reaching my breaking point in late 2020. I had reached a point of *complete* exhaustion, physically and mentally. My symptoms worsened under the weight of the professional burnout I felt and the suffering I witnessed on a daily basis. At this lowest moment, I realized I needed more than physical healing. I needed faith to guide me through. One scripture that became a beacon of hope was <u>3 John 1:2 (NLT)</u>, which says,

"Dear friend, I hope all is well with you and that you are as healthy in body as you are strong in spirit."

This verse reminded me of the importance of inner strength and trust in something greater than myself. When everything else failed, faith provided me with the resilience to persevere. It offered the peace I needed to continue the hard work of recovery.

Spirituality became a vital complement to my healing process. Through prayer, meditation, and reflection, I found the strength to let go of fear and anxiety. Gradually, as I nourished my mind and spirit alongside my body, I began to see tangible progress. Faith gave me the patience to endure when improvements were slow and incremental. It kept my hope alive when giving up seemed so much easier. This integration of science and faith ended up shaping my entire perspective on holistic healing. I learned that true wellness has to involve the mind and spirit, as well as the body. Faith, I found, helps us believe in the unseen—in the possibility of renewal even in the darkest of moments. It is a powerful force that still continues to guide me and those I serve on the path to lasting transformation!

The Founding of HOPE

The creation of HOPE—Holistic Options & Personal Empowerment marked both the culmination of my journey and a fresh start. This initiative was inspired by the realization that healing requires a combination of faith *and* science. It became clear through my own experience—both personal and professional—that conventional medicine's focus on merely symptom management often left many without true relief. In emergency care, our conventional healthcare system is unprecedented. However, in terms of chronic disease, the purpose should be to regain health or prevent illness, not just "manage symptoms." Developing this program came with its obstacles. Introducing a model that integrated functional medicine and spiritual empowerment challenged a lot of traditional thinking.

Yet, I knew from experience that addressing only the physical or spiritual aspects separately was insufficient for long-term well-being.

This program was designed to provide support for those who feel stuck, depleted, and overlooked by the conventional system.

The foundation of the program rests on six essential habits:

1. Healthy eating
2. Optimizing sleep
3. Managing stress
4. Being physically active
5. Reducing toxins, and
6. Nurturing our social connections

These habits reflect a commitment to holistic care, where healing begins by attending to the body (and person) as a whole. Through functional testing and personalized plans, it's possible to uncover hidden imbalances like hormonal disruptions or nutrient deficiencies and learn how to actively restore a person's health. Faith also plays a crucial role. I always encourage clients to integrate spiritual practices like prayer or meditation into their day. These practices offer us inner peace, resilience, and clarity—tools that can sustain progress even through the setbacks we'll undoubtedly face.

The connection between spiritual grounding and physical recovery strengthens every person's healing journey. The launch of this program during a global crisis was like fate expressing the necessity of its value.

The pandemic exposed critical weaknesses in our healthcare system and deepened the mistrust many patients already felt. It also highlighted the importance of empowering people to reclaim their well-being and to show them that there is a way for them to take their health into their own hands. My mission, started through hardship, continues today: to provide healing, transformation, and empowerment to those who need it most!

What HOPE Can Offer

When someone reaches out for help through HOPE, they are often overwhelmed by a host of chronic symptoms—exhaustion, autoimmunity, brain fog, digestive issues, or unrelenting chronic pain. Many have seemingly exhausted the solutions of conventional healthcare that appear available to them. The core philosophy of HOPE is to change that narrative by targeting root causes through functional medicine and lifestyle transformation. One of the foundational tools we use is functional lab testing. Unlike routine lab tests that focus on diagnosing specific conditions, functional tests dig deeper to evaluate how well the body's systems are working. These assessments can uncover unidentified hormonal imbalances, specific nutritional deficiencies, immune or inflammatory markers, disrupted gut microbiome, and toxin loads that may be contributing to someone's symptoms.

We start with functional lab testing, which digs beneath the surface to assess how the body's systems are actually functioning. These tests look at markers like your hormones, gut health, nutrient levels, and toxin loads—factors that conventional tests often overlook. The results help us identify what's driving a person's symptoms and give us the foundation for a more personalized approach to the *why* of their condition. From there, we move on to a personalized consultation. Here, I take the time to learn each person's full story—their medical history, their daily habits, and their story. Together, we develop a plan that's tailored to their needs. I guide them through their test results and help them take ownership of their recovery journey. A major part of that journey is lifestyle coaching. Making lasting improvements isn't easy, which is why we focus on these six core habits. These habits all work together to promote deep, lasting healing, as we cannot really be healthy if one of these habits is not maintained. Spiritual health is equally important. Chronic illness, of course, often leads to discouragement and signs of depression or anxiety, but nurturing the mind and spirit can create a renewed sense of purpose and hope!

An Invitation To Begin Your Journey!

Healing starts with a single step—and sometimes, that step is simply believing that it's possible! If you're holding this book, you may already feel weighed down by the struggle of managing an illness that just never seems to go away. You might be tired of hearing that this or that is going to help. I understand that! You may feel like you have tried *everything,* only to get worse. But I'm here to tell you that healing can happen. Not overnight, and not through a magic pill or shortcuts. It starts with small, intentional steps that build momentum. Real healing begins when you decide to stop accepting survival as your "new normal" and start thinking with "healthy" as a way of living. But where do you start?

Everything in this book has been designed to help you take those steps. One choice at a time—whether it's focusing on your sleep, changing how you eat, or simply pausing to reflect and do some mindfulness—leads to transformation. The body has an incredible capacity to heal when you support it fully. I have walked this path. I have felt the fatigue that may cloud your mind and the pain that leaves you unable to face the day. I also know how freeing it feels when those debilitating symptoms begin to lift. That's why I'm committed to guiding you through this process. Faith carried me when nothing else did. It reminded me that even when progress is invisible, it's still unfolding. I want you to trust that, too. You're not alone in this journey, and I want you to know that real healing is within reach. I have experienced this myself. I know what it feels like to be trapped in a cycle of chronic fatigue, pain, and anxiety.

And I also know the relief that comes when the body and mind begin to recover. My mission with this program is to walk alongside you, offering the tools and support needed to help you reclaim your health and well-being. I encourage you to begin today by taking one meaningful step forward. You don't have to do this alone. Transformation is possible. Healing is possible. And I am honored to be part of your journey toward lasting wellness.

PART 1

The Real Problem
And The Why

CHAPTER 1

An Introduction To Holistic Health

Hope deferred makes the heart sick, but a dream fulfilled is a tree of life.

— Proverbs 13:12 (NLT)

For years, I worked as a pharmacist, helping people manage chronic diseases such as high blood pressure, diabetes, and lung disease. My job was to dispense medications and educate my patients on how to use them effectively. However, something was missing in this picture. Week after week, month after month, I would still see the same patients, with the same struggles, stuck in a cycle of worsening symptoms while their prescription roster steadily expanded. It was frustrating—for me and for them.

My pharmacy career started in retail- "dispensing" medications, ensuring the prescribed drug was safe and appropriate for the patient. Performing a medication review with each order, looking for drug-drug interactions, allergy checks, and confirming the drug and dose were correct for the patient's age and indication being treated. The worst part was dealing with insurance plans when a medication was denied or having to switch to another drug that was less optimal for the patient's condition, because that's what was covered by their plan.

I transitioned into an acute care (hospital) setting, where I was part of a medical team working in the Critical Care Unit. My role was to assist doctors in selecting medication therapies based on clinical practice guidelines and evidence-based practices. Some of the most common reasons for CCU admissions were pneumonia, heart failure, stroke, myocardial infarction, urinary tract infections, and sepsis (a condition with multi-organ failure due to "cytokine storm," which many became familiar with during COVID). I was responsible for reviewing medications and adjusting regimens to ensure the safety, efficacy, and appropriateness of prescribed therapies. I would say that this was the highlight of my career, as I knew we were "saving lives" every day with the help of pharmaceutical interventions (aka medications).

Yet, it didn't take long until overwhelming stress, fatigue, and burnout consumed me, negatively impacting my own health. These were the primary reasons for leaving my hospital job.

My next experience was working in primary care. This opportunity allowed me to work with providers and patients in one setting, something I've always enjoyed. However, it wasn't until working in this setting that I realized how "sick" people were. Yes, it was different from the hospital, where I expected to take care of critically ill patients, but in an ambulatory care setting, it was worse because people were living with so much disease, and in my opinion, a reduced quality of life despite all the medications they were taking to treat their diseases. I was helping people "manage medications" for chronic diseases- hypertension, diabetes, chronic obstructive pulmonary disease (COPD), etc. No one was getting better, no disease was cured or reversed, more and more medications were added to treat symptoms, and it just kept getting worse. Add to this skyrocketing drug costs and subsequent insurance denials, promulgating the chronic disease epidemic.

In my final effort to continue working as a pharmacist, I tried consulting in long-term care (LTC) facilities. This was one of the most difficult positions I had. Witnessing the impact and burden of chronic disease in older adults. In 2023, the CDC estimated 76.4% of US adults reported 1 or more chronic conditions: Alzheimer's, diabetes, hypertension, lung disease, kidney disease, stroke, and cancer.[1] The chronic disease epidemic contributes to $1.4 trillion in annual healthcare costs. This also leads to increased prescribing of medications to help manage disease- the average number of medications for individuals in LTC is seven. [2]

I was spinning my wheels, feeling helpless, realizing I was unable to change a system that was focused on "sick care," not true health care, and certainly not focused on prevention of disease.

Along came COVID…and I broke (again).

This changed everything; I was no longer the pharmacist, I was the patient!

Looking back, I realize, as a healthcare provider, I was putting my patients first- I forgot to take care of my own health, and after years of neglecting my personal well-being, I had developed my own set of conditions: fatigue, anxiety, digestive issues, allergies, headaches, back pain, and unwanted weight gain.

I believe that my experience with COVID was rooted in my underlying poor health status. This virus took control of me in ways I could not imagine, and despite all my clinical knowledge and helping people manage their diseases, I was unable to help myself or climb out of the abyss. There was no "pill for my ill"; I was left without a solution.

To help myself, I started to research and explore other options. I began learning about nutrition and the incredible importance of our gut health. I learned about the interconnectedness of the mind, body, and spirit. This was not just eye-opening, it was life-changing.

I not only found solutions for myself, but I discovered an effective way to help others move beyond the endless cycle of symptom management to real and actual healing.

Reclaiming my health (and life) was not easy or quick, but this long and painful journey was necessary- a lesson for me to understand, because this is what brought me to where I am today- living and thriving again, and now I can give people HOPE, that they too can reclaim their health!

In the end, I came to the startling realization that managing illness is <u>not</u> the same as managing health.

In this chapter, you and I start that same journey. Together, we will redefine what real health means, explore the principles of holistic health, and understand why integrating the mind, body, and spirit is essential for true well-being. My hope is that you will see your health not as an absence of disease but as a vibrant, balanced way of living.

After thirty years as a clinical pharmacist, I have come to realize that our conventional healthcare system, while very effective at managing emergencies or critical care, it is unable—or perhaps unwilling—to truly address chronic disease. The system focuses on managing symptoms rather than identifying root causes, and it neglects preventive measures that could transform long-term health outcomes.

This chapter is about rethinking what health means. It's about moving beyond the "sick care" model that you may be stuck in, to embrace a proactive, integrative approach that connects your physical, mental, and spiritual well-being. Together, we will look at how these elements interact and why they are essential to achieving lasting health.

Question: What Drove My Shift From Conventional To Holistic Health?

As a pharmacist, I saw firsthand the limitations of conventional medicine. While medications might be able to chemically "manage" (or suppress) symptoms, they do not address the root cause of why you are sick in the first place. The same patients I saw would return month after month, their conditions unchanged, more medications prescribed, and their quality of life declining.

My own struggles brought this realization to life in a way I had never imagined. A diet I originally thought was healthy turned out to be the source of my mercury and copper toxicity. This imbalance disrupted everything, from my energy levels to my iron metabolism, and left me with symptoms that traditional blood tests were unable to detect.

It wasn't until I turned to functional medicine testing that I found real answers and could start to heal. This experience taught me that true health requires a proper look at <u>what</u> is happening inside the body, and what is causing the dysfunction (symptom). My energy was plummeting, I was full of inflammation, and traditional tests didn't provide any answers. Functional medicine testing, however, uncovered the imbalances I was experiencing, and addressing these changed everything for me. This experience reinforced what I already suspected: real healing requires looking at the whole person, not just isolated symptoms.

Question: What Does "Health" Really Mean?

Real health is not just the absence of disease. The World Health Organization defines it as "a state of complete physical, mental, and social well-being." True health goes further than this and requires balance between all aspects of life. It means having the energy to *live* fully (not just survive), and to have the clarity needed to think and function well, along with the resilience to face the challenges of life.

Wellness, meanwhile, is an active process. It's not something you achieve and then forget about. Rather, it is based on the daily choices you make to nourish your mind, body, and spirit. My hope is that this chapter challenges you to rethink health as something you can create and build, step-by-step, for a life of lasting wellness. That is why I will incorporate strategies for whole-body wellness, mindfulness-based stress reduction techniques, and spiritual references throughout this book while keeping in mind the power of faith in our healing journey.

Question: How Does Holistic Health Differ From Conventional Care?

Conventional care focuses solely on diagnosing disease and treating symptoms. This means they focus *on the symptom*, instead of what is causing it. Have a headache? Here's a pain reliever. High blood pressure? Well, you're prescribed medication for that, of course. High cholesterol? Here's a statin. While these treatments may be necessary for short-term management of symptoms, they do not do anything to remedy the cause of this condition. And unfortunately, providers do not have enough time, training, or incentives to prescribe nutrition and lifestyle therapies; it's too easy to prescribe a pill for it.

Holistic health—an approach that considers the whole person, including physical, mental, emotional, social, and spiritual well-being rather than just treating isolated symptoms or diseases—takes a broader view. It asks deeper questions about the causes of your symptoms. Questions about your diet, stress in your life, sleep, and even your emotional well-being. For example, chronic stress has been shown to lead to hormonal imbalances and digestive issues, which can disrupt your sleep and your immune system. Crohn's Disease, an Inflammatory Bowel Disease (IBD), is thought to have "no cure," but it is well-known that stress seems to have a powerful influence on this condition. When we address the root causes, this creates an opportunity for lasting healing. The interconnectedness of your mind, body, and spirit is central to this approach, as illustrated by <u>Luke 11:34 (ESV)</u>: *"Your eye is the lamp of your body. When your eye is healthy, your whole body is full of light."*

Question: Why Is The Connection Between Mind, Body, And Spirit So Important?

Because our mind, body, and spirit are so connected, stress doesn't just "live in your thoughts." It affects you physically, from your digestion, immune system, blood pressure, and energy levels. Faith and spiritual practice can restore balance to your life and bring a sense of calm that supports your physical *and* emotional health.

When we are in a state of constant mental or physical stress, simply loading up on a bunch of medications can be likened to throwing a wet towel over a gasoline-fueled fire pit. It's not going to put out the fire.

Holistic health recognizes these connections and encourages you to nurture all three aspects. The gut microbiome, for example, is an entire ecosystem that is vital to our health. It influences our mental health by producing neurotransmitters like serotonin and dopamine in the gut. Addressing gut health can not only improve digestion but also enhance our emotional resilience and mental clarity. By focusing on the whole person, we can create a foundation that sustains you in good health and promotes resilience.

Question: How Does Holistic Health Integrate Wellness Into Daily Life?

Holistic health isn't about making a series of dramatic overhauls to your life. Rather, it is based on small, consistent actions that build up over time to create sustainable and meaningful changes in your well-being.

It's about making choices that nourish your mind, body, and spirit each day—choices that align with your unique needs and values.

For instance, you can start with your diet. Nutrient diversity is very important to our health. Consuming fiber-rich foods promotes a healthy microbiome: increasing beneficial bacteria, gut barrier function, and metabolic byproducts that regulate mood, metabolism, and health. Eating fiber can also help reduce inflammation, yet fewer than 5% of Americans meet the daily fiber recommendation of 25–30 grams. Adding fermented foods, like kimchi, sauerkraut, or yogurt, can enhance your gut health by promoting the beneficial bacteria, while dietary sources of omega-3 fatty acids reduce systemic inflammation and support brain health.

These are practical, achievable steps toward better physical health that we can incorporate, step by step. Rest and sleep are equally critical. Regular, restful sleep restores your body and mind and enhances mental clarity and energy levels. Creating an environment that promotes good sleep—like a cool, dark, and quiet room—and reducing screen time before bed can significantly improve the quality of your rest. Furthermore, practicing calming activities such as prayer or journaling before you go to sleep can help align your mental and spiritual well-being.

Movement and exercise also don't have to mean intense workouts at the gym for hours and hours. Many daily activities, like walking, stretching, swimming, hiking, or gardening, are easy ways to fight a sedentary lifestyle and be a little more active.

Evidence shows that even moderate activity can improve our mood, reduce anxiety, fight symptoms of depression, and enhance our overall health. Finally, we can work on prioritizing moments of gratitude and reflection. Practices like mindfulness or prayer ground us in our purpose and connect us to something greater. These small, consistent habits—whether nutritional, physical, or spiritual—add up to significant changes over time, creating a life that feels balanced and whole.

Question: Why Is It Important To Understand The Difference Between "Sick Care" And True Health Care?

Our current healthcare system simply waits for a "problem to develop" before it takes any action. However, this is like seeing smoke rising from a building for (sometimes for *years)* to only call the fire department when it is engulfed in flame! This "sick care" approach focuses on making a diagnosis, then treating the symptoms (i.e., disease), rather than preventing or reversing them.

Our entire healthcare system is set up on a crisis, reactive basis. This, by default, means that we "have to be sick" to "get care." The tragedy is that most of this suffering never had to happen, as nearly 9 out of 10 cases of Type 2 Diabetes are entirely preventable![31]

True health care would prioritize prevention. It would *aim* to have us be and stay healthy. It would look into why we are getting ill, or are ill, and look at what it can do to have us be healthy again. It would address issues before they developed into serious conditions or diseases. This distinction between reactive and proactive care underscores the importance of taking charge of your well-being today.

Question: How Does Faith Influence Holistic Health?

Faith provides strength, hope, and perspective to life! Proverbs 13:12 reminds us, *"Hope deferred makes the heart sick, but when the desire is fulfilled, it is a tree of life."* Faith anchors you during challenging times and can inspire you to care for yourself better, as part of a greater purpose, and to have hope. Positive relations to religion have been shown to have a positive impact on our quality of life, especially when dealing with chronic illness.[4] Whether through prayer, scripture, or quiet reflection, faith offers a path to clarity and resilience.

Question: What Are The Core Components Of Holistic Health?

As mentioned, holistic health is rooted in three interconnected components: the mind, the body, and the spirit. Each of these aspects plays a vital role in your overall well-being, and nurturing one often strengthens the others. Together, they create a balanced and sustainable approach to health.

- **Mind (Emotional):**

Emotional well-being involves recognizing and accepting your emotions, processing and managing them, and expressing them in healthy ways. It also includes adapting to life's pressures and maintaining resilience during challenges. Chronic stress, for example, can disrupt hormones, weaken the immune system, and impact mental clarity. Practices like mindfulness, journaling, breathing exercises, and prayer can help you manage stress and foster emotional balance. The gut-brain connection further emphasizes the relationship between your mind and body, with emotional health directly influencing digestive and immune functions.

- **Body (Physical):**

Physical health relies on eating a balanced diet, exercising regularly, and getting enough restorative sleep. Diets like the Mediterranean Diet have been shown to improve the microbiome, metabolism, cardiovascular, and brain health.[5] Regular physical activity—whether it's walking, stretching, or gardening—improves cardiovascular health, reduces stress, and enhances mood. Routine health checkups and addressing symptoms early are equally important, as is avoiding risky behaviors that could compromise your well-being.

- **Spirit (Faith):**

Spiritual health involves expanding your sense of purpose and connecting with something greater than yourself. Faith provides strength and clarity during life's challenges, fostering hope and resilience. Practices such as prayer, meditation, or engaging with a supportive community can ground you and help you find meaning. Prayer is a very powerful practice, as we are reminded in 1

John 5:15 (NLT) *And since we know he hears us when we make our requests, we also know that he will give us what we ask for."*

This connection to purpose and faith supports emotional and physical health, creating a foundation for long-term well-being.

When you intentionally nurture your mind, body, and spirit, the benefits ripple through all areas of your life. Addressing stress (mind), for example, can reduce inflammation (body) and foster peace (spirit). By creating harmony among these three components, you build a resilient and fulfilling approach to health that lasts.

Question: Why Does Holistic Health Matter For Long-Term Well-Being?

One of our aims is to build resilience. Once we can determine the root causes of your symptoms, we will know what to address. When the root cause is addressed, you will, of course, feel a lot better!

But by focusing on future prevention, enhanced health, and creating a basis for maintained wellness, you can, in turn, create a foundation that supports your life for *years* to come. The gut microbiome plays a critical role here, as it functions as the basis of our entire state of health. Strengthening your gut health through proper nutrition and lifestyle changes is just one example of how holistic health supports long-term well-being.

Question: What Can You Expect As You Continue With This Book?

This book will guide you through practical steps you can take to improve your health and explain my method and how I can support you. I have been there, walked that path, and I know the way out! From understanding nutrition, utilizing functional lab testing, and applying the HOPE Method, each chapter will build on the last.

By the end, you will also have a key summary section and some questions to reflect on the tools you now have to create better health for yourself.

Health is more than the absence of disease; it's a vibrant state of physical, mental, and spiritual well-being that requires intentional daily choices. Conventional "sick care" focuses on managing symptoms after disease develops, while holistic health addresses root causes and emphasizes prevention before problems arise. Mind, body, and spirit are interconnected: stress affects your mental and physical health, poor nutrition drains your energy, and spiritual practices can restore balance to both.

True healing requires looking at the whole person, not just isolated symptoms, which is why functional testing often reveals answers that traditional tests miss. Small, consistent actions build lasting change—you don't need dramatic overhauls, just daily choices that nourish all aspects of your well-being. Faith provides strength, hope, and perspective that support both emotional resilience and physical healing during challenging times. Prevention is always better than treatment.

Before you move on, take a moment to reflect. Where do you feel strong in your health, and where do you see opportunities for improvement? Remember, change doesn't happen overnight. It starts with small, intentional actions—a healthier meal, a moment of prayer, or a commitment to rest.

The journey to holistic health is personal and transformative. Each step you take brings you closer to balance and clarity. As we continue through this book, you'll find practical tools and guidance to help you along the way. Let's move forward together.

Questions for Reflection

1. What are your most concerning health conditions or symptoms, and what would you be doing with your life if you weren't suffering from these issues?

2. Are you currently managing symptoms or addressing root causes, and which area needs more attention—your mind (emotional health), body (physical health), or spirit (faith/purpose)?

3. Have you felt stuck in the "sick care" cycle of endless appointments and medications without real improvement, and what questions about your health remain unanswered?

4. What does vibrant health look like for you personally—not just absence of disease, but the energy and vitality to live out your purpose fully?

5. What small, consistent action could you start today that would nourish your overall well-being and move you toward the balanced life you desire?

CHAPTER 2

The Chronic Disease Epidemic

*Our troubles are small. They last only for a short time. But they are
earning for us a glory that will last forever. It is greater
than all our troubles.*

— 2 Corinthians 4:17 (NIrV)

Now, more than ever, people are being diagnosed with conditions
such as diabetes, heart disease, autoimmune disorders, and neurodegenerative diseases. And yet, despite all of our advancements
in pharmaceuticals and medical technology, we are not getting
healthier, and chronic disease is on the rise. I have seen the dev-
astation of chronic disease firsthand—both in my patients and in
my family. For years, I believed medications were helping patients,
but then I started to see that people were not truly healing. Instead,
their prescriptions were just helping to manage their symptoms or
disease. Even with my advanced knowledge and understanding of
human physiology and pharmacology, I was frustrated that despite advances in medicine, we were not actually improving health
or reversing disease. As a pharmacist, I was helping people "manage chronic disease," but the reality was their symptoms persisted
and often progressed. Our diagnose-and-treat system of care re-
sulted in more medications, uncontrolled symptoms, adverse drug
effects, hospitalizations, and even surgical interventions- this was
not health care, it was "sick care".

Chronic disease has become the defining health crisis of our time. The World Health Organization (WHO) reports that chronic diseases now account for 74% [1] of deaths worldwide. Unlike acute illnesses—such as infections or injuries, which require immediate medical attention—chronic diseases develop gradually, often over years or even decades. They stem from a complex interplay of lifestyle choices, environmental exposures, and unhealthy diet, many of which go unrecognized until symptoms become severe and a diagnosis is assigned to the disorder. Yet instead of seeking out and addressing the root causes, conventional medicine responds reactively, relying on prescriptions and procedures that manage symptoms rather than resolve the underlying problem.

This results in an escalating pattern of lifelong medications, worsening symptoms, and no clear path to recovery. Patients are often told their condition is something they must "manage" indefinitely rather than something that can be improved—or even *reversed*. This approach is not just ineffective; it's unsustainable—both for the individual and for the healthcare system as a whole. Beyond the physical toll, chronic disease steals precious moments, opportunities, and peace of mind from our lives, and places a heavy financial and emotional strain on families. If medicine alone were the answer, wouldn't we be seeing fewer cases, fewer prescriptions, and more people thriving? But instead, we see a system that seems to sustain disease rather than heal it. But there is always hope. The body is designed to heal when given the right conditions.

What is health? Health is your body's natural state when barriers to healing are removed and all systems function as designed. True health is more than the absence of disease—it is restoration, renewal, and the opportunity to reclaim vitality.

In this chapter, we will examine the true scope of chronic disease, why conventional medicine is not set up to handle it, and what must change to restore health. But first, we must answer a critical question: What is disease?

Defining Disease

So what is disease? The National Cancer Institute defines it as "an abnormal condition that affects the structure or function of part or all of the body and is usually associated with specific signs and symptoms."[2] While this definition works for infections, injuries, or acute conditions, it fails to capture the complexity of chronic disease. Acute diseases—like pneumonia or a broken bone—have a clear cause and a direct way of being treated. A bacterial infection may require antibiotics. A wound might need stitches.

Once treated, the body heals. Chronic diseases, however, do not follow this pattern. They develop over years, often without any noticeable symptoms at first. They also result from multiple system failures rather than a single occurrence.

Chronic illnesses are not random occurrences. They evolve from a gradual breakdown of metabolic, immune, and hormonal balance, often fueled by harmful lifestyle factors, environmental toxins, and long-term inflammation. Yet, the way modern medicine defines and classifies disease dictates how it is treated. Too often, a diagnosis is just a label for the symptoms a person is experiencing—and not a look into *why*. If a patient repeatedly presents with high blood sugar, they may, in the end, be diagnosed with diabetes and prescribed metformin or insulin—often without looking at what is triggering the imbalance in the first place. If they have joint pain, they may be diagnosed with arthritis and given anti-inflammatories, like NSAIDs. But does anyone ever ask why the patient's blood sugar is spiking? Or why is their immune system attacking the joints? Most of the time, those questions are never asked at all.

This is why so many people end up on lifelong medications and never truly heal. Instead of identifying the underlying dysfunction, symptoms are treated as if they were the disease itself. The numbers tell the real story—more people are living with obesity, diabetes, heart disease, autoimmune disorders, and neurodegenerative conditions than at any other point in history.

- Obesity now affects over 42% of American adults, a staggering increase from past decades. Excess weight isn't just about appearance—it fuels inflammation, metabolic dysfunction, and cardiovascular disease.

- Diabetes rates have quadrupled since 1980, with 537 million people worldwide now living with the disease. Type 2 diabetes, once rare in young adults, is now common in teenagers—a direct result of diets high in sugar, chronic stress, and inactivity.

- Heart disease remains the #1 cause of death in the U.S., responsible for 1 in 5 deaths annually. We have cholesterol-lowering drugs and high-tech interventions, yet the numbers continue to climb. If these treatments were the answer, why aren't we seeing a decline?

- Neurodegenerative disorders, including Alzheimer's and early-onset dementia, are rising sharply—even in adults as young as 30 to 64. Once believed to be purely genetic, research now reveals that chronic inflammation, toxin exposure, and metabolic dysfunction play a key role in cognitive decline.

- Autoimmune diseases affect over 50 million Americans, yet many remain misdiagnosed for years. Conditions like lupus, Hashimoto's thyroiditis, and multiple sclerosis are increasing at an alarming rate, closely linked to gut health, environmental toxins, and chronic stress.

Despite more medications, more specialists, and more research than ever before, we are getting sicker. The reason is clear: we are not treating disease—we are treating symptoms. Instead of identifying what is breaking down in the body, we are chasing lab results with prescriptions.

The Root Causes of Chronic Disease

Chronic disease is also not the result of a single issue. Rather, it develops from multiple dysfunctions within the body, each one compounding the next. These imbalances do not exist in isolation, either; they fuel one another and create a cycle of worsening symptoms and deeper health decline. One of the most significant drivers of chronic disease is *metabolic dysfunction.*

Metabolic Dysfunction

This is a disruption in how the body produces, stores, and utilizes energy. Metabolism is not just about gaining or losing weight; it is the foundation of how every cell in the body functions. When this system fails, the consequences extend far beyond energy levels. At a cellular level, metabolic dysfunction happens when the body can no longer efficiently convert food into usable energy.

This leads to insulin resistance, oxidative stress, and mitochondrial dysfunction, creating a ripple effect that impacts our brain, heart, immune system, and overall health. One of the key drivers of metabolic dysfunction is the Standard American Diet, or "SAD".

The SAD or Western-style diet has increased consumption of ultra-processed foods that are high in unhealthy fats, refined sugar, and harmful chemicals like food colorants, flavorings, artificial sweeteners, and preservatives, and has been linked to chronic diseases like obesity, diabetes, heart disease, and metabolic dysfunction.

This diet also lacks essential vitamins and minerals, contributing to nutritional deficiencies in iron, calcium, magnesium, and zinc, which are associated with conditions such as anemia, osteoporosis, cardiovascular disease and hormone imbalances.

The Western diet is also low in fiber. The Dietary Guidelines for Americans (DGA) and the American Heart Association (AHA) recommend adults aim for 25-38 grams of fiber daily, depending on age and sex, with women needing around 25 grams and men around 38 grams. Although adequate intake of all types of fiber is associated with many health benefits, an estimated 95% of American adults and children do not consume the recommended amounts of fiber.[31]

Fiber also plays a critical role in maintaining our gut health and integrity. It helps feed beneficial bacteria and reduce inflammation. When our fiber intake is low, the gut microbiome is disrupted, leading to a state of imbalance (dysbiosis) between beneficial versus harmful bacteria. This microbial shift results in a deficiency of by-products, or metabolites, that are normally produced by the beneficial bacteria, such as vitamin K and B's, hormones and neurotransmitters like dopamine and serotonin, and short-chain fatty acids (SCFAs) that are critical for cellular functions both inside and outside the gastrointestinal (GI) tract. These changes to the intestinal ecosystem also contribute to gut-barrier dysfunction, where the lining of the GI tract becomes more permeable (also called 'leaky gut'), allowing harmful substances to leak into the bloodstream.

This triggers widespread immune dysregulation and chronic inflammation. While short-term inflammation is a necessary response to injury or infection, long-term, unresolved inflammation silently damages our bodily tissues, DNA, and cells. It also accelerates disease and fuels pain. The most common dietary contributors to inflammation include:

- processed foods,
- excess sugar,
- and inflammatory oils (like seed oils and omega-6s)[4]

Over time, these metabolic failures set the stage for more serious, system-wide breakdowns. The body struggles to regulate blood sugar, fat storage, and energy production.

When our metabolic function is disrupted, disease does not just "develop"—it *thrives!* Suppressing all these symptoms with medication will never restore balance to an energy system that is failing at its foundation. The only way to reverse this dysfunction is to identify what is driving it. Whether it be poor diet, chronic stress, gut dysbiosis, or toxin exposure, we must identify and correct imbalances before they progress further.

<u>Gut Health</u>

Gut health and immune regulation are deeply connected, yet they are often ignored in terms of health. The gut is not just responsible for digesting our food—it plays a direct role in our immune function, metabolism, and even hormone balance. Approximately 70-80% of our immune system resides in our gut.[5] This means that a significant portion of your body's defense against illness is concentrated in your digestive tract. The Gut-Associated Lymphatic Tissue (GALT) refers to a network of lymphoid tissues located within the gastrointestinal tract.

It plays a crucial role in maintaining gut health and protecting against infections, acting as the first line of defense against ingested pathogens. When our gut function is compromised, the immune system is triggered, which increases the risk of autoimmune disease. Conditions like Hashimoto's thyroiditis (HT), inflammatory bowel disease (IBD), and rheumatoid arthritis (RA) have all been linked to gut dysbiosis and increased intestinal permeability, also known as "Leaky Gut Syndrome."

This connection is particularly evident in thyroid health, as nearly 20% of thyroid hormone conversion, from inactive T4 to active T3, occurs in the gut. An imbalance in gut bacteria (dysbiosis) can result in lower conversion of thyroid hormones. Other causes of thyroid dysfunction have been attributed to untreated infections like *Helicobacter pylori (H. pylori)* and parasites (*Blastocystis hominus*), both have been associated with autoimmune thyroiditis conditions.[6][7]

Chronic infections, microbial imbalances, and a weakened gut lining can leave the immune system in a state of *over-activation*, simply unable to differentiate between healthy and harmful substances. As the gut barrier breaks down, toxins, bacteria, and undigested food proteins enter the bloodstream, which fuels systemic inflammation and triggers immune dysfunction. Our immune system is designed to protect us by making antibodies that fight off harmful invaders, but sometimes these antibodies resemble parts of our own cells or proteins. This look-alike effect, called *molecular mimicry*, confuses the immune system, leading it to mistakenly produce antibodies that attack our own cells or tissues. Over time, this can lead to the development of autoimmune diseases or conditions.

Instead of identifying and correcting these causes, conventional medicine often treats the symptoms with anti-inflammatory drugs like steroids or prednisone, antihistamines, and even biologics or immunosuppressing drugs like methotrexate, adalimumab (Enbrel), or infliximab (Remicade). Unfortunately, these do not address the root causes and may further weaken the body's natural defenses. The good news: once we understand this process, we can take steps to remove the trigger, calm the inflammation, and retrain the immune system.

Hormonal Imbalance

Hormonal balance is a critical factor in chronic disease, yet it is often completely dismissed or overlooked. The endocrine system (made up of glands such as the thyroid, adrenal glands, testes, and ovaries) regulates hormones that control our metabolism, energy, stress response, immune function, and reproductive health. Yet, when this system is disrupted, it sets off a chain reaction of dysfunction throughout the body. One of the most common and underestimated drivers of hormonal imbalance is chronic stress. Prolonged stress activates the hypothalamic-pituitary-adrenal (HPA) axis, the body's central stress-response system. This leads to cortisol imbalances and keeps the body locked in a constant state of high alert—the familiar 'fight-or-flight' mode. While this response is protective in the short term, ongoing activation disrupts the body's normal rhythm. Over time, these cortisol fluctuations can contribute to blood sugar instability, mood swings, sleep disturbances, persistent fatigue, and weight gain. Left unaddressed, chronic stress places a heavy burden on both the mind and body, paving the way for broader health challenges.

Many people live with exhaustion, poor sleep, and anxiety without realizing that imbalanced stress hormones may be the reason why.

I know! For years, I pushed through exhaustion, assuming it was just part of my demanding career. I lived in a constant state of stress, moving from one responsibility to the next, believing that if I just pushed a little harder, I could regain control. But no amount of sleep, caffeine, or so-called "self-care" could shake the fatigue. My energy was gone. My body hurt. My weight is increasing. My mind was foggy. And still, no doctor asked *why*. I was experiencing symptoms of anxiety, brain fog, and fatigue, all of which were connected to hormone imbalance. At the time, I had no idea that chronic stress also contributes to dysbiosis and leaky gut—two key drivers of hormone imbalance, inflammation, and the cascade of symptoms I was experiencing. Ironically, I did not consider my age or gender (aka declining hormones) as a factor in my worsening symptoms. Yet despite the obvious impact of menopause on women's health and quality of life, conventional medicine often dismisses hormone imbalance, clings to outdated fears about hormone replacement, and leaves countless women without the evaluation or treatment they deserve. This is something I had to advocate for myself in the years ahead.

Each of these dysfunctions- metabolic, gut and hormone imbalance, fuels the next and creates a cycle of disease. Therefore, simply treating your symptoms will never lead to true healing. However, finding out just what is happening with your body can be the first step in treating the imbalance that occurred in the first place.

Breaking Free from the "Symptom = Diagnosis" Trap

In conventional healthcare, the cycle of symptom management and medications can be very hard to break. This cycle continues because conventional medicine is built to focus on *managing disease*, not resolving it. But there is another way. The body is not designed to be broken. Healing is possible when we stop suppressing our symptoms and start identifying their underlying dysfunctions. This is the foundation of the HOPE Method. Through functional lab testing, we are able to pinpoint the specific imbalances that drive disease. Comprehensive panels, allow us to uncover gut infections, hormonal dysregulation, levels of toxic burden, and metabolic failures. When we then address these causes directly, the body can begin to rebuild itself.

By shifting our focus from disease management to root-cause healing, we can begin to restore what has been lost. Let us take a look at an example of how this can be done.

Case Study: The Rise of Early-Onset Dementia & Alzheimer's Disease

Dementia was once thought to be an illness of old age—something that developed in the later years of life. But that assumption no longer holds true. Younger adults, even those in their 30s and 40s, are now being diagnosed with early-onset dementia and Alzheimer's at unprecedented rates. A 2017 Blue Cross Blue Shield (BCBS) Health Index study revealed just how serious this trend has become. The study estimated that 126 million Americans between the ages of 30 and 64 are now affected by early-onset dementia or Alzheimer's disease.

These findings highlight a disturbing shift: neurodegenerative diseases are no longer just a concern for the elderly.[8] According to the Alzheimer's Association's 2019 report, an estimated 5.8 million Americans of all ages are living with Alzheimer's dementia, including 200,000 individuals under the age of 65.

This number is projected to rise to 7.1 million by 2025—a 27% increase from 2019.[9] Alarmingly, Alzheimer's is the sixth-leading cause of death in the United States, and the fifth-leading cause for those aged 65 and older. Despite advancements in medical research and treatment, deaths from Alzheimer's have more than doubled between 2000 and 2017, increasing by 145%, while deaths from heart disease have decreased by 9% during the same period. This stark contrast highlights the urgent need for a paradigm shift in how we approach, diagnose, and treat Alzheimer's disease.

Why Is This Happening?

Unlike traditional late-onset Alzheimer's, which has long been associated with aging and genetics, early-onset cases are largely driven by environmental and metabolic factors. This means that our daily choices—what we eat, how we manage stress, and the toxins we're exposed to—play a far greater role in brain health than previously believed.

Early cognitive decline has also been linked to:

- Toxin exposure
- Blood sugar imbalances
- Gut dysbiosis and leaky gut
- Chronic stress and poor sleep

This crisis raises an urgent question: If Alzheimer's and dementia are appearing decades earlier than they used to, then why aren't we addressing this sign? Instead of waiting until cognitive decline is irreversible, we must shift our focus to prevention and early intervention—before the symptoms even begin.

The Emotional and Financial Costs of Chronic Illness

Chronic disease does not just affect our body—it infiltrates every aspect of our lives. It dictates how we wake up in the morning, how we move through our day, and whether we have the energy to engage with the people we love. Chronic disease is an unrelenting presence, one that often comes with an emotional and financial burden far greater than most people realize.

<u>The Emotional Toll</u>

Living with chronic illness means waking up every day in uncertainty. Will today be a "good" day or another day lost to pain, fatigue, or brain fog? Will you be able to keep up with your commitments to your job and the family, or will symptoms force you to cancel again? Over time, this relentless unpredictability takes its toll.

- **Depression and Anxiety** – The awareness of decline, along with daily struggles, often leads to sadness, fear, and heightened anxiety.

- **Social Isolation** – Difficulties with memory and communication can strain relationships and cause withdrawal from social activities.

- **Loss of Independence** – Everyday tasks such as driving, managing finances, or preparing meals gradually become difficult or impossible, leading to frustration and loss of dignity.

- **Decline in Overall Health** – Dementia increases vulnerability to poor nutrition, infections, falls, and reduced mobility, further impacting quality of life.

It's not just the patient who suffers. Caregivers bear an invisible burden too, watching a loved one deteriorate while medical treatments provide little relief. The emotional exhaustion, grief, and helplessness can be overwhelming.

The Financial Burden

Chronic disease is also not only emotionally draining, it is financially devastating. 90% of U.S. healthcare spending, over $4.1 trillion annually[10] goes toward managing chronic disease. But where does that money go?

- **Endless Medications** – Many patients are prescribed multiple drugs for life, with costs piling up month after month.

- **Lost Income** – As health declines, so does the ability to work. Many are forced to reduce hours or leave their jobs entirely.

- **Long-Term Care Costs** – As diseases progress, patients often require in-home care, specialized medical equipment, or assisted living, adding thousands in expenses each year.

For many families, chronic illness leads to financial ruin. Even with insurance, out-of-pocket costs are crushing. Some are forced to choose between paying for treatment or covering essentials like food and rent. This is the reality of a system built on disease management—not prevention. If modern medicine were *truly* fixing chronic disease, then we wouldn't be in a crisis. Despite billions spent on treatment, the problem is only getting worse. A healthcare model that keeps people dependent on medications will never lead to true recovery.

The Functional Medicine Approach

Unlike conventional medicine, functional medicine *asks*, "Why?" It looks beyond the diagnosis and examines what is actually going on with the body. Instead of simply treating a symptom, it seeks to identify and correct the root causes of dysfunction. Functional medicine focuses on uncovering and reversing these chronic imbalances to give the body what it needs to heal and to prevent it from getting ill.

Case Example: Two Different Approaches

Consider a 45-year-old woman who has been battling persistent fatigue, anxiety, constipation, and joint pain for years. She has seen multiple doctors, undergone countless tests, and yet, no one has been able to explain why she feels this way. Each visit ends the same way—another prescription, another temporary fix, but no real answers. In the conventional approach, she is diagnosed based on her symptoms. Anti-inflammatories for joint pain. Anti-depressants for anxiety. A laxative for constipation. But no one asks *why* she is in pain or *why* she is exhausted. Instead, her symptoms are managed, not resolved. Over time, fatigue worsens, gut issues persist, and inflammation remains high. The cycle continues, leaving her dependent on prescriptions without any real improvement in her health. Now, let's take the functional approach. Instead of masking symptoms, the goal is to uncover what is actually driving her symptoms in the first place. Advanced testing is done to assess:

- **Nutrient levels**—is she deficient in key vitamins and minerals needed for energy and tissue repair?

- **Gut health**—is there underlying dysbiosis, leaky gut, or an undiagnosed infection contributing to systemic inflammation?

- **Toxic burden**—are heavy metals, environmental toxins, or chemical exposures causing inflammation and fueling her joint pain?

- **Hormonal balance**—are her adrenal glands depleted? Is thyroid function sluggish? Are estrogen and progesterone imbalanced?

Her functional lab tests reveal gut dysbiosis, heavy metal toxicity, and hormone imbalance—issues that conventional medicine never tested for. Instead of prescriptions, this woman would be given a targeted plan to restore gut integrity, remove toxins, rebalance hormones, and strategies to manage stress.

Within months, her pain could decrease, her energy return, and she would no longer rely on medications to get through the day. One approach keeps her trapped in an endless cycle, and the other restores function and eliminates the need for pharmaceutical intervention altogether.

Key Takeaways

Chronic disease is no longer the exception—it is the norm. Conditions like obesity, diabetes, heart disease, neurodegenerative disorders, and autoimmune conditions are rising at an alarming rate, despite medical advancements and increased healthcare spending. If our current system were truly working, these numbers would be declining. Instead, they continue to climb. One of the greatest failures of modern medicine is its focus on symptom suppression rather than true healing.

Patients are placed on lifelong medications, managing their disease instead of resolving it. This failure is now becoming even more obvious with the rise of early-onset dementia and Alzheimer's. Once considered diseases of old age, these conditions are now appearing in adults as young as 30 to 64, largely driven by chronic inflammation, metabolic dysfunction, and environmental toxins. This isn't just a matter of bad luck or genetics—our daily choices play a far bigger role in long-term brain health than we once believed. Beyond the physical burden, chronic illness devastates lives financially and emotionally. The cost of long-term medications, doctor visits, and lost wages can bankrupt families, while the mental toll of pain, isolation, and uncertainty creates an ongoing cycle of stress and despair.

But there is another way. Functional medicine shifts the focus from disease management to true healing. By addressing gut health, inflammation, toxicity, nutrient imbalances, and hormonal dysfunction, it restores the body's natural ability to heal. The question isn't, "What drug do I need?"—it's "*Why* is my body struggling, and what can I do to fix it?"

Questions for Reflection

The way we think about health determines the choices we make. Real healing starts with asking better questions—the kind that make us challenge what we have always been told and reconsider what we accept as "normal."

Take a moment to reflect on what you've learned in this chapter and how it may apply to your own experience.

1. Do you see patterns in your own health that may be connected—fatigue, joint pain, weight gain, digestive issues?

Have you ever been told these were just part of aging or stress?

2. Have you ever received a diagnosis but felt like no one explained what was actually causing your condition?

3. Think about the medications you or a loved one takes regularly. Were they prescribed as a long-term solution, or just to manage symptoms?

4. What steps have you taken (if any) to look beyond prescriptions and into the root causes of your health concerns? What obstacles have held you back?

5. After reading this chapter, do you see your health differently? What is one thing you can do today to shift from symptom management to real healing?

The journey to healing begins with asking the right questions—and being willing to seek the answers. Here is a question only you can answer:

Are you willing to stay on the same path—relying on a system that keeps you in maintenance mode—or are you ready to take control of your health? Are you ready to start asking why your symptoms exist instead of just treating them? The next chapter will take this conversation even deeper—into one of the most critical (and overlooked) factors in chronic disease: the gut. Research has shown that gut health affects nearly every chronic illness, influencing metabolism, immunity, inflammation, and even brain function. If you don't fix your gut, you can't truly fix your health. Healing begins with understanding—and now, you have that knowledge. The next step is applying it. Are you ready?

CHAPTER 3

All Disease Begins In The Gut

*How you made me is amazing and wonderful. I praise you for that.
What you have done is wonderful. I know that very well.*

— Psalm 139:14 (NIrV)

The gut is one of the most powerful and complex systems in the body, designed not just for digestion but for maintaining our immune balance, metabolic function, and neurological health. Yet, when this system is compromised, it can become the root cause of many chronic diseases. For centuries, healers have understood the gut's foundational role in health. Modern science now confirms that gut health influences everything from the state of our metabolism and immune resilience to mental well-being and degree of systemic inflammation. Like the roots of a tree, a strong gut provides stability and nourishment. But when the gut microbiome is imbalanced, or the gut lining becomes permeable, the effects spread throughout the entire body, leading to autoimmune disorders, metabolic dysfunction, and chronic inflammation. In this chapter, we will explore the critical role of the gut microbiome, uncover what disrupts gut health, and identify how to restore balance for long-term wellness.

Hippocrates' Wisdom and Modern Science

"All disease begins in the gut." – Hippocrates.

More than two thousand years ago, Hippocrates, the Father of Medicine, made this statement. Today, cutting-edge science has confirmed that the gut plays a central role in nearly every aspect of our health. The microbiome is defined as the collection of all microbes, such as bacteria, fungi, viruses, and their genes, that naturally live on and inside our bodies. Notably, the gut microbiome has been linked to immune function, brain health, metabolism, and even chronic disease.

What Hippocrates understood intuitively, modern research is now proving at the molecular level. For decades, conventional medicine has treated the body as a grouping of separate systems. If you have issues with your stomach, the stomach is treated. Yet, functional medicine has brought us back to a core truth: health cannot be "compartmentalized." All systems influence each other. Hippocrates emphasized whole-body healing, and we now know that inflammation, hormone imbalances, and autoimmune conditions often originate in the gut.

Hippocrates also taught that lifestyle determines the outcome of health. He advocated for proper nutrition, stress reduction, and movement, principles that align perfectly with what we now understand about chronic disease prevention. Modern medicine generally promotes pharmaceuticals over prevention or health. Yet, a growing body of research confirms that dietary changes, microbiome balance, and lifestyle interventions can reverse or prevent many chronic illnesses. Hippocrates may not have known about the microbiome or inflammatory markers, but his intuition was correct!

Modern medicine is only now catching up, confirming that the root of most chronic diseases lies in gut health.

The Human Microbiome: An Overview

The human microbiome is one of the most complex and influential ecosystems within the body. Composed of trillions of bacteria, viruses, fungi, and other microorganisms, it plays a central role in digestion, immunity, metabolism, and hormone regulation.

The microbiome has been the focus of extensive scientific study in recent years. From 2007 through 2016, the National Institutes of Health supported the Human Microbiome Project (HMP), a groundbreaking initiative designed to generate resources for the comprehensive characterization of the human microbiome and to explore its role in health and disease. The HMP's work has significantly advanced our understanding of how microbial communities interact with the human host, influence biological processes, and contribute to both wellness and illness. Its findings have provided a foundation for ongoing research into how these microbial ecosystems can be shaped to support better health outcomes.[1]

In an average human body, the number of microbial cells is nearly ten times more than human cells. This means that we HUMANS are 70-90% microbial, approximately 30 trillion cells are human cells, but an astounding *100 trillion cells* are microbial.[2] While the majority of these microbes reside in the gut, particularly in the large intestine, they also inhabit our skin, mouth, respiratory tract, and other mucosal surfaces, working in harmony with the body to maintain balance and resilience. The human microbiome may also weigh as much as 5 pounds!

These microbes are generally not harmful to us; in fact, they are essential for maintaining health. For example, they produce certain vitamins that we do not have the genes to make, break down our food to extract nutrients we need to survive, teach our immune systems how to recognize dangerous invaders, and even produce helpful anti-inflammatory compounds that fight off other disease-causing microbes. An ever-growing number of studies have demonstrated that changes in the composition of our microbiomes correlate with numerous disease states, raising the possibility that manipulation of these communities could be used to treat disease.

Human microbial communities exist in various locations, such as the respiratory system, skin, oral cavity, vaginal area, and gut. Microbial diversity, or the range of all these different kinds of organisms, differs throughout the gastrointestinal tract due to changes in pH, oxygen, bile, mucus, and digestive function. The highest bacterial load is in the large intestine (10^{12}/gm in the colon), where there is typically no oxygen (anaerobic environment) and the pH is slightly acidic to neutral.

A healthy microbiome is not made up of only the presence of beneficial bacteria, but the diversity of those bacteria. A rich and varied microbial population helps regulate inflammation, synthesize essential nutrients, and support our immune defense.

Several bacterial species common in the large intestine (e.g., *Bacteroides*, *Bifidobacterium*, and *Enterococcus*) are known to synthesize vitamins. B-group vitamins such as B2 (riboflavin), B3 (niacin), B5 (pantothenic acid), B6 (pyridoxine), B7 (biotin), B9 (folate or folic acid), and B12 (cyanocobalamin) are water-soluble vitamins that are abundant in the diet but are also produced by gut bacteria. It is also estimated that up to half of the daily vitamin K requirement is likewise supplied by gut bacteria.[3]

However, when our microbial balance is disrupted, a state known as *dysbiosis,* the effects influence the entire body. Research now links imbalances in the microbiome to obesity, diabetes, cardiovascular, neurological disorders and even autoimmune diseases.[4]

Dysbiosis can impair the integrity of the gut lining. This protective barrier with tight junctions between cells becomes porous or permeable, a condition known as *"leaky gut"*. This increased permeability allows toxins and undigested food particles to enter the bloodstream, triggering an immune response to these antigens or foreign substances (i.e., food proteins, toxins, bacteria). This gives further rise to inflammatory mediators (cytokines and immune cells) trying to combat the invading substance that overstimulates the immune system, resulting in chronic inflammation throughout the body.

I know this was a lot of information to take in, but it is important that you get the full picture. Despite its complexity, the microbiome is not a fixed system, it is constantly evolving based on the dietary and lifestyle choices we make. This means that by prioritizing gut health, we have the ability to shape our microbiome and, in turn, influence long-term health.

Case Study: When Gut Health Transforms Chronic Pain

I recently treated a patient who came to me with severe, persistent low-back pain and migraines that had plagued her for years. She had tried everything: chiropractic care, physical therapy, and multiple pain management approaches, but nothing provided lasting relief. Her pain was so debilitating that her sleep was impaired, and she couldn't work effectively or enjoy time with her family.

What conventional approaches had missed was the root cause. Through comprehensive testing, we discovered that a "leaky gut," a parasitic infection, and multiple food sensitivities (gluten, dairy, and eggs) were driving systemic inflammation and contributing to her symptoms. Rather than simply treating the pain, we implemented a strategic two-phase approach: nourish first, then detox.

We began by supporting her gut lining by eliminating food sensitivities, optimizing nutrient absorption, and strengthening her immune system before addressing the parasitic infection. This sequence was crucial; attempting to eliminate pathogens from a weakened system often fails and can worsen symptoms.

The results were remarkable. Within weeks of completing the protocol, she experienced marked improvement in both her migraines and back pain. For the first time in months, she woke up without that familiar aching sensation. Her energy returned, her sleep improved, and she could engage fully in her daily activities again.

This case perfectly illustrates how seemingly unrelated symptoms often trace back to gut dysfunction. When we address the root cause rather than just managing symptoms, the body's inherent healing capacity can be restored.

Commensal/Keystone Bacteria and Gut Microbiome Insights

Within the ecosystem of the gut microbiome, certain bacteria serve as keystone species (organisms that have a disproportionately large impact on their ecosystem relative to their abundance). These commensal or keystone species are microorganisms, primarily bacteria, that reside on or in the human body, like the skin, oral cavity, and gut, without causing harm and often provide benefits like aiding digestion and boosting the immune system. In our gut, these are essential bacteria that uphold balance, protect the intestinal lining, and regulate immune response. Much like keystone species out in nature, which maintain the stability of an entire ecosystem, these microbes determine whether the gut functions as a source of health or a driver of disease. Some examples of keystone bacteria are:

- Akkermansia muciniphila

- Lactobacillus

- Bifidobacterium

Each has a unique influence on preserving our gut health. *Akkermansia* specializes in strengthening the gut lining by generating mucus-derived sugars and metabolic products that support the growth and energy needs of other gut microbes. It also promotes mucosal health and mucus production, maintaining the protective layer that separates intestinal cells from harmful invaders. These functions help maintain a "tight" gut barrier, which prevents any unwanted substances (like undigested food) or bacterial invaders from leaking into the bloodstream. Low levels of *Akkermansia* have been linked to obesity, metabolic dysfunction, and inflammatory disorders, reinforcing its role as a crucial guardian of gut integrity. [5]

Lactobacillus is another key protector that contributes to immune regulation and an efficient digestive system. This bacterium produces lactic acid, which creates an acidic environment that inhibits the growth of harmful bacteria while supporting beneficial microbes. They produce beneficial metabolites like hydrogen peroxide, nitric oxide, short-chain fatty acids (SCFAs), and bacteriocins (antimicrobial peptides), which contribute to gut health. Some Lactobacillus strains help modulate immune responses and reduce excessive inflammation that can lead to food intolerances, food allergies and autoimmune conditions.[6]

People with irritable bowel syndrome (IBS) have been shown to have lower levels of Lactobacillus. This deficiency dysbiosis has been linked to increased gut sensitivity, contributing to the classic symptoms of IBS such as abdominal pain, bloating, and altered bowel habits.

Meanwhile, *Bifidobacterium* is important in gut resilience by producing short-chain fatty acids (SCFAs), which reduce inflammation and nourish the cells of the colon.[7]

These bacteria are especially important in early life, where they aid in digestion and help infants develop a balanced immune system, protecting them from infections and allergies.

Bifidobacterium infantis produces folate (vitamin B9), which is essential for various bodily functions, including red blood cell production and DNA synthesis. A loss of bifidobacteria at an early age (due to antibiotic exposure, c-section, formula-fed) can cause a wide range of disorders. Specifically, a reduction in the abundance of *Bifidobacterium* in infants has been shown to increase the prevalence of obesity, diabetes, metabolic disorders, and all-cause mortality later in life.[8]

In adults, a decline in Bifidobacterium levels has been associated with irritable bowel syndrome (IBS), depression, and metabolic disorders.[9][10][11] Therefore, a well-functioning microbiome depends on the presence of these keystone species. Without them, the gut becomes vulnerable, which sets the stage for chronic disease.

The Two Major Bacterial Phyla

These keystone bacteria can be classified into different *phyla* (large biological groupings used to classify organisms based on shared characteristics). Two *phyla* predominantly dominate the human digestive tract, including the mouth, nose, throat, and colon: gram-negative *Bacteroidetes* and gram-positive *Firmicutes*. These phyla make up about 90% of the gut microbiome. An abnormal amount of one or both *phyla* may indicate an imbalance in the normal microbial community of the gastrointestinal tract.

Bacteroidetes are gram-negative bacteria that ferment polysaccharides and other indigestible carbohydrates, producing short-chain fatty acids (SCFAs) such as butyrate, which have multiple beneficial effects in the gut. These bacteria are believed to support microbial balance, maintain barrier integrity, and contribute to neuro-immune health. High levels may be associated with reduced digestive capacity or constipation.

One example is *Bacteroides fragilis* (*B. fragilis*), a complex bacterium that can act as both a commensal (beneficial) organism and a pathogen (an organism that can cause disease), depending on its location and the host's condition. While it is generally part of the normal gut flora, it can cause infections if it enters the bloodstream or surrounding tissues.[12]

The *Firmicutes* phylum consists of gram-positive bacteria that primarily dominate the upper gastrointestinal tract, though some are also found in the lower GI tract. This phylum includes several important genera (groups of closely related bacteria with similar traits) such as *Bacillus, Lactobacillus, Enterococcus, Staphylococcus, Streptococcus, Roseburia* spp., *Faecalibacterium prausnitzii*, and *Clostridia* spp.

Notably, *Roseburia, Faecalibacterium prausnitzii,* and *Clostridia* are major butyrate producers and tend to be more dominant in the large intestine.

Metabolites produced by these bacteria help maintain host health and support essential metabolic, neurologic, and immune functions.

Dysbiosis and the Firmicutes: Bacteroidetes Ratio (F/B Ratio)

When the gut microbiome becomes imbalanced, the effects extend far beyond the intestinal tract. Altered production of bacterial metabolites has been linked to metabolic disease, cardiovascular problems, digestive disorders, neurodegenerative conditions, and even cancer.

Dysbiosis is also associated with obesity development. In particular, a higher *Firmicutes-to-Bacteroidetes ratio* (F/B ratio), primarily driven by an increase in Firmicutes, promotes excess energy extraction and storage from food, disrupts appetite regulation, and fuels inflammation linked to insulin resistance, type 2 diabetes, and other metabolic disorders, while low ratios have been seen in inflammatory bowel disease. [13] [14]

Gut microbes break down indigestible carbohydrates and produce metabolites that promote health by regulating metabolism, strengthening the immune system, and protecting the intestinal barrier.

SCFAs, in particular, are vital for health, as they not only aid digestion but also help regulate blood sugar, influence hormone secretion, and maintain the integrity of the gut lining.

- **Butyrate** is the preferred energy source for intestinal cells, fueling repair and reducing inflammation.

- **Butyrate** supports intestinal barrier integrity, reduces intestinal inflammation, promotes motility, enhances fatty acid oxidation, inhibits tumor cell progression, and fosters a balanced microbiome.

- **Acetate** is the most abundant SCFA. It supports cholesterol synthesis and appetite regulation, maintains energy balance and metabolic homeostasis, and resists oxidation and mitochondrial stress.

- **Propionate** supports intestinal barrier integrity, impacts energy balance, hepatic glucose production, and cholesterol metabolism. It is involved in appetite regulation and has been proposed as a biomarker for Irritable Bowel Syndrome (IBS).[15]

The gut works continuously "behind the scenes" to produce key compounds that keep the body functioning. Bile acids, neurotransmitters such as dopamine and serotonin, SCFAs, and vitamin metabolites are all microbial byproducts with important roles in digestion, metabolism, and immune regulation.

In short, everything in the body is connected to the gut. When the gut thrives, these metabolites work in harmony, keeping our systems balanced. But when that balance is disrupted, the consequences can be far-reaching. The key is not just to manage our symptoms but to restore the body's natural ability to heal.

What Breaks the Microbiome?
(Disruptors of Gut Health)

Diet, medications, stress, and environmental toxins are some of the biggest disruptors of our gut health, as they shift the microbiome from a state of resilience to one of dysfunction.

When these disruptors take hold, beneficial bacteria diminish, harmful microbes flourish, and the gut barrier begins to break down. One of the most damaging influences on gut health is the Western or Standard American Diet (S.A.D.), loaded with processed seed oils, sugar, and artificial sweeteners and additives. Highly refined carbohydrates, excessive sugars, and unhealthy fats fuel gut dysbiosis, as they feed harmful bacteria while starving the beneficial microbes that maintain gut balance.[16]

Artificial sweeteners like aspartame and sucralose disrupt microbial diversity, while preservatives and emulsifiers damage the intestinal lining, potentially leading to "leaky gut" and systemic inflammation. Over time, consuming these promotes inflammation, weakens our gut's integrity, alters the microbiome, and sets the stage for chronic disease.[17] [18]

The dietary influence on our microbiome is profound, as eating even one high-fat meal results in a large die-off of gram-negative bacteria. This leads to a release of endotoxins from their cell walls. These endotoxins, like lipopolysaccharide or LPS, increase the permeability of tight junctions, allowing toxins to permeate the gut barrier and enter systemic circulation. Once in the bloodstream, LPS interacts with immune cells, releasing a pro-inflammatory response that causes chronic inflammation in virtually *every tissue in the body*. LPS endotoxin can induce symptoms of inflammation, fever, leukopenia, and damage to blood vessels, finally leading to hypotension and septic shock.[19]

LPS can also cross the blood-brain barrier and induce an inflammatory response, which is known to cause harmful effects on brain function, such as memory impairment and neurological disorders. [20]

Medications and Our Gut

Now, while medications can be necessary, many come at a high cost to our gut health. Antibiotics, for instance, wipe out harmful *and* beneficial bacteria. This creates microbial imbalances that can take months or even years to recover!

However, non-antibiotic drugs may also dramatically change the gut microbiome and ultimately lead to impaired health outcomes. Proton pump inhibitors (PPIs), like omeprazole and pantoprazole, are commonly prescribed for acid reflux to reduce stomach acid. These drugs create an environment where bacteria can thrive (referred to as opportunistic or overgrowth of bacteria).

The use of PPIs is associated with decreased bacterial richness and profound changes in the gut microbiome, and these microbial changes are linked to a less healthy gut ecosystem. Remarkably, greater microbial alterations have been associated with PPI users than in those who do not use them.[21] Nonsteroidal anti-inflammatory drugs (or NSAIDs), like ibuprofen and aspirin, are known to erode the gut lining, increasing intestinal permeability and inflammation, especially with long-term use.

Overuse of these medications can severely disrupt gut function, yet they are among the most frequently prescribed drugs worldwide.

Stress and Our Gut

Beyond diet and medications, the gut is highly sensitive to stress. Chronic stress elevates cortisol, a hormone released by the adrenal glands. High levels of cortisol promote an imbalance in gut flora (dysbiosis), reducing beneficial bacteria such as Lactobacillus and Bifidobacterium. This worsens intestinal motility (how food is moved through the gut), promoting bloating, cramping, and malabsorption. Cortisol also alters our microbial balance, degrades the gut barrier, and weakens our immune response.

Our gut has been referred to as the "*second brain*". The gut-brain axis (GBA) is a bidirectional communication network between the central nervous system (brain) and the enteric nervous system (gut nervous system or ENS), influencing digestion, mood, and overall health, with the gut microbiota playing a significant role.[22][23]

Recent advances in research have described the importance of gut microbiota in influencing these interactions. This interaction between microbiota and GBA appears to be *bidirectional,* namely through signaling *from* the gut *to* the brain via neural, hormonal, and immune pathways. In other words, approximately 80 to 90 percent of the neurons in the gut carry information *from* the gut *to* the brain.[24] Which is why people say, "Go with your gut feelings", as our gut is communicating primarily *to* our brain.

Our Nervous System and Digestion

The parasympathetic nervous system, our "rest-and-digest" mode, led by the vagus nerve, turns digestion on. It boosts saliva and gastric juices, coordinates motility, and prompts bile and pancreatic enzymes, while improving gut blood flow and mucus. Together, these actions protect the intestinal barrier and microbiome and make digestion and nutrient absorption efficient.

Stress flips the body into sympathetic "fight-or-flight," dialing digestion down. Saliva, stomach acid, and enzyme output fall; blood is shunted from the gut; motility becomes erratic, setting the stage for reflux, bloating, constipation, or urgency. Over time, stress hormones, like cortisol and adrenaline, further degrade the gut barrier and disrupt microbial balance. A brief pre-meal pause, slow, deep breaths, expressing gratitude, and thorough chewing can help restore parasympathetic tone and prepare the body for proper digestion.

Environmental Toxins

Meanwhile, environmental toxins, from pesticides in our food to heavy metals in our water, introduce a steady stream of inflammatory triggers that burden the liver and gut detoxification pathways. When these disruptors persist, the gut lining becomes compromised, and toxins leak into the bloodstream. From here, inflammation spreads throughout the body. The result? A cascade of health issues ranging from autoimmune disease to metabolic disorders and cancer. Understanding these threats is the first step in breaking the cycle of gut damage because, without removing the disruptors, true healing cannot begin.

The Conditions: Leaky Gut, Dysbiosis, and Metabolic Endotoxemia (ME)

The body is designed to maintain balance, but when gut integrity is compromised, an array of dysfunction follows. Leaky gut, dysbiosis, and metabolic endotoxemia are three conditions that often develop when this delicate system breaks down! Although distinct from each other, they are deeply interconnected, each fueling the next in a cycle that promotes inflammation, immune dysfunction, and chronic disease.

"Leaky Gut": When the Barrier Fails

As said, the gut lining acts as a selective filter that absorbs nutrients while keeping harmful substances out. But when this barrier becomes damaged, it loses its ability to protect us. "Leaky gut" is a disorder in which the intestinal barrier permeability is altered. This allows undigested particles of food, toxins, and microorganisms to migrate into the bloodstream and interact with the immune system. Tiny openings develop between the intestinal cells (like holes in Swiss cheese), and the immune system, sensing foreign invaders where they don't belong, mounts an attack. The result is chronic inflammation, food sensitivities, and a heightened risk of autoimmune disease.[25][26]

Dysbiosis: The Gut Microbiome Out of Balance

A healthy gut relies on our microbial diversity working together to support digestion, immune function, and metabolism. Dysbiosis occurs when this balance is lost. Beneficial bacteria decline, while others take the opportunity to overgrow, pathogenic strains take up residence, and produce toxins that further damage the gut lining. This disruption impairs our digestion, triggers the immune system, promotes inflammation, and alters how the body actually metabolizes (takes in and digests) nutrients.

The Western and high-fat, low-fiber diets often contribute to dysbiosis.[27] This often leads to more bacterial toxins and inflammation, along with fewer beneficial microbes like *Akkermansia*. As a result, the body produces fewer key metabolites, including vitamins, hormones, and short-chain fatty acids (SCFAs) such as butyrate, which are essential for health.

Metabolic Endotoxemia: Inflammation from Within

Perhaps the most alarming consequence of gut dysfunction is Metabolic Endotoxemia (ME). This occurs when toxic Gram-negative bacterial fragments, called lipopolysaccharides (LPS), escape from the gut into the bloodstream. Under normal conditions, these endotoxins remain contained, but when leaky gut and dysbiosis are present, they infiltrate our circulation and trigger widespread inflammation. When LPS is released into our circulation, this induces a secretion of proinflammatory cytokines, nitric oxide, and eicosanoids (anti-inflammatory and immune signaling molecules). LPS in the blood leads to a systemic inflammatory response that may progress to multi-organ system failure or sepsis, carrying a high risk of mortality.[28]

While persistent, low-grade LPS in the blood promotes chronic inflammation and the progression of disease, affecting multiple tissues like the liver, heart, adipose tissue (fatty tissue), our muscles, and arteries.[29][30] Perhaps most concerning is the fact that LPS can cross the blood-brain barrier, which can cause neuroinflammation and cognitive impairment.[31]

These three conditions, as said, are connected: Leaky gut allows toxins to enter the bloodstream, which fuels inflammation. Dysbiosis disrupts microbial harmony, weakening gut integrity and diminishing production of beneficial metabolites. Metabolic endotoxemia *amplifies* all the damage, driving systemic inflammation and chronic disease.

The cycle continues until the root cause is addressed. As you can see, we cannot just take a pill and "get better" on a broken gut. Leaky gut also follows a very predictable path, with triggers that include stress, toxins, pathogens, drugs, and infections. Left unnoticed, leaky gut progresses, resulting in chronic inflammation and immune response, which ultimately leads to systemic disease and very poor health. All healing begins with understanding. The gut is not just a digestive organ—it is the foundation of whole-body health.

Poor Digestive Health as a Condition: H. pylori and Hypochlorhydria

Digestion begins in the mouth, but continues in the stomach, where powerful acids further break down the food we eat, activate enzymes, and eliminate harmful bacteria before they can enter the intestines. When acid production in the stomach is compromised, digestion weakens, opportunistic microbes thrive, and nutrient deficiencies follow. Two of the most overlooked contributors to poor digestive health are *Helicobacter pylori* (H. pylori) infections and hypochlorhydria (low levels of stomach acid). Although these factors are very different, they both disrupt our stomach function and prime the body for nutrient deficiencies and chronic disease.

H. pylori: A Hidden Cause of Gut Dysfunction

H. pylori is a gram-negative (outer membrane composed of lipopolysaccharides (LPS), spiral-shaped bacterium that burrows into the stomach lining, weakening its protective barrier and triggering inflammation. This infection is surprisingly common, estimated to affect over half of the world's population, yet many people remain undiagnosed.[32] Over time, *H. pylori* can lead to chronic gastritis, ulcers, acid reflux, and even stomach cancer. One of the most concerning effects of *H. pylori* is its ability to suppress stomach acid production. The bacterium produces urease, which is an enzyme that neutralizes stomach acid by converting urea to ammonia, a mechanism employed to survive in the acidic environment of the stomach. While many associate acid reflux with *too much* stomach acid, *H. pylori* often causes the opposite problem, reducing acid levels to the point where digestion slows down and the food just sits there, undigested in the stomach, regurgitating up the throat.

Hypochlorhydria: The Silent Digestive Breakdown

Low stomach acid, or hypochlorhydria, is another widespread but often ignored condition. Many people mistakenly believe that acid reflux is caused by excess stomach acid, leading them to take acid-reducing medications like proton pump inhibitors (PPIs). In reality, low stomach acid is often the real culprit. A healthy stomach maintains a highly acidic environment with a pH between 1.5 and 3.5. This acidity serves multiple critical functions:

- Eliminates pathogens in food

- Aids in the digestion and absorption of nutrients (especially iron, zinc, calcium, and vitamin C)

- Activates pepsin for protein breakdown

- Enables vitamin B12 absorption through intrinsic factor

- Stimulates the release of bile and digestive enzymes[33]

Hypochlorhydria can develop from multiple causes beyond H. pylori infection. Common triggers include medications (particularly antibiotics and PPIs), chronic stress, poor diet, eating too quickly or "on-the-go," aging, and bacterial overgrowth.

Each of these factors can disrupt the stomach's ability to produce adequate acid, compromising digestive function. When acid levels drop, digestion slows. Proteins remain undigested, creating an environment where pathogenic bacteria thrive. This not only increases the risk of infections like *H. pylori* and small intestinal bacterial overgrowth (SIBO) but also leads to poor absorption of critical nutrients (iron, magnesium, calcium, zinc), potentially resulting in health issues like anemia (from iron deficiency) or weakened bones (from calcium deficiency). Both *H. pylori* infections and hypochlor-hydria disrupt digestion at its core. When stomach function fails, food is not properly broken down, nutrients are not absorbed, and gut bacteria shift into imbalance. The effects are far-reaching: poor digestion weakens immunity, fuels inflammation, and contributes to metabolic disorders.

The Gut's Role in Metabolic Health

While metabolism is often thought of in terms of calories in versus calories out, its function is far more complex. The gut microbiome acts as a "metabolic control center." The bacteria in the gut play a key role in breaking down the food we eat, extracting nutrients, and producing short-chain fatty acids (SCFAs) like butyrate, acetate, and propionate, and many other gut-derived hormones. These compounds help regulate our production of energy, improve insulin sensitivity, and reduce inflammation. They also stimulate the release of hormones that regulate hunger, such as glucagon-like peptide-1 (GLP-1), ghrelin, and leptin, which control our appetite and feelings of hunger and satiety.[34]

Patients with metabolic disorders often have a lowered microbial diversity and an overgrowth of *Firmicutes* bacteria that are more efficient at breaking down complex carbohydrates, having greater energy extraction from food, thus promoting weight gain even though the calories we eat remain the same.[35]

A diverse, well-balanced microbiome supports these metabolic processes and helps the body maintain a healthy weight and steady blood sugar levels. However, when the gut microbiome becomes imbalanced, our metabolism begins to break down.

This shift alters *how* the body stores fat and uses energy, and contributes to insulin resistance, an increased accumulation of fat, and chronic inflammation.

Key Takeaways

Here are some key takeaways for you to remember:

- Every system in the body, from the immune response to our metabolism (and even brain function), is influenced by the trillions of microbes that make up the gut microbiome.
- When this ecosystem is thriving, it promotes good digestion, strengthens our immune defense, regulates inflammation, and makes it possible for us to take in essential nutrients. But when gut health is disrupted, the consequences ripple throughout the *whole* body (not just the gut), which increases the risk of chronic disease.

The microbiome is not a random collection of bacteria; it is an intricate network where specific keystone species play a crucial role in maintaining this balanced ecosystem. Beneficial bacteria like *Akkermansia muciniphila* and *Lactobacillus* help protect the gut lining, regulate immune response, and prevent harmful microbes from taking over. Their presence is essential for preventing conditions like leaky gut, dysbiosis, and metabolic endotoxemia, gut imbalances that drive inflammation and chronic illness.

Yet, modern life is just *filled* with sources of gut disruptors that threaten our health. And most people have no idea! Processed foods, chronic stress, environmental toxins, and medications such as antibiotics and acid blockers can alter the microbiome and compromise gut function.

Over time, these disruptions impair our digestion, alter the immune system, and contribute to metabolic dysfunction. Infections like *H. pylori* and conditions such as low stomach acid compromise health by altering nutrient absorption and digestive function. It is clear: gut health is not an isolated factor; it is the key to whole-body wellness.

Questions for Reflection

The way we care for our health is shaped by what we believe about our bodies. If we see symptoms as "random," we tend to treat them as isolated problems. But when we recognize that everything in the body is connected, we begin to ask different questions—questions that lead to real answers.

Take a moment to reflect on what you have learned in this chapter and how it applies to your own health.

1. What is one change you can make today to support your gut microbiome? Could it be adding more whole foods, reducing processed ingredients, or finding ways to manage stress?

2. How have your diet and stress levels influenced your digestion and overall health? Have you noticed any patterns, like bloating after certain meals, fatigue after a stressful day, or cravings that seem hard to control?

3. Do you experience symptoms like brain fog, joint pain, poor sleep, or low energy? Could these be signals of an imbalanced gut rather than random discomforts?

4. What steps can you take to reduce exposure to gut-disrupting toxins and medications? Are there alternatives you haven't considered?

5. How does understanding the gut's role in overall health shift the way you approach self-care? Does it change how you view your health challenges and the solutions available to you?

This chapter has looked at the science, disruption, and restoration of gut health. By taking proactive steps, we can begin to reverse dysfunction, prevent disease, and honor the incredible system our digestion truly is. Small, intentional changes, like nourishing our body, reducing stress, and addressing gut health, can lead to long-term transformations. As we move forward, we will look at how these gut imbalances are linked to chronic conditions throughout the body. From metabolic dysfunction to autoimmune disease, the next chapter will uncover how the gut's influence extends far beyond digestion and what steps can be taken to restore true health.

CHAPTER 4

Gut Imbalances And Chronic Disease

Bless the Lord, O my soul, and forget not all His benefits,
who forgives all your iniquities, who heals all your diseases.

— Psalm 103: 2-3 (MEV)

The body was designed with an incredible ability to maintain balance and restore itself. Yet, in today's world, chronic illness is more common than ever. Many people struggle with ongoing fatigue, digestive discomfort, hormonal imbalances, and inflammatory conditions without realizing that the gut is at the center of it all.

Approximately 80% of the immune system resides in the gut, where it plays a central role in regulating your immune response. It helps your body handle the constant stream of microbes and food particles you're exposed to every day. It teaches your body to tolerate what's safe while fighting off harmful germs, helping to prevent infections.

Research shows that when the gut microbiota becomes imbalanced, a state known as dysbiosis, it can disrupt immune regulation and contribute to cardiovascular diseases, cancers, respiratory disorders, inflammatory bowel diseases, type 2 diabetes, obesity, allergies, and colorectal cancer.[1][2] Additional factors such as infections, antibiotics, toxin exposure, low-fiber diets, circadian rhythm disruption, and psychological stress can impair gut barrier integrity, allowing bacteria and their components to enter circulation and trigger systemic, low-grade inflammation.[3]

When the gut is in balance, it helps regulate digestion, immunity, metabolism, and even brain function. But when it becomes compromised, the effects extend far beyond the digestive system. Imbalances in gut bacteria and damage to the gut lining can disrupt the body's natural processes, making it harder to absorb nutrients, fight infections, and keep inflammation in check. Over time, this can contribute to a wide range of chronic health challenges.

This chapter explores how gut imbalances contribute to chronic disease and why restoring gut health is a foundational step toward healing. We will examine the connection between the microbiome, inflammation, and metabolic health, and explore how targeted strategies can support healing and long-term wellness.

Metabolic Syndrome: Obesity and Diabetes

Metabolic syndrome is not simply a matter of excess weight or elevated blood sugar reflects a cluster of interconnected physiological changes that place the body at significantly higher risk for chronic disease. This condition is defined by the presence of at least three of the following: abdominal obesity, insulin resistance or elevated fasting glucose, high blood pressure, high triglycerides, and low HDL cholesterol.

Together, these markers signal underlying metabolic dysfunction and a heightened risk for cardiovascular disease, stroke, and type 2 diabetes. A growing body of evidence shows that metabolic syndrome is closely tied to gut health. Dysbiosis, particularly an increased *Firmicutes* to *Bacteroidetes* ratio (F/B ratio), has been associated with obesity, insulin resistance, cardiovascular disease, and systemic inflammation.[4]

One of the critical links between gut dysbiosis and metabolic syndrome is metabolic endotoxemia.[5] High-fat, low-fiber diets, poor microbial diversity, and other disruptors can increase intestinal permeability, allowing bacterial components such as lipopolysaccharides (LPS) from gram-negative bacteria to pass into the bloodstream.[6] Once in circulation, LPS binds to immune cell receptors, triggering the release of pro-inflammatory cytokines (TNF-α, IL-1β, IFN-γ). This persistent, low-grade inflammation impairs insulin signaling, alters lipid metabolism, and promotes adipose tissue dysfunction, key drivers in the progression of metabolic syndrome.

Importantly, this inflammatory state does not remain confined to the gut. Systemic inflammation from endotoxemia contributes to vascular dysfunction, hypertension, and atherosclerotic plaque development, while also influencing brain signaling related to appetite and energy regulation.[7] Over time, the combination of dysbiosis, increased gut permeability, and immune activation creates a self-reinforcing cycle that perpetuates metabolic imbalance and elevates the risk of serious chronic disease.

The gut microbiome does far more than help digest food, it also has a major influence on metabolism and weight regulation. Studies in animals have shown that when gut bacteria from an obese donor are transferred to germ-free mice, the mice tend to gain weight even if their diet does not change.[8][9][10][11] There is also real-world evidence of this effect in people. One published case described a woman who received a fecal microbiota transplant (FMT) to treat recurrent *Clostridium difficile* infection. The treatment worked, but the donor, though healthy, was overweight. In the months after the procedure, the woman developed new-onset obesity.[12] This case has raised important questions about how much the donor's gut bacteria can influence the recipient's metabolism. It also shows why careful donor selection is so important, especially for patients who may already be at risk for metabolic health issues.

Despite being linked to all of these metabolic diseases, the gut also has the power to reverse or heal. Beneficial bacteria produce short-chain fatty acids (SCFAs), such as butyrate, which improve insulin sensitivity, support fat metabolism, and lower inflammation. However, people with obesity and diabetes often have a deficiency or absence of bacteria that produce SCFA and stimulate the release of appetite-regulating hormones like GLP-1, leptin, and ghrelin, key messengers that signal appetite and satiety, making it harder to feel satisfied after eating.[13] [14] Maintaining a diverse and balanced gut microbiome helps keep these hormones in balance, which supports healthier eating patterns, steadier blood sugar levels, and more effective weight management.

Beyond gut bacteria, nutrient status also plays a powerful role in metabolic health. Vitamin D, in particular, has been closely tied to insulin sensitivity, weight regulation, and inflammation control. Research suggests that maintaining a serum 25(OH)D level above 32 ng/mL (80 nmol/L) supports optimal immune and metabolic function.[15] Low Vitamin D levels are strongly linked to a higher risk of diabetes and metabolic syndrome, with studies showing that the risk increases as serum Vitamin D concentrations decrease.[16] [17] Without enough Vitamin D, the body has a harder time maintaining glucose control, regulating immune response, and keeping inflammation in check, three key factors in preventing insulin resistance and metabolic dysfunction.

The Gut-Heart Connection

The connection between gut health and heart disease runs deeper than most people realize. While high cholesterol, elevated blood pressure, and lifestyle habits are well-known contributors, the gut microbiome quietly plays a powerful role in cardiovascular health. An imbalanced gut can fuel chronic inflammation, disrupt blood sugar regulation, and damage the lining of blood vessels, all of which set the stage for heart disease. One of the key culprits in this process is a weakened gut barrier, often referred to as "leaky gut." When this barrier becomes compromised, harmful substances (LPS endotoxin) can pass into the bloodstream, triggering widespread immune responses. The resulting inflammation contributes to arterial stiffness, plaque buildup, and high blood pressure, factors that significantly raise the risk of heart attack and stroke.[18] [19]

Beyond this, certain gut bacteria metabolize dietary compounds like choline and carnitine, found in red meat and eggs, into a substance called trimethylamine (TMA). In the liver, TMA is converted into trimethylamine N-oxide (TMAO), a compound shown to promote vascular inflammation, atherosclerosis, thrombosis, heart failure, and kidney fibrosis. Elevated TMAO levels are now recognized as a major risk factor for cardiovascular disease.[20] Fortunately, the gut can also be part of the solution. Beneficial bacteria help regulate cholesterol metabolism, reduce inflammation, and support overall heart function. Diet plays a crucial role in shaping the gut microbiome. Reducing consumption of processed meats and increasing fiber-rich foods can help shift the microbiome away from TMAO-producing bacteria and toward microbes that promote heart health.[21]

Neurodegenerative and Mood Disorders: Alzheimer's, Parkinson's, Anxiety, and Depression

The gut and brain are in constant conversation through what is known as the gut–brain axis (GBA), a communication network in which signals travel in both directions, but about 80% of the traffic actually goes *from* the gut *to* the brain. One of the main highways for this exchange is the vagus nerve, which carries information from the gut's environment to influence brain function and mood. The trillions of microbes in the gut play an active role in this process. They produce metabolites, including hormones, neurotransmitters, vitamins, and short-chain fatty acids (SCFAs), that send chemical messages to the brain. These signals can shape everything from mood and motivation to memory and focus.[22]

When the gut barrier becomes compromised, a condition often called "leaky gut," bacterial byproducts and toxins can slip into the bloodstream. This can spark an immune response that reaches the brain and overstimulates microglia, the brain's immune cells. Chronic microglial activation fuels neuroinflammation, which has been linked to cognitive decline, memory issues, and a higher risk of neurodegenerative conditions like Alzheimer's and Parkinson's disease.[23]

The gut's influence on brain health is not limited to inflammation. It also produces a large share of the body's key neurotransmitters, about 90% of serotonin and 50% of dopamine are made in the gut. When the microbiome is imbalanced, this production is altered, potentially leading to symptoms such as anxiety, depression, mood swings, and brain fog, even in people who otherwise live a healthy lifestyle.[24]

Polyphenols, natural compounds found in fruits, vegetables, tea, and wine, can help bridge the gap between gut health and brain function. Once consumed, polyphenols are fermented by gut bacteria and are transformed into beneficial metabolites. These metabolites include short-chain fatty acids (SCFAs), tryptophan, tyrosine, and brain-signaling molecules like dopamine, serotonin (5-HT), norepinephrine, and epinephrine. These compounds help regulate neurotransmission, reduce inflammation, and support the brain's stress response. In addition, polyphenol metabolites have antioxidant properties, fight inflammation, and improve mitochondrial function, critical factors in protecting the brain from degenerative damage.[25, 27] By enhancing nerve synaptic plasticity and reducing oxidative stress, polyphenols help improve cognitive function and slow down the progression of neurodegenerative diseases. Supporting the gut microbiome through a polyphenol-rich diet and targeted probiotics offers a powerful way to protect brain health.

Another area of research showing benefits in mood and cognition is with specific probiotics called *psychobiotics*. The term psychobiotic is defined as *a live organism, usually a type of bacteria, that, when ingested in adequate amounts, can produce a health benefit related to mental health.* [26] Essentially, they are probiotics that can impact mood, cognition, and overall mental well-being through their interaction with the gut microbiota.

Psychobiotic strains like *Lactobacillus* and *Bifidobacterium* not only boost beneficial neurotransmitters but also reduce stress hormones and ease symptoms of anxiety and depression. Ultimately, caring for your gut can be a key step in improving mental clarity, emotional resilience, and long-term brain function.[26]

The Gut-Lung Axis:
Respiratory Health and COVID-19

Although the gut and lungs function in separate parts of the body, they are tightly connected through the immune system, a relationship known as the gut-lung axis. This connection became especially significant during the COVID-19 pandemic, when researchers discovered that imbalances in gut health could worsen respiratory outcomes.

When SARS-CoV-2 virus enters the body, it typically infects the upper respiratory tract. However, in individuals with a disrupted gut microbiome, the integrity of the gut barrier is weakened. This allows the virus to move from the lungs into the gastrointestinal tract, where it binds to ACE2 receptors in the gut. This can cause gastrointestinal symptoms (nausea and vomiting) and further compromise the body's defenses.

Once the virus crosses the damaged gut barrier and enters systemic circulation, it triggers an uncontrolled immune response. This widespread inflammation, often referred to as a *cytokine storm*, can lead to multiorgan failure and severe complications in COVID-19 patients.[28] The more the gut barrier is compromised, the more likely it is that microbial products and the virus itself will leak into the bloodstream, amplifying inflammation and contributing to poor outcomes.[29] By contrast, a healthy gut microbiome helps maintain the integrity of the gut barrier, limiting viral entry and controlling inflammation. In a balanced gut, regulatory T cells help prevent immune overactivation and reduce the risk of systemic inflammation. During the pandemic, it became clear that patients with healthier gut microbiota were better equipped to fight off infection and avoid complications such as pneumonia, blood clots, and sepsis.[30]

Autoimmune Conditions: Thyroid, Lupus, and Others

Around 70–80% of the body's immune system resides in the gut, within a network called gut-associated lymphoid tissue (GALT). This is the largest mass of lymphoid tissue in the body, made up of immune cells like B and T lymphocytes, macrophages, and antigen-presenting dendritic cells. GALT is on constant alert; it defends against harmful pathogens while maintaining tolerance to beneficial microbes and dietary food antigens.

The gut microbiome plays a critical role in this immune activity. Microbial metabolites and food antigens stimulate the GALT's immune cells to produce immunoglobulin A (IgA), the body's most abundant antibody. Secretory IgA acts like a shield for the mucosal lining, blocking microbial invasion and keeping the immune system in balance with friendly bacteria.

The gut's mucus layer, produced by intestinal goblet cells, is another essential part of immune defense. This protective coating separates the inner gut lining from the outside world. Without enough mucin, bacteria can reach the epithelial surface, sparking intestinal inflammation. Healthy commensal bacteria also contribute by digesting food, maintaining gut-barrier function, regulating immune responses, and producing vitamins, neurotransmitters, and short-chain fatty acids.

When this gut–immune system partnership is disrupted, as in dysbiosis or leaky gut, it can set the stage for autoimmune conditions, diseases where the immune system mistakenly attacks the body's own tissues.[31] Autoimmunity can affect almost any organ, but the thyroid is one of the most common targets.

In Hashimoto's thyroiditis (HT), the immune system attacks thyroid cells, reducing thyroid hormone, ultimately slowing metabolism and leading to symptoms like fatigue, weight gain, and sensitivity to cold.

On the other hand, Graves' disease triggers an overactive thyroid, which then floods the body with hormones that speed up the heart rate and lead to anxiety, weight loss, and heat intolerance.

Although their effects are opposite, both conditions have been linked to immune dysregulation due to pathogens in the gut. Bacterial infections like *Helicobacter pylori (H. pylori)* and parasites (*Blastocystis hominis)* [32], [33] can trigger the immune system, increasing the production of antibodies to fight infection, but mistakenly "mimic" proteins that are similar to the thyroid cells- a condition known as *molecular mimicry.*

Molecular mimicry happens when the immune system makes antibodies to fight an infection, but those antibodies also recognize similar features on the body's own tissues. Because the invader and our cells look alike, the immune system can attack healthy tissue, which may lead to autoimmune disease.

Some autoimmune diseases, like lupus, are more complex and unpredictable. Lupus can target multiple organs at once, including the skin, joints, kidneys, heart, and brain, with symptoms ranging from mild rashes and joint pain to severe organ damage. Unlike thyroid conditions, lupus tends to flare in cycles, with symptom-free periods followed by sudden inflammation. Triggers such as stress, infections, or even sunlight can provoke these flares, making the disease difficult to manage; however, newer insights into the microbiome provide hope for the prevention and management of lupus.[34]

Other autoimmune conditions have their own distinct patterns.[35] Rheumatoid arthritis attacks the joints, causing persistent pain, stiffness, and swelling that worsen over time. Multiple sclerosis targets the protective sheath around nerves, disrupting communication between the brain and body and leading to symptoms like muscle weakness, fatigue, and vision problems. Psoriasis accelerates skin cell turnover, creating thick, scaly patches that can cause both physical discomfort and emotional distress.

Despite their differences, most autoimmune diseases share common underlying triggers. Gut imbalances, chronic stress, environmental toxins, and nutrient deficiencies can all play a role in setting off immune system dysfunction.

Another contributing factor to the development of autoimmune disease is leaky gut. A biomarker of increased gut permeability is *zonulin*, a protein that regulates the tight junctions between intestinal cells or colonocytes.[36] When zonulin levels rise, the gut barrier becomes more permeable or "leaky", which allows bacteria, toxins, and undigested food particles to leak into the bloodstream. This leakage activates the immune system and increases the likelihood of antibody production and autoimmune conditions.

Stress hormones can further intensify inflammation and leaky gut, which makes symptoms more severe and recovery more difficult. Environmental toxins, such as pesticides, heavy metals, and chemical pollutants, can also interfere with immune signaling, increasing the risk of mistaken attacks on healthy tissue. Even diet can likewise impact its progression. For some people, certain foods may help calm inflammation, while for others, those same foods have developed antibodies that trigger inflammatory or delayed-allergic type reactions.

Hope Through Testing and Observation

For too long, healthcare has been built on guesswork. If you have pain, you are given a painkiller. If you have high blood pressure, you're given medication to lower it. But what is actually causing the problem? *Why* is your body struggling in the first place? Instead of getting real answers, many people are given prescriptions and sent on their way, only to return months later with more symptoms and more medications.

In functional medicine, we aim to uncover the root cause instead of treating symptoms. We stop the cycle of temporary fixes and use precise tools to reveal hidden imbalances in the gut, immune system, and metabolism.

Targeted Tests for Gut-Related Chronic Disease

- **Intestinal Permeability Assessment** - This measures zonulin and occludin, proteins that regulate gut barrier integrity. High levels indicate leaky gut, which allows toxins and food particles to enter the bloodstream, fueling food sensitivities and autoimmune conditions like Hashimoto's, lupus, and rheumatoid arthritis.

- **Plasma Endotoxin Test** - This detects lipopolysaccharides (LPS) in the blood, a marker of metabolic endotoxemia. Elevated LPS is linked to obesity, insulin resistance, and systemic inflammation, which tells us that gut dysfunction is driving disease progression.

- **Environmental and Chemical Exposure** – Assesses exposure and evaluates the impact of environmental toxicants, heavy metals, pesticides, and mycotoxins on mitochondrial function, neurologic function, and important metabolic pathways impacting gut health, neurotransmitter metabolism, detoxification capacity, and nutritional status. Identifying toxins can provide a more accurate and targeted evaluation of an individual's overall health risks as well as therapeutic options to reduce risks.

- **Comprehensive Stool Analysis** - This goes beyond microbiome testing, measuring secretory IgA (immune response), digestive function, inflammation, and the presence of beneficial as well as pathogenic bacteria, parasites, or yeast. It reveals whether dysbiosis, infections, immune dysfunction, increased permeability (zonulin), or gut inflammation are contributing to chronic disease.

Even with lab results, your daily experience matters. Keeping a gut health journal that tracks digestion, energy, mental clarity, skin health, and inflammatory symptoms helps connect lab findings with real-world patterns. Many people discover that certain foods, stressors, or habits directly trigger their symptoms, insights that no blood test alone can provide.

Lifestyle Shifts That Heal

Gut health does not improve with temporary efforts. It improves with consistency. The choices made each day, what we eat, how we move and sleep, and the way we manage stress, either support healing or perpetuate dysfunction. These are not trends. They are core physiologic needs. The microbiome is responsive to the environment. When the environment improves, so does the body's ability to digest, repair, defend, and regulate.

Food as Medicine

Microbial health begins with food. A fiber-deficient diet is one of the most common and most correctable drivers of dysbiosis and inflammation. The average intake in the U.S. is under 15 grams per day. The minimum needed to support gut function and microbial balance is twice that! Soluble fiber, from lentils, oats, and cooked vegetables, supports the growth of bacteria that produce short-chain fatty acids, critical for immune regulation and gut lining integrity. Insoluble fiber, found in leafy greens and raw vegetables, improves motility and prevents overgrowth of harmful microbes. Both are necessary.[37]

Polyphenols, found in foods like green tea, blueberries, and pomegranate, act as microbial modulators. Once metabolized by gut bacteria, they produce compounds that reduce inflammation and support the gut-brain axis. A lack of dietary diversity limits this benefit. Fermented foods provide live bacteria. Kimchi, sauerkraut, kefir, and plain yogurt (when unpasteurized and free from additives) introduce probiotic strains that can enhance barrier function and reduce bloating. But probiotics are only part of the picture. Prebiotics, such as fibers found in garlic, onions, leeks, and asparagus, are the fuel these bacteria require to survive. A therapeutic diet doesn't need to be extreme. It needs to be diverse, nutrient-dense, and anti-inflammatory. What matters most is not what is removed temporarily, but what is sustained over time.

Eliminating Gut Disruptors

You cannot heal what is constantly being harmed. Gut restoration depends not only on what you add, but what you remove. Ultra-processed foods, industrial seed oils, and added sugars drive microbial imbalance and immune dysregulation. These foods are engineered to bypass satiety signals, alter blood sugar, and feed inflammatory pathways. They have no place in a therapeutic diet. Beyond food, chemical exposures degrade the gut environment. Pesticides, food dyes, artificial sweeteners, and preservatives impair microbial diversity and weaken mucosal defenses. Many of these compounds are still approved for consumption despite known effects on gut permeability and immune function.

Alcohol, chronic NSAID use, and long-term antibiotics are other common disruptors. Each has a measurable impact on microbial ratios and increases the risk for fungal or bacterial overgrowth. If the goal is repair, the environment must change. That includes the grocery list, the pantry, and the daily routine.

Prioritizing unprocessed, nutrient-dense, organic whole foods is not restrictive—it's necessary. For many patients, simply removing what is irritating the gut is what finally allows healing to begin.

Healthy Fats and Omega-3s

The gut lining depends on adequate fat for structural repair and inflammatory regulation. Patients on low-fat diets or consuming only processed fats often have compromised mucosal integrity. Omega-3 fatty acids, particularly EPA and DHA, modulate inflammation at the cellular level. They reduce pro-inflammatory cytokines, support immune balance, and improve conditions such as intestinal permeability and autoimmune reactivity.[38] These are found in cold-water fish (salmon, sardines, mackerel), flaxseed, chia seeds, and walnuts. Monounsaturated fats like olive oil, avocado, and raw nuts also contribute to microbial health by reducing oxidative stress in the gut. These fats help regulate insulin sensitivity, lipid metabolism, cell wall integrity, intestinal immunity, and inflammatory response. Fats are not the problem. The wrong fats are.

Movement, Stress, and Microbiome Balance

Gut motility is governed by the nervous system. Physical movement and stress management are essential, not optional, for gut health.[39] Exercise increases microbial diversity, enhances insulin sensitivity, and supports intestinal transit.[40] It doesn't need to be intense. Walking, strength training, and stretching. All of these stimulate vagal tone and help move digestion forward. Chronic stress shifts the body into a sympathetic-dominant state, reducing blood flow and acid production in the digestive tract, slowing motility, and impairing immune response. Elevated cortisol weakens the gut barrier and disrupts sleep, hormone function, and microbial balance. Restoring parasympathetic tone through deep breathing, prayer, journaling, or consistent sleep rebuilds this connection. Sleep is also where the body performs its most important repair work. Without it, no gut protocol is effective.[41]

Turning to Scripture in Chronic Illness

Chronic illness can be both physically draining and emotionally overwhelming. When symptoms linger and answers remain elusive, it is easy to feel defeated. Yet faith offers a different perspective; it reminds us that we are not alone in our struggles.

Hope, rooted in faith, can be a powerful form of healing in itself. It encourages us to care for our bodies with intention, which starts with recognizing that we are fearfully and wonderfully made.

Many people view faith and science as opposing forces, but in truth, they are deeply connected. The same God who designed the intricate systems of the body also gave us the tools, knowledge, wisdom, and research to understand how those systems work. Holistic health means embracing both prayer and medicine as vital parts of the healing process. Today, we understand that restoring microbial balance is essential for reversing inflammation and chronic disease. Fasting, a spiritual practice with deep biblical roots, is now recognized for its physical benefits, including gut healing and improved metabolic resilience. Faith does not stand in opposition to science; it enhances it. When we pursue healing, we can draw from both biblical wisdom and scientific insight, trusting that they work together to restore the body. Healing is not a straight path, and it often requires patience, trust, and intentional effort.

It means leaning on God's promises while taking practical steps through nutrition, stress management, and medical care to support our well-being.

Even when progress feels slow or medicine offers limited answers, faith remains a constant source of strength. It reminds us that we are never alone in our experience. In every step of the healing process, God is present.

Key Takeaways

Throughout this chapter, we have discussed how gut health is deeply connected to chronic disease. From metabolic syndrome and heart disease to neurodegeneration and autoimmune conditions.

However, healing is completely possible. By restoring gut balance, we can:

- Improve metabolism and insulin sensitivity, reducing the risk of obesity and diabetes.

- Support cardiovascular health, lowering inflammation, and preventing arterial damage.

- Enhance brain function and emotional well-being, reducing the risk of neurodegeneration and mood disorders.

- Regulate the immune system, calming autoimmune activity and strengthening resilience.

- Prevent and reverse chronic inflammation, a key driver of disease progression.

Questions for Reflection

Take a moment to reflect on your personal health process:

1. What signs of gut imbalance have you personally experienced, and how have they affected your daily life?

2. What specific changes to your diet or lifestyle can you implement immediately to start improving your gut health?

3. How does the gut's role in regulating inflammation change the way you think about chronic disease?

4. What functional lab tests might provide the best insight into your own gut health, and how can they help guide your next steps?

5. How can faith and scientific understanding work together to support your path to healing?

Understanding how the gut influences everything from heart disease to diabetes gives us a clearer picture of why symptoms persist despite conventional care. Yet knowledge alone is not enough — lasting change requires a deeper reason to take action. This is where your WHY comes in. Without it, efforts often feel scattered and unsustainable. With it, every choice gains purpose and momentum. In the next chapter, we'll explore how to uncover your WHY and use it as the driving force for transformation.

CHAPTER 5

Finding Your Why

Joyful is the person who finds wisdom,
the one who gains understanding.

— Proverbs 3:13 (NLT)

For so many people, health feels like a battle they just cannot win. They do what they are told—visit their doctor and follow the standard advice—but instead of feeling better, they remain stuck. Their energy is drained, symptoms persist, and each new prescription seems to lead to another one. It is a frustrating cycle—but what if the real issue is not the symptoms themselves? What if the missing piece is not just another medication or another diet but something deeper? This is where your WHY becomes essential. Without a clear WHY, all efforts become scattered, motivation fades, and old habits often fall back into place. But when you truly understand what is at stake, your choices begin to change. Your WHY is the key that turns short-term effort into lasting transformation. Maybe it's the prospect of regaining your energy to keep up with the kids. Maybe it is the promise of breaking free from medications and reclaiming control over your body again. Or maybe it's the notion that you could simply feel like yourself again—strong, vibrant, and in charge of your own well-being. Whatever it is, finding your WHY is the first step toward real, lasting change. In this chapter, we will discuss how to uncover your WHY, why functional medicine provides a new path forward, and how taking ownership of your health is the most powerful decision you can make.

The Limitations of Conventional Healthcare

As we have already talked about, medicine today is built for crisis care. If you have a heart attack, break a bone, or need emergency surgery, the system works exactly as it should—quickly, organized, and effectively. But when it comes to chronic disease, this system fails us. People who are struggling with chronic exhaustion, joint pain, digestive issues, or hormonal imbalances often find themselves trapped in a cycle of "patch-up" care. This is not the fault of the individual doctor, it is the way the system has been designed. Conventional medicine excels at treating acute illness, where problems have a clear cause and an immediate solution, according to the textbooks. Chronic disease, however, does not fit this model. Conditions like autoimmune disorders, metabolic dysfunction, and chronic inflammation develop over years and are influenced by how we eat, stress levels, toxins, and microbiome imbalances. They present with many signs, indications, or "warnings" long before they are at a level where they might be diagnosed as an illness. In conventional care, many patients are left wondering why they are still exhausted despite following their doctor's recommendations. They ask why their body feels off balance when every test says they are "fine." They often end up realizing (too late) that they are not getting better; they are getting worse. Therefore, true healing begins when you understand what conventional medicine was never meant to address.

The Power of Asking Questions

Healing begins with curiosity! Too often, people are too quick to accept a diagnosis without questioning it—or their physician. They may be told they have IBS, high blood pressure, or Type 2 diabetes, but rarely does anyone explain *why* this happens in the first place.

A diagnosis is not an answer; it is a label. It simply names the condition but leaves the cause unknown, which makes true healing impossible to reach. This is where asking the right questions becomes essential. When did your symptoms first appear? Was there a specific event, illness, or life change that triggered them? Symptoms do not happen at random, even if it might seem that way. A stressful period at work, a change in your diet, loss of a loved one, disrupted sleep, or underlying hormonal shifts all contribute to how you feel, whether or not the connection is obvious to you. Most people are not thinking about these links when they feel unwell. That is why identifying patterns is part of what I do as a provider. Another critical question to ask is: *"Can this condition be reversed or cured?"*

Conventionally, care is guided by what is known as the *Standard of Care*—a system of diagnostic and treatment protocols based on guidelines from several regulatory organizations. This refers to the "basic checklist" most doctors follow: the tests they order, the treatments they offer, and the medications and procedures they're expected to stick to are all pre-arranged, no matter who the patient is, their history, or their current condition. It's meant to diagnose disease, rule out an emergency, and then move things along efficiently. But here's the problem: once all the boxes are checked off, you're handed a prescription, and it ends there. Take chronic fatigue, for example. If you tell your doctor you're tired all the time, they might order a few standard labs—blood count, thyroid hormones, and maybe a metabolic panel. If everything comes back "normal," that's usually the end of the conversation. But feeling tired all the time isn't fine—and "normal" test results often rely on a diseased average population.

However, what those basic labs *don't* check is your nutrient status, gut function, inflammation, hormone fluctuations, or toxic load. Therefore, the most obvious cause of your fatigue may not have even been considered.

This is why asking questions matters—real questions, not just "What's wrong with me?" but "What did you test for?", "Why?", "What does this rule out?" or "What else should I know about?" Too often, people walk out of an appointment assuming that everything important has been looked at and that their physician knows everything that needs to be known. But that is not always the case. In the Standard of Care, a basic set of tests is considered appropriate for the average patient and the average case. This is just how the system is built. So if your labs came back "normal" and you were told everything looks fine—even though you still feel awful—it does not necessarily mean everything is "in your head"! It probably just means that the tools used did not find the obvious cause. You are not expected to know how to read lab results or design your own treatment plan. But you *can* ask what was included in the testing and what was not. You can ask whether your nutrient levels are checked or whether the evaluation looked at your gut health, hormone balance, inflammation, or toxic exposures. Rather than seeking explanations on the internet, you should ask your doctor specific questions to understand what was actually evaluated. For example:

- *"Can you walk me through which lab markers were tested and what they ruled out?"*

- *"Were any of these results borderline, or just considered 'normal' based on the reference range?"*

- *"Were things like nutrient levels, inflammation markers, or hormone balance part of this panel?"*

- *"If these tests do not explain my symptoms, what else might we need to look into?"*

These kinds of questions are not confrontational—they are practical, and you have a right to ask. They can help you understand what was included in your care and where further investigation might be appropriate. This is not about doubting your provider but understanding the limits of the system they are working in. The standard of care is not "wrong"—it is just too narrow. And once you understand that, you are in a better position to advocate for care that goes beyond symptom management. After all, better questions lead to better conversations, better decisions, and better outcomes. Perhaps the most important question of all: *Have I accepted my condition as "normal"?* Many people do, and they just assume their condition is just part of normal aging, that their bloating is "just how their body works," or that anxiety and brain fog are inevitable. But none of these things are normal: they are signals! And when you start asking "Why," you begin to break free from the cycle of symptom suppression.

"Test, Don't Guess" – Functional Testing as a Compass

When it comes to health, guessing is dangerous!. Yet, this is exactly what often happens when doctors rely on standard lab tests that only detect disease once it has fully developed. As I mentioned earlier, functional medicine takes on a different approach. Functional testing is a powerful tool because it can identify hidden dysfunctions that conventional labs often overlook. A person who is struggling with anxiety and insomnia might be prescribed a standard pharmaceutical without anyone checking whether their cortisol level is out of balance.

These tests all provide the small, missing pieces of the puzzle. Some of the most revealing functional tests include:

- **Mineral Levels & Toxic Elements Analysis**– Minerals are the building blocks of metabolism. An imbalance, too much calcium, too little magnesium, can disrupt energy production, brain function, and hormone balance. Functional lab testing can also detect toxic metals like lead and mercury, which interfere with cellular function, damaging vital organs like your brain, kidneys, and liver.

- **Comprehensive Stool Analysis** - The gut is the foundation of health, housing 70% of your immune system and producing vitamins and neurotransmitters that affect mood and cognition. A comprehensive stool test can reveal bacterial imbalances, parasites, yeast overgrowth, inflammatory and immune markers, and digestive dysfunction that standard testing completely misses.[1] Since gut health impacts everything from nutrient absorption to immune function, this test often uncovers the root cause of many chronic symptoms.

- **Adrenal & Stress Hormone Testing** – Chronic stress wreaks havoc on the body, but standard lab tests don't assess how well your adrenal glands are functioning. Measuring the adrenal stress hormones, cortisol and DHEA, can reveal if your brain-body connection or hypothalamus-pituitary-adrenal axis (HPA axis) is dysregulated, leading to symptoms of chronic fatigue, poor sleep, inflammation, and immune dysfunction.

- **Nutrient Deficiency Panels** – Vitamins and amino acids fuel every system in the body. Deficiencies in vitamin D, B12, iron, or magnesium can mimic conditions like depression, brain fog, and chronic fatigue. Without testing, many people are left treating symptoms when the real issue is a nutritional imbalance.

Consider this case as an example: A patient comes in with relentless fatigue, brain fog, and poor sleep. She has been tested for thyroid disease multiple times, but her results were always "OK." No one looks deeper into her case, as the tests all say she's "fine." But a closer look with functional lab tests might reveal something obvious: a common gut infection, H. Pylori – creating an environment of low stomach acid that impairs digestion of protein and reduces absorption of nutrients like iron and B12– resulting in deficiencies so severe they are starving her cells of the raw materials needed for production of hormones, neurotransmitters and essential nutrients required for energy, cognition, and stable mood. Once those are corrected, her energy could begin to return. Her mind would clear, and she might begin to sleep better. She could finally feel like herself again. There is a strong connection between low levels of B vitamins and higher rates of depression, anxiety, and stress. In other words, deficiencies do not just drain the body—they also disrupt the mind.[2]

Shifting from Passive to Active Health Management

Generally, healthcare is set up as a "passive" experience. You visit your doctor, receive an evaluation, are given their findings, and are told what to do. However, healing requires *active* participation in your care. Chronic diseases and poor health are also "lifestyle diseases," in many cases, and simply taking a pill, yet not changing anything about how we live, will not address the condition. The most successful patients are often the ones who take control of their health, seek a deeper understanding, and engage in their care with intention. Of course, when your *why* is determined, and you see that you *can* understand your health and take action to improve your condition, the process itself becomes easier to confront. The shift from passive to active health care starts with three key steps:

1. Understand Your Test Results – Know Your Numbers

Most patients are handed their lab reports filled with numbers, acronyms, and reference ranges, but almost no actual explanation. If a result falls "within normal limits," it does not always mean *optimal*, and it definitely does not mean *nothing is wrong*. Here's how to take control of your results—without needing a medical degree:

- Ask your doctor: "What does this result mean in the context of how I feel?" You are not just asking if it's "in range"—you are asking what it says about your current state of health. A value at the lower or higher end of the reference range is often associated with symptoms (i.e., not an optimal level).

- Request a printout or summary of the key labs from your visit. If something was tested, you should know what it was and why.

- If your report does not include a reference range, ask your doctor what the "normal" range is so you understand where you are and have a better idea of the optimal level or target, which is typically in the middle of the reference range.

- Circle any values that are borderline (high or low)—even if the lab did not flag them. Numbers can be technically normal while still showing dysfunction, especially if they are trending up or down over time.

- Keep a folder (digital or physical) with all of your lab results so you can track any patterns. Changes over time can matter more than isolated numbers from one test.

Here is why this matters: Let us say your thyroid panel shows a Thyroid Stimulating Hormone (TSH) value of 3.9; the normal reference range for TSH is generally considered to be between 0.4 and 4.0 mIU/L. You are told that your thyroid level is "normal"; however, it is recognized that a TSH level above 4.0 mIU/L may indicate hypothyroidism (underactive thyroid). So even though the lab says normal, you still feel exhausted, cold, and foggy, and no one has explained why. Or take vitamin D. The minimum cutoff for deficiency might be 30 ng/mL, but for immune and cardiometabolic health, many practitioners aim for levels at or above 50.

This isn't just a preference—it's based on solid research. Studies consistently show that optimal vitamin D concentrations above 30 ng/mL are essential for reducing cardiovascular disease and all-cause mortality, with many health benefits requiring levels between 40 to 50 ng/mL.[3] When researchers examined thousands of adults, they found that higher vitamin D levels provided significantly better protection against diabetes, heart disease, and metabolic dysfunction [4]. That's why updated clinical guidelines now recommend much higher vitamin D supplementation of 800 to 2000 international units per day in adults who want to ensure a sufficient vitamin D status, although higher doses may be needed to achieve 25(OH)D, concentrations of 30 to 50 ng/mL (75 to 125 nmol/L).[5] If your result is 32, it technically passes—but it may not be enough to support your immune system, metabolic, or cardiovascular health. Understanding your labs in the context of your symptoms can change everything. The goal is not just to "pass" a test here but to understand what your body needs to function well.

2. Ask Better Questions

When your physician says everything looks normal, but you still feel unwell, try these practical approaches:

- Bring a written list of your top three concerns to stay focused

- Ask directly: "What else could be causing these symptoms?"

- Request: "Can you explain why you don't think these symptoms are related?"

Being precise can help both of you focus on what matters most, help you better understand what is being considered and what this means, and enable you to make more informed decisions.

3. Track Your Progress Over Time

To track your progress, you can use a simple method that is easy to maintain:

- Keep a basic symptom journal in a notebook or phone app

- Rate major symptoms from 1-10 each week (not daily, which is often too frequent)

- Note any major diet, medication, or lifestyle changes you make and when

- Take dated photos of visible symptoms like skin issues

This is why re-testing is so valuable. When you immediately feel better, it's normal to think everything is handled. However, if symptoms persist or you have not achieved your goals, retesting is always recommended to ensure the root causes have been addressed.

Alternatively, this might be a time to consider exploring other functional labs that help to identify food sensitivities or toxic exposures from mold, pesticides, chemicals, or heavy metals- as these have been linked to many diseases that can keep you from achieving optimal health. This practical tracking gives you more objective information to work with instead of relying on how you feel in the moment. When you can show yourself that your headaches have decreased from weekly to monthly occurrences after eliminating certain foods, you provide valuable data that might otherwise be missed.

Taking Responsibility for Your Healing

Many people begin to start out with excitement, eagerness to make a change, and full of hope, but when progress begins to feel slow, or you run into a challenge, it can be hard not to question whether what you're doing is working. This is when your WHY matters most! Your WHY is what keeps you going when motivation fades or when the going gets tough. It reminds you of *why* you started— why you chose to prioritize your health, why you said no to another path, and why you committed to finding real solutions. Trusting the process also relies on the understanding that healing is not always linear: oftentimes, because chronic conditions evolve over years, healing is gradual. It doesn't happen magically overnight but occurs through small wins, small betterments, and small achievements, bit by bit. There will be ups and downs, moments of frustration, and times when you feel like nothing is changing. But every small step—every healthy meal, every restful night, every effort to reduce stress—is moving you forward.

Taking responsibility for your health means shifting your mindset. Instead of chasing quick fixes or temporary motivation, you must build a lifestyle that supports healing in the long run. This means:

- Being consistent even when progress feels slow. True healing happens over time, not overnight.

- Owning your choices. Every action, from the food you eat to the way you manage stress, contributes to your well-being.

- Seeking support without giving up control. Working with practitioners is valuable, but your health is ultimately in your hands.

Healing is not just physical—it is emotional and spiritual, too. When setbacks happen, lean into your faith, rather than frustration. Trust that your body was designed to heal and that every effort you make *is* leading you toward restoration and optimal health!

Common Roadblocks to Finding Your WHY

For many, the most challenging part of healing is simply taking the first step! The desire to feel better is very clear—especially when we feel miserable all the time. Yet when it comes to identifying a clear sense of purpose, many people feel stuck. It can all seem like too much; too much change, too much to decide on, and too many choices. This can cause a person to "freeze up," and this kind of hesitation often stems from the mental and emotional barriers that can make it so difficult to move forward.

Fear of Change

Change is rarely comfortable, even when it's necessary, and it often feels way easier to stick with familiar habits—eating the same foods, following the same routines, and continuing with the same medications—because they provide a sense of safety. Even when those habits no longer support well-being, their familiarity can be reassuring. For many, the fear is not just about failure, "What if I try and it doesn't work?", but also about success. "What if I do feel better, and now I have to maintain it?" These fears are understandable. But meaningful change does not have to be immediate or overwhelming. It starts with one manageable shift. From there, momentum builds naturally.

Feeling Overwhelmed

In today's world, the abundance of health advice can feel more paralyzing than empowering. One source recommends eliminating carbohydrates, another to only eat meat, while other sources encourage 3-day water fasts, from one day to the other. All of this data often results in confusion and total inaction. When everything feels urgent, the best way forward is to simplify things. And here, I can be of great assistance to you. Rather than attempting to overhaul everything at once, try to choose one small, sustainable habit to focus on. It might be drinking more water, taking a brief walk each day, or cutting back on processed foods. Try to experiment with some healthy foods, new recipes, and new ways of being active. These consistent, achievable actions all form the foundation for lasting progress.

Doubt in Alternative Approaches

Some people have spent years relying solely on conventional medicine and have been taught that if something is not diagnosed through traditional tests, it must not be real or legitimate. So how can you know if my approach is "the best"? Well, you can't! However, any approach that supports your body's natural ability to heal, that supports overall health, and that empowers you in understanding your health and how you can take charge of your own path is "good." And here, the HOPE Method can definitely supply just that: Hope and empowerment!

The other mindset makes it difficult to explore new approaches, even when conventional treatments aren't working. After all, you have most likely been where you are and have done what you're doing for a while now. If you have been stuck in the same cycle for years, it may be worth asking: *What if there is another way?* After all, functional medicine does not reject conventional care; it builds upon it.

Reframing Your Mindset Around Health

What you believe about your body can directly influence how it heals, often in ways that are not immediately apparent. At all times, a quiet dialogue is taking place between your thoughts and your biology. At times, it is subtle, and at other times, it is a lot more pronounced! When we are ill, it is easy to slip into a mindset that assumes this is just how life will be from now on. However, that belief can shape how your body responds, how you interpret your symptoms, and whether you continue searching for solutions or "give up." Some people do not even realize that they have adopted an identity centered around being unwell.

After months or years of dealing with fatigue, pain, or other chronic symptoms, the language becomes automatic. "I'm just someone with a weak immune system." "It's my genes," or "This is just how my body is." Those phrases might *feel* factual, but they can quietly reinforce a sense of permanence—one that discourages growth or change. That is not to say you should ignore what you are feeling. Pain and discomfort are real, and so is frustration. But viewing your body only through the lens of dysfunction makes it harder to recognize signs of progress. Shifting that perspective begins with how you talk to yourself. A small change in language—from "I'm always exhausted" to "I am feeling better every day"—can create space for healing. It softens the edges of hopelessness. There's also growing evidence that expectation influences biology. The placebo effect has been well-documented and has served as an example of how belief itself can produce measurable physical changes. The opposite is also true: when we expect failure or decline, the body often follows suit. None of this means illness is imagined. It means the mind and body are not separate, and healing does not respond only to medication or diet but to mindset as well.

Key Takeaways

As you reflect on this chapter, try to keep the following in mind—not just as concepts, but as tools to help you take real steps forward:

- **Finding your WHY provides clarity and direction.**

  Without a clear WHY, it is easy to fall into the trap of starting strong and fading fast. But when you know what is at stake—whether it is getting off medications, being present for your family, or simply feeling like yourself again—you stop relying on motivation and start building momentum. Your WHY keeps you anchored when things get hard, and it reminds you that the work you are doing is about something bigger than short-term goals.

- **The right questions lead to the right answers.**

  If you do not ask, you will never know what has been missed. Most conventional care follows a set pathway: standard labs, standard diagnoses, and standard treatments. But that does not mean everything relevant has been evaluated.

Asking *what was tested, why it was chosen,* and *what was ruled out* allows you to uncover what may have been overlooked—and begin identifying the true drivers of your symptoms.

- **Functional testing fills in the blanks.**

  When standard labs come back "normal" but you still feel unwell, it is often because those labs were designed to detect disease, not dysfunction. Functional testing goes further. It can reveal nutrient deficiencies, hormone imbalances, toxic burdens, and stress patterns that affect how your body actually functions on a daily basis. This is not about testing for the sake of testing—it is about getting the information needed to take targeted, effective action.

- **Knowledge empowers action.**

  When you understand what is going on in your body—not just in abstract terms, but in actual data—you are no longer guessing. You stop relying on symptom suppression and start making strategic choices that support healing. That might mean changing how you eat, when you sleep, what supplements you take, or how you manage stress—but now you are doing it with purpose, not out of frustration.

Questions for Reflection

Now, take a moment to reflect on where you are in your healing process. Answer these questions honestly because they will help you uncover the next step forward:

1. Have I taken ownership of my health, or am I waiting for someone else to "fix" me?

2. What symptoms have I ignored or dismissed as "normal"? Many people assume fatigue, bloating, or brain fog are just part of life. What have you been tolerating that may be a sign of imbalance?

3. What tests have I had done? Have they looked beyond basic panels? Standard labs do not always tell the full story. Have you explored functional testing to uncover deeper issues?

4. What is my WHY for wanting to heal? What is my ultimate goal?

5. How can I start applying this knowledge today to take the next step in improving my health? What is one action—big or small—that you can take today to move toward healing?

Moving Forward – From WHY to HOW

Clarity creates momentum! Understanding why you need to take control of your health can be the first breakthrough. It shifts your mindset, fuels your motivation, and helps you make better choices. But knowing your WHY is just the beginning. The next step is to turn that motivation into action. Real transformation happens in the small, consistent decisions you make every day. What you eat, how you sleep, and how you manage stress are daily choices that can determine whether your body moves toward healing or stays stuck in dysfunction. This is where we go from mindset to strategy. In the next chapter, we begin exploring the Six Healthy Habits, starting with the foundation of all healing: Nutrition as Medicine. Food is more than fuel—it is information that speaks directly to your cells.

The right nutrients can reduce inflammation, balance hormones, detoxify harmful substances, and restore energy in ways no prescription ever could. You've taken the first step by uncovering your WHY. Now, let us look at how we can use that motivation to transform your health—one habit at a time.

PART 2

The Six Healthy Habits

CHAPTER 6

Food As Medicine

But he answered, "It is written, Man shall not live by bread alone, but by every word that comes from the mouth of God."

— Matthew 4:4 (ESV)

Long before modern medicine became the standard of care, food was recognized as the primary healer. "Let food be thy medicine and medicine be thy food." As said by Hippocrates, this powerful phrase captures the fundamental connection between nutrition and health that has been understood for centuries. However, somewhere along the way, we lost this truth. The modern approach to food is no longer about nourishment but about convenience, profit, and marketing. Instead of eating for health, people are consuming ultra-processed, chemically altered foods that barely resemble real nutrition. And the consequences are undeniable! The rates of obesity, Type 2 diabetes, heart disease, digestive issues, and autoimmune conditions have soared because we are feeding these diseases rather than our health. Many people still think of nutrition in terms of calories, dieting, and weight loss, but food is so much more than that. Every bite we take sends instructions to our cells, either fueling energy and healing or driving inflammation and dysfunction. Food is information. It tells the body what to do, how to function, and whether to thrive or decline.

At its core, Hippocrates' wisdom highlights several key principles that remain relevant today. Prevention is truly the best medicine, and a healthy diet acts as preventative medicine in itself. By providing the body with essential nutrients, wholesome food strengthens the immune system, enhances organ function, and fosters overall well-being. Beyond prevention, good food nourishes not only the physical body but also the mind! Optimal nutrition directly benefits our mental health, cognitive state, and emotional well-being. Good quality, nourishing food is a vital component of holistic healthcare. The healing power of food just cannot be overstated. Yet, despite this power, food is often entirely overlooked in conventional medicine. Today, med students in the U.S. generally spend as little as *21 hours* [1] out of a 4-6,000 hours 6,000-hour-long curriculum over 4 years on nutrition. So, instead of addressing signs of nutritional deficiencies that may lead to chronic disease (or drive it!), general physicians are set up to "diagnose and treat." This represents a significant departure from Hippocrates' integrative approach to healthcare, which combined treatments with lifestyle interventions, including nutrition, to optimize patient outcomes. So, in this chapter, we will uncover the hidden deficiencies in modern diets, expose how the food industry manipulates what we eat, and explore the healing potential of whole, nutrient-dense foods. Because true health isn't found in a prescription bottle—it starts with what's on your fork.

What You Don't Know You're Missing – Essential Nutrients

Many assume they are getting the nutrients they need. They eat a variety of foods, take some multivitamins, maybe a supplement here and there, and believe they are covering their bases. But despite their best efforts, nutrient deficiencies are widespread—and often go undiagnosed. The reason? In truth, our modern food supply is just not what it used to be. Industrial farming has stripped the soil of its essential minerals, and processed foods are loaded with preservatives, additives, and chemicals. Even whole foods today contain fewer vitamins and minerals than they did decades ago. A study looked at 43 different garden crops between 1950 and 1999, noted a steady erosion of key nutrients—calcium dropped by around 16%, iron by some 15%, protein by roughly 6%, and riboflavin (vitamin B2) tumbled a startling 38%! [2] Many people are unknowingly "running on empty," struggling with fatigue, brain fog, hormonal imbalances, and weakened immunity, all due to missing nutrients.

Essential nutrients cannot be synthesized by the body and, therefore, must be supplied from the food we eat. These nutrients serve three critical functions: they provide energy, contribute to body structure, and regulate chemical processes within the body. Nutrients are broadly classified into *macronutrients* and *micronutrients*, each group playing a key role in maintaining our health. Macronutrients are required in larger amounts and include carbohydrates, proteins, and fats. Carbohydrates, in their simplest form as glucose, regulate blood sugar and provide immediate energy. These are, for instance, found in vegetables, fruits, grains, and legumes. Proteins break down into amino acids, aiding in tissue growth and repair while synthesizing DNA, hormones, enzymes, and neurotransmitters. We can obtain protein from animal sources like meat, seafood, and dairy or plant sources such as beans, legumes, nuts, and seeds. Fats, composed of fatty acids, are stored as energy and contribute to our endocrine function, immune health, and cellular structure. Healthy sources include both animal fats from dairy, eggs, and meat, and plant-based options like nuts, seeds, avocados, and olive oil.

Micronutrients, needed in smaller quantities but no less important, include vitamins and minerals. Water-soluble vitamins like B vitamins (B1, B2, B6, B12), vitamin C, pantothenic acid, biotin, and folic acid must be regularly consumed as they aren't stored in the body. Fat-soluble vitamins (A, D, E, K) can be stored in fatty tissues. Essential minerals like calcium, phosphorus, magnesium, iron, and potassium, along with trace elements such as zinc, selenium, iodine, and copper, are vital for countless bodily functions. What many don't realize is that the body often sends warnings when we are deficient in nutrients. Severe hair loss can signal low iron levels, which also cause fatigue, headaches, and feeling cold. A "burning" sensation in the feet or tongue often indicates B12 deficiency, which can also lead to balance issues and cognitive impairment if left untreated. Wounds that heal slowly might point to vitamin C deficiency, while bone pain can be a sign of vitamin D deficiency. Even something as concerning as an irregular heartbeat could be related to calcium deficiency, as calcium regulates our heartbeat.

And if your night vision deteriorates, you might be lacking vitamin A, which is crucial for eye health. Some of the most concerning deficiencies include Vitamin D; many Americans are deficient in this crucial vitamin. Vitamin D deficiency has become a global health epidemic, yet its far-reaching impact on metabolic, cardiovascular, immune regulation, and cancer prevention is often overlooked in conventional medicine.

Optimal levels of Vitamin D (above 30-50 ng/mL) have been shown to reduce the risk of various health conditions, including all-cause mortality, Alzheimer's Disease, autoimmune and allergic diseases, cancer, cardiovascular disease (CVD), COVID-19, diabetes (T2DM), and hypertension.[3] Studies consistently show that people with higher vitamin D levels experience significantly lower rates of heart disease, metabolic dysfunction, immune disorders, and several types of cancer.[4] The mechanism involves vitamin D's role in regulating over 1,000 genes, modulating immune responses, and supporting cellular function throughout the body.[5]

Table: Optimal 25(OH)D Concentrations for Various Health Outcomes

Health Outcome	Optimal 25(OH)D Level (ng/mL)	Type of Evidence
All-cause mortality	>30 ng/mL	Observational studies
Alzheimer's disease and dementia	>25 ng/mL	Meta-analysis
Breast cancer	>60 ng/mL	Observational studies
Colorectal cancer	30-40 ng/mL	Meta-analysis
Cardiovascular disease	>30 ng/mL	Observational studies
COVID-19 mortality	>60 ng/mL	Retrospective studies
Diabetes mellitus type 2	>50 ng/mL	RCT analysis
Gene expression	>40 ng/mL	Clinical trial
Hypertension	>40 ng/mL	Observational studies
Preterm delivery	>40 ng/mL	Observational studies

Adapted from Grant, W.B., et al. A Narrative Review of the Evidence for Variations in Serum 25-Hydroxyvitamin D Concentration Thresholds for Optimal Health. Nutrients 2022. [3]

Unfortunately, conventional medicine typically considers vitamin D levels above 30 ng/mL as "sufficient," which falls far short of the optimal levels research shows are needed for disease prevention and immune function. Most people require maintenance doses of 800-2,000 IU (of vitamin D3 daily to achieve these therapeutic levels, [6] rather than the minimal 600-800 IU recommended by standard guidelines.

The **magnesium depletion score (MDS)** is a practical tool that helps identify individuals at risk for magnesium deficiency based on common risk factors. [7]

Your MDS is calculated by adding points for the following factors:

Factor	Criteria	Points
Diuretic Use	Current use	1
Proton Pump Inhibitor (PPI) Use	Current use	1
Kidney Function (eGFR)	60–90mL/(min·1.73 m²)	1
	<60 mL/(min·1.73 m²)	2
Heavy Alcohol Consumption	Present	1
Total Possible Score		0–5

MDS Risk Categories:

- **Low risk (0-1 points):** Minimal magnesium depletion risk

- **Moderate risk (2 points):** Increased risk of cardiovascular and metabolic complications

- **High risk (3-5 points):** Significantly elevated risk of all-cause mortality, cardiovascular disease, metabolic syndrome, and stroke

Research shows that individuals with higher MDS scores face dramatically increased health risks. Those with high MDS scores (3-5 points) have up to 92% increased risk of cardiovascular mortality and 58% increased risk of all-cause mortality compared to those with low scores. [8] This is particularly concerning because the medications contributing to magnesium depletion—diuretics and PPIs—are among the most commonly prescribed drugs in America.

Fiber, found in plant foods, is key to gut health, detoxification, and metabolic balance. Without it, digestion slows, toxins accumulate, and blood sugar becomes unstable. Omega-3 fatty acids are anti-inflammatory fats that are critical for our brain health, mood stability, cell membrane function, and heart function. Deficiencies are linked to anxiety, depression, and chronic inflammation. B vitamins are essential for our energy production and nervous system health. Deficiencies in these often manifest as fatigue, brain fog, and low metabolism. Iron, as a last point, is needed for oxygen transport and cellular energy. Deficiencies can lead to weakness, dizziness, and poor concentration. But many imbalances based on nutritional deficiencies are entirely correctable, and through nutrient-dense foods, we can restore what's missing—and allow the body to heal from within.

The Problem With The Food Pyramid

For decades, we have been guided by nutritional advice that has inadvertently contributed to our chronic disease epidemic. In 1992, the USDA introduced the Food Guide Pyramid, which placed bread, cereal, rice, and pasta as the foundation of a "healthy diet," recommending a staggering 6-11 servings *daily!* This guidance puts processed grains at the center of the American diet while relegating vegetables, fruits, and proteins to smaller portions of our daily intake. What many do not realize is that this pyramid wasn't built purely on nutritional science. It was heavily influenced by agricultural economics and food industry lobbying.[9] Government subsidies made wheat, corn, and soy the most heavily produced and cheapest crops, so naturally, they formed the foundation of official dietary recommendations. This "grain-heavy approach" served economic interests more than health interests, driving consumption of cheap, shelf-stable carbohydrates.

Meanwhile, healthy fats—critical for our hormone balance, brain health, and metabolism—were unfairly vilified and placed at the tiny tip of the pyramid with the advice to "use sparingly." This misguided fear of fat led to an explosion of fat-free products that compensated for their lack of flavor by adding sugar, refined carbohydrates, and artificial ingredients. Over the years, the government has updated these guidelines—moving from the pyramid to MyPyramid in 2005 and then to MyPlate in 2011—but the damage has already been done. Generations of Americans learned to prioritize grain-based foods and avoid fats, leading to dramatic increases in the consumption of processed foods.

The consequences have been profound! Americans now consume foods that are calorie-dense but nutrient-poor. So, instead of supplying the body with essential vitamins, minerals, and fiber, the typical diet floods the system with refined sugars, inflammatory fats, and artificial ingredients. This creates metabolic dysfunction, damages the gut, and causes systemic inflammation—the foundation of most modern diseases. A better approach focuses on whole, nutrient-dense foods rather than processed alternatives. The Harvard Healthy Eating Plate provides a more balanced perspective, emphasizing vegetables and fruits as the foundation, with whole grains (not refined!) as a supporting role alongside healthy proteins. Nutritious fats from olive oil, avocados, nuts, and fish are encouraged rather than feared. The Mediterranean diet, which is consistently ranked as one of the healthiest diets, follows similar principles. It prioritizes plant foods, includes moderate amounts of fish and seafood, limits red meat, and emphasizes healthy fats like olive oil.

This way of eating has been shown to reduce inflammation, support gut health, and lower the risk of cardiovascular disease, cancer, neurodegenerative conditions and all-cause mortality. [10] When we step away from misleading guidelines and return to real, whole foods, our body responds with increased energy, better digestion, improved mood, and reduced inflammation. The solution isn't to count our servings or follow a specific diet with "replacement foods" but to choose quality, minimally processed foods that provide the nutrients our bodies actually need to thrive.

Big AG and The Tobacco Industry's Sugar-Coated Influence on Our Health

Most people believe that public health guidance about nutrition comes from unbiased scientific research. Honestly? Much of it was shaped by profit-driven corporations—particularly the tobacco industry, which masterfully manipulated America's eating habits when its primary product faced increasing scrutiny. As regulations tightened around cigarettes in the mid-20th century, tobacco giants needed new markets to maintain their enormous profits. Their solution was both brilliant and devastating: apply their expertise in addiction to processed foods. Companies like Philip Morris, best known for Marlboro cigarettes, acquired food conglomerates such as Kraft and General Foods, bringing their sophisticated understanding of human cravings into our kitchens.

What made the tobacco industry uniquely dangerous in food production was its advanced knowledge of addiction mechanisms! For decades, they had studied precisely how to make cigarettes more addictive, manipulating nicotine delivery to maximize dependence. When they entered the food industry, they brought these tactics with them, creating what some researchers call "the bliss point"— the *perfect* combination of salt, sugar, and fat that triggers intense pleasure responses in the brain while overriding natural satiety signals. The tobacco industry's food scientists engineered products that stimulated cravings and encouraged overeating.

They developed sophisticated formulations to enhance "mouthfeel," ensure products dissolved at specific rates to maximize flavor delivery, and created textures that required minimal chewing—allowing consumers to eat faster and consume more before feeling full. These weren't just delicious foods; they were scientifically designed to be difficult to resist and nearly impossible to consume in moderation. At the same time, the sugar industry was fighting its own battle against emerging research. By the 1960s, scientific evidence was mounting that sugar—not fat—was the primary driver of heart disease and metabolic dysfunction. Facing potential regulation, the Sugar Research Foundation (now the Sugar Association) paid Harvard researchers to publish reviews dismissing sugar's harmful effects while emphasizing the dangers of dietary fat.[11]

These industry-funded studies profoundly shaped our public health policy for decades. The demonization of fat led to an explosion of low-fat products filled with sugar to maintain palatability. Americans dutifully avoided egg yolks, butter, and meat fat while unwittingly consuming unprecedented amounts of refined sugar and processed carbohydrates. Not coincidentally, rates of obesity, diabetes, and metabolic syndrome began their dramatic climb upward during this same period. The consequences of this corporate manipulation continue today. To point is not to assign blame but to reclaim control over our food choices. When we recognize how our preferences have been deliberately engineered to benefit corporate interests, we can begin making truly informed decisions about what we eat. Real health comes from whole, unprocessed foods—not the strategically formulated products created by companies with expertise in addiction.[12]

Mindful Eating – How, Where, and When to Eat

What we eat matters, but how we eat is just as important. In a world of "on the go," "take away," drive-ins, and food that is eaten in front of a TV or while we stare at our phones, constant distractions, and late-night snacking, many people unknowingly sabotage their digestion, metabolism, and nutrient absorption. Food should nourish the body, but when eaten in a stressed-out or distracted state, it can trigger bloating, blood sugar crashes, and inflammation. Mindful eating is the practice of slowing down, engaging with your food, and optimizing digestion. Portion control is not the dominating aspect. Rather, allowing the body to fully absorb and utilize nutrients is. When we eat with awareness, we support gut health, regulate metabolism, and prevent common digestive issues.

Our digestive system works most efficiently when we are in a parasympathetic—or "rest and digest"—state. This is the opposite of the sympathetic "fight or flight" response that stress triggers. When we eat while we are stressed, the body diverts energy away from digestion. This leads to decreased stomach acid production, reduced enzyme activity, and poor nutrient absorption. The digestive process actually begins in the mouth, where saliva and enzymes start breaking down food. The stomach then produces acid (HCl) that continues protein digestion while protecting against pathogens. From there, food moves to the small intestine—the primary site of nutrient absorption—where specialized structures called villi and microvilli dramatically increase absorption surface area to extract nutrients needed for energy, tissue development, and cellular repair.

Try to follow these basic points:

- **Eat in a Relaxed State** – Take a few deep breaths and say a prayer before eating to activate the parasympathetic nervous system. Avoid eating when you feel rushed, anxious, or overwhelmed. This simple practice can significantly improve your digestive function by ensuring adequate stomach acid and enzyme production.

- **Chew Your Food Thoroughly** – Digestion begins in the mouth, and thorough chewing sends signals throughout the digestive tract to prepare for food! When we eat too quickly, we force the stomach to work harder, breaking down larger food particles. Try to chew each bite 20-30 times before swallowing to support the entire digestive process.

- **Avoid Eating in Front of Screens** – Multitasking while eating—scrolling through social media, watching TV, or answering emails—leads to "mindless overeating" and poor digestion. Distracted eating reduces satiety signals, causing people to consume more calories without realizing it. Instead, focus on the flavors, textures, and experience of the meal.

- **Respect Your Circadian Rhythm** – The body's metabolism follows a natural rhythm of daytime and nighttime. Eating late at night, when digestion slows, can lead to blood sugar imbalances, fat storage, and disrupted sleep. The body is most efficient at processing food earlier in the day—so prioritizing meals before sunset supports hormonal balance and metabolic health.

Another aspect of mindful eating involves being aware of what's in your food. Learning to read nutrition labels helps you make informed choices about what you're putting in your body. Here's what to focus on:

Serving Size – This is listed at the top of every label. Remember that all nutrition information is based on one serving—if you eat multiple servings, you'll need to multiply all values accordingly.

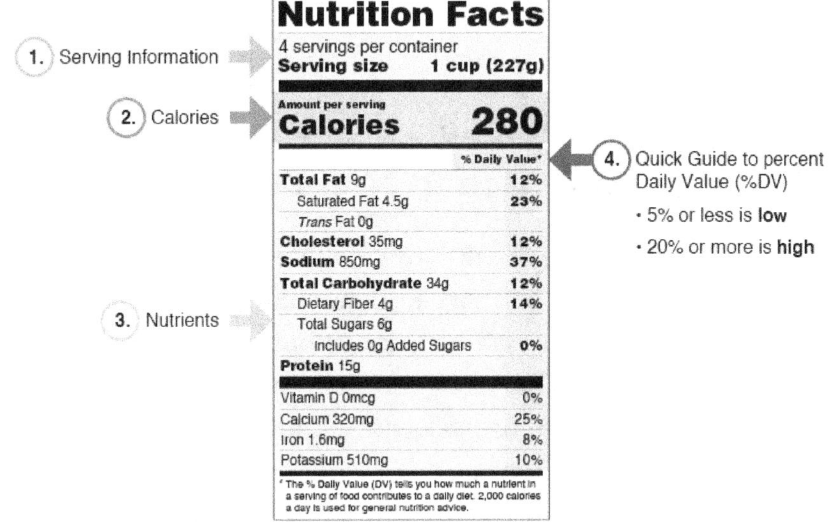

Calories – While not the only important factor, calories provide information about energy content. Be aware that "low-calorie" doesn't automatically mean "nutritious."

Nutrient Information – Look beyond just calories to the actual nutrient content. Pay attention to macronutrients (fats, carbohydrates, protein) and micronutrients (vitamins and minerals). The fiber content is particularly important for digestive health.

Percent Daily Values (%DV) – These tell you how much a nutrient in a serving contributes to a daily diet based on 2,000 calories. As a general guide, 5% or less is considered low, while 20% or more is high. This can help you quickly identify foods high in beneficial nutrients or those high in nutrients you may want to limit.

Mindful eating is not about restricting how you eat but focusing on eating to fully benefit from your food. When we slow down, chew our food properly, respect the body's natural satiety signals, and make informed choices about our food, we improve digestion, stabilize energy, and prevent metabolic dysfunction. These small but powerful practices transform the act of eating from a mindless activity into a nourishing experience that supports overall health.

The Functional Medicine Approach to Nutrition

Conventional medicine relies on prescriptions and symptom management rather than prevention. Functional medicine takes a different approach—it sees food as the foundation of health, not an afterthought. It asks: What does the body need to function optimally? What imbalances are silently leading to disease? Rather than a one-size-fits-all diet, we can create personalized nutrition plans based on genetics, gut health, and metabolic function. Some people thrive on more healthy fats, while others need a diet higher in clean carbohydrates.

By identifying unique nutritional needs, healing becomes precise and effective. The gut microbiome is key in this approach. Dysbiosis—characterized by decreased microbial diversity, loss of beneficial bacteria, and overgrowth of harmful microbes—has been linked to numerous health conditions. As mentioned earlier, gut imbalances can drive everything from metabolic disorders (obesity, Type 2 diabetes) to autoimmune conditions (celiac disease, rheumatoid arthritis, inflammatory bowel disease), cardiovascular problems (hypertension, atherosclerosis), neuropsychiatric disorders (depression, Parkinson's, Alzheimer's), and even certain cancers. This is why we focus so much on supporting your gut health through nutrition! For those with autoimmune conditions, specific nutritional approaches can help manage inflammation and support immune balance. The Autoimmune Protocol (AIP), for instance, is basically a very targeted version of the Paleo diet that's been fine-tuned for autoimmune conditions.

The idea is that certain foods—even ones considered "healthy" in a typical diet—might trigger inflammation or immune flare-ups if you are genetically susceptible. AIP aims to calm down that process by carefully removing common food items and then gradually testing them back into the diet to see which ones cause trouble.

This temporarily removes potential inflammatory triggers like nightshades, eggs, nuts, and seeds while emphasizing nutrient-dense foods like bone broth, organ meats, and fermented vegetables to support gut healing. For those with cardiovascular concerns, the Mediterranean diet, which is rich in olive oil, fatty fish, vegetables, and modest amounts of wine, has consistently shown benefits for heart health, blood pressure, and cholesterol levels. Metabolic conditions like insulin resistance and diabetes often respond very well to lower-carbohydrate approaches that emphasize protein, healthy fats, and non-starchy vegetables. Meanwhile, conditions related to detoxification challenges may benefit from cruciferous vegetables (broccoli, kale, cabbage) that support liver function, along with adequate hydration and fiber to eliminate toxins.

Environmental toxins are another critical consideration! As mentioned, glyphosate (the active ingredient in Roundup) is widely used in agriculture across the United States and has been linked to microbiome disruption, increased inflammation, and various health conditions, including cancer.

Similarly, toxic metals like lead, cadmium, arsenic, and mercury can be found in many common foods—even baby foods!—and have been associated with developmental issues, neurological damage, and chronic disease.

To minimize exposure to these harmful substances, the Environmental Working Group (EWG) offers valuable resources through the Healthy Living App.[13] This tool can help you identify foods with the lowest pesticide residues (the "Clean Fifteen") and those with the highest contamination levels (the "Dirty Dozen"), allowing for more informed shopping choices. The app also provides information on food additives, personal care products, and household cleaners, making it easier to reduce the overall toxic burden. For individuals with autoimmune conditions, specialized dietary approaches like the Autoimmune Protocol (AIP) can provide additional guidance for identifying and eliminating potential inflammatory triggers. [14]

Food packaging is another often-overlooked source of toxins! In functional medicine, we advise avoiding plastics (especially those marked with recycling codes 3, 6, and 7, which may contain hormone-disrupting chemicals), aluminum cans lined with BPA, and non-stick cookware coated with PFAS chemicals as much as possible. Better alternatives include glass containers, stainless steel, unbleached parchment paper, and cast-iron or ceramic cookware. No matter your condition or where you start, true wellness begins with restoring the body's natural ability to function optimally through targeted nutrition, toxin reduction, and support for the body's innate healing processes.

Key Takeaways

Every meal is an opportunity—to fuel healing or feed disease! The way we nourish our bodies impacts everything from our energy levels to our long-term health. Food is far more than just fuel—it is information, sending signals that can either restore balance or contribute to dysfunction. Throughout this chapter, we have explored the undeniable power of nutrition. As you process what you have learned, keep these key insights in mind:

Food has the power to heal or harm. Whole, nutrient-dense foods supply the body with what it needs to thrive, while processed, artificial ingredients disrupt balance and fuel chronic illness.

As Hippocrates wisely noted, *"Let food be thy medicine and medicine be thy food."* This isn't just ancient wisdom—modern research continues to confirm the profound impact our food choices have on our physical and mental well-being.

The Standard American Diet is a major driver of disease. Designed for convenience rather than nourishment, it is packed with sugar, unhealthy fats, and additives that disrupt metabolism and gut health. The research is clear—dysbiosis (an imbalanced gut microbiome) has been linked to numerous chronic conditions, including autoimmune disorders, metabolic diseases, cardiovascular problems, and even neuropsychiatric conditions.

How we eat is just as important as what we eat. Eating in a rushed or distracted state impairs digestion, while mindful eating enhances nutrient absorption, stabilizes blood sugar, and improves overall health. Remember that our bodies were designed to be in a parasympathetic "rest and digest" state during meals for optimal nutrient utilization.

Functional medicine prioritizes food as a tool for healing. Instead of suppressing symptoms with medications, it identifies underlying imbalances and restores health through personalized nutrition and lifestyle adjustments. This approach recognizes that each person has unique needs and imbalances requiring individualized solutions.

Questions for Reflection

Now, take a moment to assess your own habits and beliefs about food. Reflect on these questions:

1. Am I maybe missing key nutrients in my diet? Have I experienced symptoms like fatigue, poor concentration, brain fog, or frequent illness that could point to deficiencies?

2. How have my environment and upbringing shaped my eating habits? Do I eat out of convenience, cultural norms, or emotional triggers rather than nutritional needs?

3. What small but meaningful change can I implement today? Could I swap out processed snacks, increase my intake of whole foods, or adjust my meal timing to better support my metabolism?

4. Have I been influenced by misleading nutrition advice? Have I avoided certain foods based on outdated or commercialized health messaging rather than actual science?

5. How does my faith or mindset shape my relationship with food? Do I see eating as a way to fuel and care for my body, or has it become a source of stress, guilt, or emotional comfort?

However, your journey back to health doesn't stop with nutrition. Food is a powerful tool, but even the most nutrient-rich diet cannot fully support the body without another critical factor: restorative sleep. In the next chapter, we will take a look at the power of sleep, what sleep actually is, and what happens when we sleep.

CHAPTER 7

The Transformative Power Of Sleep

"Come to Me, all you who labor and are heavily burdened, and I will give you rest."

— Matthew 11:28 (MEV)

Sleep is not just a biological need but a foundation of health that most of us sacrifice first. In today's world, we give up sleep for deadlines, phone scrolling, and streaming. This sacrifice costs us dearly. During sleep, your body repairs itself, restores balance, and resets systems. While you rest, your body regulates hormones, repairs cellular damage, and clears brain toxins. Without good quality of sleep, just like without proper food, your health cannot last. When we close our eyes at night, we acknowledge our physical limits. This chapter shows how sleep heals your body from within. You'll discover how proper rest builds resilience, balances hormones, and restores emotional stability. The goal isn't simply more sleep, but better sleep—the kind that allows your body to heal properly.

What Happens When You Sleep?

Sleep moves through several distinct stages, each playing a specific role in restoring your health. These stages create a pattern that supports healing and renewal. Your body alternates between REM (rapid eye movement) sleep and non-REM sleep. Non-REM sleep divides into three stages—N1, N2, and N3—each with different brain activity patterns and body functions. A complete sleep cycle lasts about 90 minutes, and your body needs 4-6 cycles each night for full restoration. Light sleep begins the process.[1] During the first stage (N1), your body relaxes. Your heartbeat slows, muscles loosen, and your brain shifts from alertness to calm. Brain activity changes from alpha waves (brain waves associated with relaxed wakefulness, measuring 8-13 Hz) to the slower theta waves (4-7 Hz waves that indicate light sleep). Many people dismiss this stage, but it serves as your essential transition between wakefulness and deeper sleep.

The second stage (N2) brings sleep spindles and K-complexes to your brain patterns. Sleep spindles are brief bursts of rapid brain activity (12-14 Hz) that appear as short squiggles on brain wave readings. These spindles strengthen memory and learning pathways by forming new connections between brain cells. K-complexes are sudden, sharp waveforms followed by a slower wave—essentially a quick spike followed by a deep valley in brain activity. These K-complexes help you stay asleep despite noise and assist in memory processing. This stage prepares your body for the deeper healing that follows.

Deep sleep (N3) brings the most significant repair work. During this stage, your brain produces slow delta waves (high-amplitude, low-frequency waves of 0.5-4 Hz). Your tissues rebuild, muscles recover, and your immune system strengthens. Your body releases growth hormone during this time, supporting renewal and reducing inflammation. Without enough deep sleep, healing remains incomplete, leaving you vulnerable to illness and fatigue. Your body repairs tissues, strengthens bones and muscles, and boosts immunity during this stage. This is also when sleepwalking and night terrors typically occur.

REM sleep offers different benefits. Your brain becomes highly active, processing emotions and organizing memories. While your brain activates in patterns similar to wakefulness, your body remains still, most muscles temporarily paralyzed (a condition called atonia) except for your eyes and breathing muscles. This muscle paralysis prevents you from acting out your dreams and protects you from injury. During REM sleep, most dreaming occurs as your brain processes experiences, connects new learning, and handles emotional events. REM sleep builds mental resilience and emotional balance for your day ahead. Each stage plays a vital role in health. Sleep isn't just wasted time being unconscious: it is essential recovery time. Understanding these stages helps explain why the quality of sleep matters so much for healing and wellness.

The Short Sleep Crisis

Sleep is not optional. It's not a luxury you can sacrifice for productivity, entertainment, or convenience. The evidence is overwhelming and alarming: insufficient sleep directly fuels the development and progression of chronic diseases that are killing and disabling millions of Americans. Across the United States, more than one-third of adults consistently sleep less than the recommended 7 hours per night.[2] In some states, like Massachusetts, this figure reaches 33.2% of the adult population—that's more than 1 in 3 people systematically destroying their health through sleep deprivation.[3]

The geographic patterns reveal that this crisis spans every region, with some areas showing nearly 40% of adults living in chronic sleep debt. When you look at a map of short sleep prevalence, you're looking at a map of preventable chronic disease waiting to happen.

The Centers for Disease Control and Prevention has issued a clear warning that should alarm every American: insufficient sleep has been directly linked to the development and management of our most deadly chronic diseases. According to CDC data, people who consistently sleep less than 7 hours per night face significantly higher risks for:[4]

- **Type 2 Diabetes**: Sleep deprivation disrupts how your body processes glucose and responds to insulin, creating the perfect conditions for diabetes to develop.

- **Heart Disease**: Your cardiovascular system depends on sleep for repair and regulation. Without adequate rest, blood pressure rises, inflammation increases, and your heart works harder just to keep you alive.

- **Obesity**: Sleep loss hijacks the hormones that control hunger and satiety, driving you to eat more while your metabolism slows down.

- **Depression and Anxiety**: Mental health deteriorates rapidly without sufficient sleep, as your brain loses its ability to process emotions and stress effectively.

- **Cancer**: Growing evidence links chronic sleep deprivation to increased cancer risk, particularly colorectal, breast, and prostate cancers.

- **Cognitive Decline**: Your brain literally can't clean itself properly without adequate sleep, leading to memory problems and increased dementia risk.

Data from Massachusetts provides a stark example of how sleep deprivation translates into real health consequences. Among adults in the state, those sleeping less than 7 hours per night show dramatically higher rates of chronic conditions:[5]

The relationship between sleep and chronic disease creates a vicious cycle that's difficult to break. Sleep deprivation doesn't just increase your risk for one condition; it sets up a domino effect that can devastate multiple body systems simultaneously. Looking at the CDC data analyzing prevalence of chronic conditions among short sleepers versus adequate sleepers, the differences are striking--sleeping less than <7 hours per night is associated with increased risk for obesity, diabetes, high blood pressure, coronary heart disease, stroke, frequent mental distress, and all-cause mortality.[6]

Sleep disruption attacks your health on two fronts: immediate consequences that you feel right away, and long-term damage that builds silently until it becomes life-threatening. Short-term consequences include increased stress responsivity, physical pain, reduced quality of life, emotional distress, mood disorders, and significant cognitive, memory, and performance deficits.

Long-term consequences for otherwise healthy individuals who continue sleeping poorly include hypertension, dyslipidemia, cardiovascular disease, weight-related issues, metabolic syndrome, type 2 diabetes, and colorectal cancer. Research shows that all-cause mortality increases significantly in people with chronic sleep disturbances.[7]

Sleep problems rarely happen alone. When researchers studied how different behaviors affect chronic disease, they found that sleep deprivation clusters with other health-destroying habits like smoking, poor diet, physical inactivity, and chronic stress.[8] These behaviors work together to accelerate disease development. The study showed clear evidence linking these modifiable behaviors to increased illness and death from chronic conditions.

This means when you shortchange sleep, you often start making other poor health choices too. You reach for more caffeine, skip exercise because you're tired, eat more sugar for quick energy, and handle stress poorly. One bad habit feeds another, creating a downward spiral that becomes harder to break the longer it continues.

However, this crisis is almost entirely preventable. Unlike genetic predispositions or environmental toxins, sleep is largely within your control. Every night, you have the opportunity to give your body the restoration it desperately needs to fight off chronic disease.

Understanding Our Biological Clock

The body runs on an internal rhythm that guides when you feel alert and when you need rest. This natural cycle, your circadian rhythm (from Latin "circa" meaning "around" and "diem" meaning "day"), affects your energy, metabolism, and overall well-being. This internal clock follows a 24-hour pattern, responding to light, food, and daily activities. From the moment you wake, your circadian rhythm begins working. Morning light signals your body to rise, triggering the release of cortisol. This is a hormone that boosts alertness and energy. This natural surge helps start the day focused and engaged. Throughout the day, energy shifts in predictable patterns, preparing for periods of activity and rest. Evening darkness triggers melatonin release, signaling it's time to wind down. This prepares you for deep, restorative sleep. The suprachiasmatic nucleus (SCN), a small cluster of about 20,000 neurons in the hypothalamus, acts as your master clock. It receives signals directly from light receptors in your eyes and coordinates timing for vital processes—from sleep-wake cycles to hormone release and temperature changes.

The SCN communicates with other brain regions and tissues to synchronize your body with your environment.

Your circadian rhythm affects more than just sleep. It regulates body temperature, digestion, and hormone release, aligning these processes for optimal daily function. When this rhythm stays in sync, sleep comes naturally, energy remains steady, and your body works efficiently. When disrupted, everything suffers—sleep fragments, energy fluctuates, and simple tasks feel challenging. Modern life works against this natural clock. Evening screen time exposes you to blue light (light wavelengths between 450-495 nm) that confuses your brain, delaying melatonin production and making sleep difficult. Missing morning sunlight weakens your natural energy signals, causing daytime sluggishness. Late dinners disrupt your body's nighttime preparations, interrupting the natural wind-down process.

Several key brain structures control your sleep. The hypothalamus (a small region at your brain's base) contains cell groups that regulate sleep and wakefulness. The brainstem (connecting your brain to your spinal cord) manages transitions between sleep and wake states. Sleep-promoting cells in these regions produce GABA (gamma-aminobutyric acid), a neurotransmitter that calms arousal centers and helps initiate sleep by inhibiting brain activity. The thalamus (a walnut-sized structure in the center of your brain) normally relays sensory information to your brain's cortex. During most sleep stages, it quiets down, blocking external stimuli. During REM sleep, it activates again, sending signals that create dreams. The pineal gland (a tiny pine cone-shaped gland deep in your brain) produces melatonin when darkness falls, signaling sleep onset.

When your circadian rhythm falls out of alignment, health suffers. Sleep fragments, energy fluctuates unpredictably, and long-term wellness declines. Living in harmony with your natural clock—rising with light, winding down with darkness, and keeping consistent rest patterns—brings deeper sleep, clearer thinking, and greater resilience.

The Impact of Poor Sleep on Health

Poor sleep undermines your body's ability to function properly. Restless nights weaken the systems designed to protect and restore you. The effects start subtly but eventually reshape how you feel, think, and live.

Your metabolism suffers first. Sleep resets our energy systems, but disrupted rest impairs how the body processes and stores energy. This leads to weight gain, ongoing fatigue, and increased diabetes risk. The body becomes less efficient at processing nutrients, controlling appetite, and maintaining a healthy weight. Occasional tiredness can develop into deeper metabolic problems affecting every aspect of your day.

Research shows that sleep deprivation directly alters hunger hormones, decreasing leptin, the hormone produced by fat cells that signals fullness, while increasing ghrelin, the hormone from the stomach that stimulates appetite.[9] [10] In controlled studies, individuals restricted to four hours of sleep experienced an 18% drop in leptin, a 28% rise in ghrelin, along with 24% greater hunger and 23% stronger appetite. Carbohydrate cravings also increased by 33% during sleep loss, helping explain why tired people tend to overeat.[11] Even moderate sleep restriction has been shown to increase daily snack consumption by about 220 calories,[12] demonstrating how inadequate sleep reshapes not only how much we eat, but also what and when we choose to eat. Over time, these disruptions in appetite and metabolism highlight the critical role of sleep in energy regulation, and show how chronic sleep loss can contribute to weight gain and obesity.[13] [14]

During sleep, the body strengthens defenses, repairs tissues, and creates immune cells. When sleep is shortened or becomes lighter, the immune system weakens. Your defenses decline, leaving you more vulnerable to infections and slower to heal. This creates on-going fatigue and lingering illness, where minor infections take much longer to overcome.

Your brain pays the heaviest price. Sleep allows your brain to process emotions, organize memories, and clear out toxins. Without this essential rest, mental clarity fades significantly. Focus becomes difficult, memory weakens, and emotional control feels increasingly elusive. Clear thinking, decision-making, and emotional management gradually diminish, leaving persistent mental fog.

The connection between sleep and brain health runs deeper than most people realize. A study following older adults found that shorter sleep duration was directly linked to faster decline in executive function and processing speed through increased cardiovascular disease risk.[15] When you don't sleep enough, your heart health suffers, and that damaged cardiovascular system can't properly support your brain function.

Even more concerning, research tracking over 4,400 adults found that people sleeping 6 hours or less had higher levels of amyloid-β buildup in their brains—the toxic protein associated with Alzheimer's disease.[16] Short sleep duration was linked to memory problems, while both too little and too much sleep were associated with depression, higher body weight, and cognitive decline across multiple areas of thinking.

Cancer risk increases with poor sleep. Sleep disorders don't just make you tired—they can contribute to life-threatening diseases. Recent research specifically links sleep problems to colorectal cancer development.[17] Sleep deprivation disrupts your metabolism, throws off your gut bacteria balance, and triggers chronic inflammation—all factors that can lead to cancer growth. This connection helps explain why maintaining good sleep isn't just about feeling rested; it's about preventing serious disease. Moreover, poor sleep creates a cascade of problems throughout your entire body. Sleep disturbances affect your hypothalamus, triggering stress hormone release that leads to elevated cortisol and other damaging chemicals. Your muscles lose glycogen storage capacity, your digestive system develops problems, and your cardiovascular system responds with hypertension, heart problems, and irregular rhythms.[18] Your endocrine system becomes dysfunctional, leading to insulin resistance, obesity, and metabolic syndrome. When one system fails, others follow.

Hormones and Sleep - How Sleep Regulates Everything

Cortisol, our primary stress hormone produced by the adrenal glands, responds immediately to sleep quality. In healthy patterns, cortisol peaks in the morning, giving energy and alertness to start your day. It gradually decreases throughout the day, allowing you to wind down during the evening. When sleep suffers, cortisol stays elevated, creating constant body stress. This leads to persistent fatigue, heightened anxiety, and feeling constantly on edge without a clear cause. Over time, this imbalance reduces your resilience against illness and emotional challenges. Cortisol follows a daily rhythm; a normal pattern shows levels are highest in the early morning after waking and gradually decline to their lowest point in the evening. This pattern, known as a diurnal rhythm, helps regulate alertness and sleep.

Melatonin plays a crucial role in our sleep. This hormone, produced primarily by the pineal gland, signals when the body should rest, responding to natural light and darkness. Sleep disruption impairs melatonin production, making falling and staying asleep harder. The effects extend beyond restless nights to a disrupted body rhythm, leaving you confused and fatigued. Without enough melatonin, even when you sleep, rest feels incomplete, leaving your mind foggy and body unrefreshed.

Melatonin shows strong daily patterns, with high levels at night and low levels during the day. Your brain's master clock sends signals through several pathways, ultimately reaching your pineal gland, which produces melatonin in darkness. Short-term supplementation with melatonin may help reduce the time needed to fall asleep, increase sleep duration, and improve sleep quality. It may also help maintain proper sleep-wake cycles, especially when sleep is disrupted or when experiencing jet lag.

Growth hormone serves as a powerful restorative factor in the body. Released primarily during deep sleep by the pituitary gland, it supports muscle repair, fat metabolism, and cellular regeneration. This natural repair system restores strength and vitality nightly. Growth hormone is released in pulses, aligning with the deeper sleep cycles. When deep sleep decreases, growth hormone levels drop significantly. The body then struggles to rebuild tissues, muscles recover more slowly, and overall repair suffers. Over time, this erodes your strength and resilience.

Thyroid-stimulating hormone (TSH), released by the pituitary gland to regulate metabolism, also responds directly to sleep quality. TSH reaches its highest levels during the night and its lowest during the afternoon. TSH levels have been shown to decrease during the deepest sleep phases. This normal, pulsatile pattern is a key part of the body's biological clock and allows TSH to respond to internal and external cues to maintain thyroid hormone equilibrium.

Hormone balance affects far more than biological processes: it shapes how you feel every day, influencing your energy, emotional stability, metabolism, and body function. Sleep provides the foundation for this delicate balance. Without good sleep, all systems struggle. With good quality of sleep, the body aligns, heals, and strengthens naturally. Health builds during those quiet hours when your body restores what daily life depletes.

Common Sleep Disruptors

Getting good sleep takes more than just going to bed at a decent time. It requires conditions that allow deep rest to take place. Many common habits undermine sleep quality. Screen usage and devices before bed rank amongst the worst offenders! Phones, tablets, and TVs emit blue light that tricks the brain into thinking it's daytime, and tells it to stay awake. This light specifically blocks melatonin production, the key hormone preparing the body for sleep. Even brief screen time before bed significantly delays natural sleep signals and makes falling asleep more difficult. Over time, this habit progressively damages sleep quality, causing restlessness and mental fog. Alcohol also tricks you into thinking you'll sleep well. You might fall asleep faster because alcohol is a depressant, but the quality of sleep suffers.[19] You will wake up more often, spend less time in deep sleep, and miss out on critical REM sleep when your brain processes emotions and consolidates memories. Even when you think you've slept through the night after drinking, your body and brain haven't actually recovered properly.

Eating too close to bedtime also causes sleep problems. The digestive system stays active when the body should be winding down. When your blood sugar spikes, then drops during the night, you often wake up and struggle to fall back asleep. This is especially true with heavy meals or sugary snacks, which keep you tossing and turning instead of moving through normal sleep cycles. When you eat matters almost as much as what you eat when it comes to getting good sleep. Irregular sleep schedules confuse your internal clock. Your circadian system needs consistency. Going to bed and waking up at different times sends mixed signals to your brain about when to release sleep and wakefulness hormones. With unpredictable patterns, your body struggles to time these processes properly. This inconsistency damages sleep quality, creating cycles of exhaustion and erratic energy levels.

Certain medications also alter natural sleep patterns. Benzodiazepines (a class of medications including Valium and Xanax that enhance the effect of GABA in the brain), prescribed for anxiety and insomnia, may chemically help you stay asleep, but they change the architecture of sleep by reducing the time spent in the deepest, most restorative stages of sleep. They increase the threshold for waking up during deep sleep. While this prevents you from waking up at night, it often *costs* restorative sleep quality. Many antidepressants disrupt REM patterns, sometimes causing REM behavior disorder (a condition where the normal muscle paralysis during dreams fails), allowing physical dream enactment.[20]

Sleep disorders undermine the quality of rest even when the duration of sleep seems adequate. Sleep apnea (a disorder where breathing repeatedly stops and starts during sleep) causes breathing interruptions during deeper stages of sleep, preventing sufficient time in restorative phases. This leads to exhaustion during the day, despite apparently adequate hours of sleep.

Conditions like narcolepsy (a chronic sleep disorder causing overwhelming daytime drowsiness and sudden "sleep attacks") disrupt the normal progression of sleep, causing premature REM entry and preventing complete restoration. These disruptors might seem minor individually, but together they create significant barriers to healing sleep. Recognizing them starts your improvement. While perfect sleep habits rarely fit with life's demands, understanding what undermines your rest can help you make better choices.

How to Reclaim Deep, Healing Sleep

The research is clear: you need 7-8 hours of quality sleep to prevent chronic disease and maintain health. Start by setting clear boundaries around the use of technology in the evening. Choose a specific cutoff time: ideally, 1-2 hours before bed, when you turn off all devices and put them in airplane mode to eliminate EMF exposure. If you must use devices earlier in the evening, wear blue-blocking glasses to filter out sleep-disrupting blue light. Replace the screen time with calming activities: lower your lighting, read a book, or simply enjoy the quiet time as you fall asleep. Make this transition consistent every night to signal the body that the day is ending. This practice creates a mental quiet that invites deeper rest.

Create a simple bedtime routine. After you stop using screens in the evening, create a simple bedtime routine that the body will learn to recognize. Select 2-3 activities that calm you: a warm shower, journaling, some light stretching, brief reflection time, or prayer. Taking time for prayer or quiet spiritual reflection can be particularly powerful for releasing the day's concerns and finding peace before sleep. The specific activities matter less than consistency. Do the same steps in the same order each night until the body automatically begins to relax when the routine starts.

Be strategic about stimulants and evening habits. Even the best bedtime routine fails if stimulants remain in your system. So, be mindful about caffeine by setting a firm cutoff no later than early afternoon. Swap out evening snacks for sleep-supportive options, such as calming herbal teas or a magnesium supplement. You can also explore aromatherapy with essential oils like bergamot, chamomile, or lavender to help relax the body and prepare for restful sleep.[21] Choosing quiet activities instead supports your natural evening wind-down. Try to focus on supporting sleep signals established through your other habits rather than on restrictions.

Create space for mental release. Despite good preparation, sleep often eludes us when the mind keeps processing daily stress. Create space for a bit of mental release before sleep. Choose one simple practice for your nightly routine: Write down a few lingering thoughts or concerns to address tomorrow, or practice a few minutes of slow breathing with extended exhales, naturally activating your parasympathetic nervous system (your "rest and digest" system that calms the body). This nightly "letting-go" teaches your mind and body that rest is both safe and necessary.

Align with your natural rhythm. Additionally, try to align your daily habits with the natural rhythm of things. Morning sunlight exposure—just 10-15 minutes—helps regulate these sleep-wake cycles by signaling the brain to suppress melatonin and increase alertness hormones. This morning light anchors your entire day's hormonal patterns. Avoid daytime napping, which can disrupt your nighttime sleep drive and make it harder to fall asleep when you need to. Turn your bedroom into a sleep haven. Create a sleep environment that's dark, cool (around 65-68°F), quiet, peaceful, comfortable, and clean for optimal sleep stage cycling. Use blackout curtains or an eye mask to block all light sources—even small amounts of light can disrupt melatonin production. Remove or silence anything that creates noise disturbances.

Exercise at the right time. Regular physical activity improves sleep quality, though timing matters. Exercise during the day or early evening (not right before bed) helps regulate sleep cycles and increases deep, restorative sleep time. Movement enhances natural restoration by creating the right kind of physical fatigue. Incorporate stress management and relaxation techniques into your daily routine as well.

Know when to seek help. For ongoing issues with sleeping, it is a good idea to consult a healthcare provider about possible underlying causes like sleep apnea, restless legs syndrome (a condition causing uncomfortable sensations in the legs and an irresistible urge to move them), or hormonal imbalances. Non-pharmacologic therapies, such as cognitive behavioral therapy for insomnia (CBT-I), are a structured program that helps identify and replace thoughts and behaviors causing sleep problems, and often works better than medication for long-term improvement.[22]

Also, approach sleep medications cautiously! While medications like benzodiazepines and melatonin help temporarily, many alter our natural sleep architecture and may decrease time spent in the critical restorative stages. If medication becomes necessary, try to use it as a short-term solution under medical guidance while building more sustainable sleep habits.

Key Takeaways

Good quality sleep does more than rest your body. It creates a foundation for healing, resilience, and emotional balance. When sleep becomes a priority, your body finds its natural rhythm, energy stabilizes, and your mind handles challenges more effectively. When sleep suffers, imbalances develop, affecting every health aspect. But even small, consistent changes can restore what's lost and invite the body back to deep, healing rest. Consider these essential points:

- Sleep forms a cornerstone of health, influencing everything from metabolism to emotional regulation. Without sufficient quality sleep, healing slows and resilience weakens.

- Your body's natural rhythms guide energy and rest cycles. Honoring these patterns through consistent habits—reducing evening screen time, establishing calming routines, and maintaining regular sleep hours—restores balance and improves sleep quality.

- Small, intentional changes create significant results over time. Simple shifts, practiced consistently, transform restless nights into deep, restorative sleep.

- True rest requires letting go of control and trusting that your body knows how to restore itself during night hours.

Questions for Reflection

Reflect honestly on your sleep patterns. These questions guide you toward better rest and improved health:

1. What habits might be disrupting my sleep? Which patterns, like late-night screen time, irregular sleep times, or consuming caffeine late in the day, stand between me and quality rest?

2. Am I truly making sleep a priority, or sacrificing it for work, entertainment, or stress management? What adjustments would better support my sleep needs?

3. What simple evening routine could signal my body that it's time to wind down and prepare for sleep?

4. What one change can I implement tonight that would invite deeper rest and begin creating healthier sleep patterns?

5. How can I release daily worries before bed, trusting that tomorrow brings a fresh perspective?

Better sleep doesn't require an overnight transformation—it begins with awareness and small, consistent steps that honor the body's need for restoration. Each choice strengthens your ability to heal and build resilience for the day ahead. Yet resilience is tested not only by how well we sleep but also by how we respond to stress. In the next chapter, we'll explore practical strategies for managing stress in ways that protect your health, restore balance, and sustain long-term vitality.

CHAPTER 8

Managing Stress For Resilience

Give all your worries and cares to God, for He cares about you.

— 1 Peter 5:7 (NLT)

Most of us accept stress as part of modern life, but its impact on health is profound. It weaves itself into our daily routines, relationships, and responsibilities. While our bodies are designed to handle brief moments of stress, like reacting to danger or meeting an urgent deadline, prolonged stress is entirely different. When stress becomes chronic, it shifts from a temporary challenge to a silent disruptor, affecting physical strength, emotional balance, and overall vitality.

The body's stress response is a remarkable system built for survival. In the short term, it sharpens focus and prepares the body to react. But when stress lingers, it keeps the body in a constant state of high alert, draining essential resources. Sleep becomes restless, digestion falters, and the immune system weakens. Even moods and emotions suffer, creating a cycle that feels impossible to break. Over time, stress can erode health in ways that aren't always immediately visible, through persistent fatigue, increased irritability, or an unexplained sense of unease.

Yet, stress itself is not the enemy. It is our response to it that shapes its influence on our well-being. When unmanaged, stress disrupts our internal balance. But when we learn to navigate it, we can protect our bodies, restore emotional strength, and regain clarity of mind. This chapter explores stress from the inside out, examining how it affects the body at a cellular level. Most importantly, we'll look at how to cultivate resilience, not as a temporary fix but as a lasting way to protect health and strengthen emotional well-being. Because when we change how we handle stress, we change how we live.

Chronic Stress: A Disruptor of Health

While we may think of stress as a negative force, it is actually the body's natural way of protecting us. In small, short-lived doses, stress sharpens focus, strengthens motivation, and helps us meet challenges. It's the burst of energy that gets us through an urgent deadline or a dangerous situation. But when stress stretches beyond those moments, when it lingers day after day, it stops being helpful and starts breaking down the body.

This shift happens when the body's stress response system, designed for temporary survival, becomes stuck in overdrive. The hypothalamic-pituitary-adrenal (HPA) axis kicks into gear, flooding the body with hormones like cortisol and adrenaline. These hormones are meant to help in a crisis, but when they remain elevated over time, they quietly chip away at health. Chronic stress often leads to more inflammation in the body. This happens because stress hormones activate the immune system to release chemicals, which trigger the release of inflammatory proteins, known as *cytokines.*

The body reacts to ongoing stress as if it's under constant threat, keeping the immune system on high alert. Over time, this can lead to a low-grade, persistent inflammatory state, damaging tissues, impairing the gut lining and contributing to conditions like heart disease, stroke, cancer and diabetes.[1]

Chronic stress profoundly affects the gut microbiome, influencing both physical and mental health. The HPA axis is a key stress-response system involving the brain and adrenal glands. When chronic stress leads to HPA axis dysregulation, it causes prolonged elevation of cortisol and other stress hormones like adrenaline.[2] These hormones directly impact gut function and microbiota composition.

Stress-driven changes in the microbiome also weaken the gut barrier by damaging tight junctions, allowing bacteria and bacterial byproducts to "leak" into the bloodstream, lymph nodes, and other organs. This translocation fuels systemic inflammation, which in turn has been linked to stress-related neuroinflammatory conditions, including psychiatric disorders such as depression.[3]

This connection shows how stress creates effects throughout the body. Chronic stress may reduce stomach acid production (hypochlorhydria), altering the stomach's ability to effectively break down food and kill pathogens. This leads to dysbiosis—a microbial imbalance in the gut—as well as decreased absorption of nutrients like calcium, iron, and zinc. Elevated cortisol levels disrupt the intestinal barrier function. This disruption, often called "leaky gut," allows toxins, bacteria, and undigested food particles to leak into the bloodstream, triggering immune responses and inflammation.

Stress changes the balance of gut bacteria, reducing beneficial bacteria like Lactobacillus while increasing potentially harmful ones. This imbalance affects digestion, immune function, mood and overall health.[4]

The Gut-Brain Superhighway: Understanding the Vagus Nerve

The vagus nerve is one of the key components of the parasympathetic nervous system, often called the "rest and digest" system. It is the longest cranial nerve, running from the brainstem to various organs, including the heart, lungs, and digestive system. It regulates gut function and communication between the gut and brain.[5][6]

When chronic stress occurs, it can reduce vagal tone, meaning the vagus nerve becomes less effective at moderating the body's stress response. The vagus nerve normally helps reduce inflammation, promote digestion, and regulate mood, but prolonged stress can impair vagal activity, leading to sustained inflammation in the body, particularly in the brain.[7]

The vagus nerve also affects gut motility and helps trigger bowel movements after eating. Stress can interfere with these digestive processes, leading to issues like constipation, bloating, or diarrhea, common in stress-related gut disorders such as irritable bowel syndrome (IBS).

The Enteric Nervous System: Our "Second Brain"

The Enteric Nervous System (ENS) is a complex network of neurons embedded within the walls of the gastrointestinal tract. Often called the "*second brain*," it can function independently from the central nervous system while constantly communicating with the brain. The ENS regulates digestion, gut motility, and secretion of gut hormones. It also links the gut microbiome to brain function through the gut-brain axis.

Stress can alter how the ENS functions, making the gut more sensitive to stimuli. This leads to heightened sensations of pain, bloating, and discomfort, often seen in stress-related conditions like IBS and other functional gastrointestinal disorders. Chronic stress disrupts the two-way communication between the gut and brain via the ENS and vagus nerve. The brain sends signals to the gut, influencing gut microbiota composition, motility, and secretion, while the gut sends signals back to the brain, affecting mood and cognitive function. When this communication is disrupted, it increases susceptibility to mental health conditions like anxiety, depression, and cognitive impairments. Gut-derived signals, including those from short-chain fatty acids (SCFAs) produced by gut bacteria, can influence brain activity, neurotransmitter production, and mood regulation.[8] Extending this connection, emerging evidence shows that prenatal stress disrupts the microbiome, impairs gut-barrier function, and amplifies inflammation, factors that can reshape brain development and elevate lifelong mental-health risks.[9]

Over time, the brain becomes less adaptable, and feelings of anxiety or emotional exhaustion can take root.

The vagus nerve and ENS work together to communicate between the gut and brain. Chronic stress disrupts this communication loop, affecting not only digestive processes but also mood and cognition. This dysregulation contributes to long-term effects on mental health, such as depression and anxiety, which are often associated with gastrointestinal disturbances.[10]

Techniques for Stress Reduction

Managing stress is not about eliminating every challenge but learning how to support the body, mind, and spirit when stress arises. This approach looks at the whole person and provides practical ways to reduce the impact of stress.[11] It is about choosing small, consistent actions that build resilience over time, creating space for the body to rest and recover. One simple yet effective practice is mindfulness. When life feels overwhelming, the mind often races toward everything that could go wrong. Mindfulness helps bring attention back to the present moment. It is about noticing how the body feels, observing thoughts without judgment, and simply being aware of what is happening right now. This pause calms the nervous system and helps break the cycle of worry. Research shows that regular mindfulness practice reduces cortisol levels by an average of 20% and lowers inflammatory markers like C-reactive protein and interleukin-6, the same markers that rise during chronic stress.[12] Even a few minutes of focused attention, like watching the breath or feeling the warmth of sunlight, can bring a sense of calm. Over time, practicing mindfulness teaches the brain to respond to stress with more clarity and less reactivity.

Breathwork is another evidence-based tool that helps ease the stress response. When we are anxious, the breath becomes shallow and fast, signaling to the body that danger is near. But slowing the breath can shift the body out of that survival mode. The Box Breathing Technique, inhaling for four counts, holding for 4, exhaling for 4, and holding for 4, has been shown to activate the parasympathetic nervous system within 60-90 seconds. This "rest and digest" mode allows the body to move out of stress response and into healing mode. Deep, steady breaths reduce heart rate, blood pressure, and muscle tension while increasing heart rate variability, a marker of resilience. Breath is always with us, making it an accessible tool for calming stress anytime, anywhere.

Movement is also essential for stress management. The body holds stress in ways we don't always notice, tight shoulders, a clenched jaw, or tension in the back.

Exercise can reduce the levels of stress hormones like adrenaline and cortisol while stimulating the production of endorphins, natural mood elevators that create feelings of well-being. Walking in nature has been shown to reduce mental fatigue, lower stress hormone levels, and improve mood more effectively than walking in urban environments. Walking through forest areas decreases negative moods of "depression, anxiety, anger, fatigue, and confusion" while improving positive mood.[13] It's not about intensity but about presence, moving in a way that feels good, helping the body reset and recharge.

When movement becomes a regular part of life, it teaches the body how to release stress rather than store it. Writing can be another effective release. Thoughts often swirl in the mind, growing heavier the longer they're left unspoken. Studies show that expressive writing for just 15-20 minutes, 3-4 times per week, reduces stress hormone levels and improves immune function.[14] Putting thoughts down on paper gives them somewhere to go. Journaling doesn't need to be structured or formal; it can be as simple as writing down what feels heavy or what feels hopeful. For some, keeping a gratitude list helps shift focus toward what is good and steady, even in stressful times. These practices don't erase problems, but they give the mind a new way to process them.

Each of these techniques, whether practiced alone or combined, offers a pathway to reduce stress and build resilience. They are not complicated, nor do they require drastic life changes.

Instead, they are simple, accessible habits that can be woven into daily routines, offering calm in moments of chaos and strength in difficult seasons.

Building Emotional Resilience

Stress will always be a part of life, but how we respond to it makes all the difference. Emotional resilience is what allows us to face challenges, adapt to them, and come through stronger. It is not about avoiding difficulties but learning how to move through them without losing balance. Resilience is not something we are born with; it's something we build, step by step, through intentional habits and small choices.

It starts with self-awareness. Understanding how stress shows up in the body and mind helps break its hold. Maybe it's a tightness in the chest, irritability that flares up too easily, or nights spent tossing and turning. Recognizing these signals is the first step toward change. Chronic stress can manifest differently in each person; some experience digestive complaints, others develop tension headaches or muscle pain, while others notice cognitive changes like forgetfulness or brain fog. Research shows that chronic stress can disrupt the gut microbiota, weaken gut-barrier function, increase intestinal permeability and promote inflammation. These biological shifts may help explain why some individuals remain stress-resilient, while others become more susceptible, as stress-driven microbiome changes likely influence mood and emotional regulation.[15] Self-awareness also means knowing what triggers stress. It could be an overloaded schedule, difficult relationships, or even internal pressures we place on ourselves. When we know our patterns, we can start to shift them, responding with intention instead of habit.

Boundaries are another key part of resilience. It can feel difficult to say no, but constantly saying yes to every demand is a direct path to burnout. Healthy boundaries are about protecting energy and knowing when to step back. It's not selfish, it's necessary. Whether it's limiting work hours, creating quiet spaces for rest, or reducing time spent with people who drain energy, setting boundaries is an act of self-care. It teaches the mind and body that rest is allowed, and that not every demand deserves attention.

Perspective also shapes resilience. Challenges can feel overwhelming, but they can also be opportunities for growth. Reframing how we view stress does not change the circumstances, but it changes how we experience them. Instead of asking, "Why is this happening to me?" we can ask, "What can this teach me?" That shift in perspective does not take away pain, but it opens the door to learning and strength. It helps us see beyond the struggle and focus on the growth it can produce. Rest is a requirement for resilience. The body cannot function well when it is always running on empty. Studies highlight that poor sleep quality directly affects stress hormone regulation, inflammation levels, and metabolism.[16] Intentional rest, whether it is through quality sleep, quiet reflection, time in nature, prayerful meditation, or simply taking a break, helps the mind and body recover. It is a way of telling ourselves that we matter, that health matters, and that there is strength in pausing. Rest creates space for clarity, balance, and renewal.

Nutrition and Stress Resilience

The connection between food and stress is often overlooked, but what we eat affects how the body responds to stress. Research demonstrates how stress alters gut function, affecting nutrient absorption, digestion, bacterial balance, and inflammation levels, all of which influence our resilience to further stress.[17]

Eating in a peaceful, calm manner stimulates digestion and supports optimal nutrient absorption. This "eating hygiene" helps activate the parasympathetic nervous system, allowing the body to properly process nutrients and maintain microbial balance and gut health.

One of the simplest ways to support the body is by focusing on anti-inflammatory foods. Stress naturally increases inflammation, and without the right nutrients, that inflammation lingers and spreads. Foods like leafy greens, berries, nuts, and fatty fish contain compounds that help the body calm this response. Specific foods rich in polyphenols—plant compounds with anti-inflammatory properties—include berries, green tea, dark chocolate, turmeric, and colorful vegetables. Research shows these polyphenols not only reduce oxidative stress but also support beneficial gut bacteria, creating a healthier microbiome that better regulates the stress response.[18] They are packed with antioxidants and essential nutrients that reduce internal stress signals, supporting both physical health and emotional well-being. Adding more of these to daily meals doesn't require a drastic change, just small, consistent choices that give the body what it needs to heal and stay resilient.

Following an anti-inflammatory diet (AID) provides support for managing stress-induced inflammation and supporting overall health.[19] Processed foods, especially those high in refined sugars, fuel inflammation. These foods disrupt the gut microbiome, reducing beneficial bacteria while allowing inflammatory species to flourish. They send blood sugar levels on a rollercoaster, increasing feelings of anxiety, fatigue, and irritability. Artificial sweeteners like saccharin, sucralose, and aspartame increase the ability of gut bacteria to form biofilms, structures that can protect harmful bacteria and increase inflammation.

Studies have shown that stress and poor diet create a vicious cycle, where stress triggers unhealthy food cravings, and highly processed, high-fat foods further impair microbiota diversity and inflammatory regulation. Excess sugar also drives cortisol production, which keeps the body in a constant state of alert. Avoiding sugary snacks, fast foods, and highly processed meals helps keep hormones steady and moods more balanced. Replacing these with whole, nutrient-rich foods gives the body a fighting chance to handle stress with strength.

Certain nutrients are especially important when it comes to managing stress. Magnesium, for instance, is known as nature's calming mineral. It regulates the nervous system, helping to ease tension, reduce muscle tightness, and support deeper sleep. When magnesium levels are low, stress feels heavier, and the body has a harder time relaxing. Research has confirmed that magnesium deficiency contributes to chronic low-grade inflammation and is a risk factor for cardiovascular disease, hypertension, and diabetes. Adults should aim for 320-420mg daily, but up to 50% of Americans don't meet these guidelines.[20] Foods like spinach, almonds, and avocados are excellent sources, and including them regularly can make a noticeable difference.

B vitamins are another critical source of support for stress management. They help regulate energy production and ensure that the brain functions smoothly. When stress is high, the body burns through B vitamins quickly, leading to feelings of fatigue and mental fog. Replenishing these vitamins through whole grains, legumes, and leafy greens keeps energy steady and helps the mind stay sharp. It's a simple but effective way to give the body what it needs during challenging times.

Omega-3 fatty acids also deserve special attention. These healthy fats, found in fatty fish like salmon, flaxseeds, and walnuts, are known for reducing inflammation and supporting brain health. These fatty acids help stabilize mood, reduce anxiety, and protect against the long-term effects of stress on the brain. Focusing on SMASH fish (salmon, mackerel, anchovies, sardines, herring), which are higher in omega-3s and lower in mercury, can help reduce health risks and mortality, with benefits for pain, inflammation, cardiovascular health, cognitive function, and immune regulation.[21]

Supporting gut health through probiotics, prebiotics, and postbiotics provides another avenue for stress resilience. Probiotics are beneficial live bacteria found in fermented foods like yogurt, kefir, sauerkraut, and kimchi. Prebiotics are the fiber-rich foods that feed these beneficial bacteria, including garlic, onions, leeks, asparagus, and bananas. Postbiotics are the metabolic compounds produced by beneficial bacteria, including short-chain fatty acids that support gut barrier function and reduce inflammation.[22]

Some beneficial bacteria are termed "psychobiotics" because they produce neurotransmitters like dopamine and serotonin, directly supporting mood regulation and mental well-being. This highlights the connection between gut health and mental health, making gut support an important component of stress management.[23]

These nutrition choices do not have to be complicated. It is about choosing foods that bring life and energy rather than those that drain it. It is about noticing how meals make the body feel, energized and focused, or sluggish and inflamed. By paying attention to these patterns, it becomes easier to make better choices, ones that strengthen resilience rather than weaken it. Because food isn't just about hunger, it's about health. It is a daily opportunity to support the body through stress, to send signals of safety and balance, and to build a foundation that allows strength to grow. Every bite is a choice, and when we choose well, we choose health.

Detoxifying Your Environment

The environment we live in every day can also trigger stress. The air we breathe, the products we use, and even the spaces we inhabit can all influence how our bodies respond to stress. Research identifies toxin exposure as one of the six major root causes of chronic disease.[24] When the body is constantly fighting against toxins, it becomes harder to find balance. Supporting health means not only managing internal stress but also reducing the external pressures that weigh the body down.

One of the simplest ways to reduce environmental stress is by minimizing chemical exposure. Many everyday products, like cleaning supplies, cosmetics, and air fresheners, are filled with synthetic chemicals that place an extra burden on the body's natural detox systems. Harmful chemicals can be classified into six categories: highly fluorinated chemicals (PFAS), antimicrobials, flame retardants, bisphenols and phthalates, certain solvents, and heavy metals.[25] These chemicals do not just disappear.

Over time, they accumulate, forcing the body to work harder to eliminate them. This constant internal effort can heighten stress responses, leading to fatigue, headaches, and hormonal imbalances.

Environmental toxins directly damage the gut microbiome, leading to disruptions in the balance between beneficial and harmful bacteria. Certain chemicals, including glyphosate (found in Roundup herbicide), have been shown to promote dysbiosis and damage the tight junctions between intestinal cells, increasing gut permeability, or "leaky gut." This allows toxins and partially digested food particles to enter the bloodstream, triggering systemic inflammation and immune responses that further tax the body. Chronic stress and toxin exposure together create a powerful strain on the gut and immune system. Disrupting the microbiome weakens both gut and brain barriers, fueling inflammation that affects not only physical health but also mood and mental well-being.[26]

Choosing organic foods and natural alternatives, like plant-based cleaners, fragrance-free skincare, and simple home remedies, lightens that load. Simple ingredients like vinegar, baking soda, and essential oils can clean effectively without introducing harmful chemicals into your environment.

The quality of the air and water we consume matters just as much. Poor air quality can irritate the lungs, increase inflammation, and trigger stress responses without us even realizing it. Mold exposure in water-damaged buildings can trigger systemic inflammation, disrupt gut function, and compromise immune regulation. Investing in air purifiers, especially for bedrooms or living spaces, helps create a cleaner environment that supports deeper rest and better breathing. Similarly, clean water is essential. Tap water can contain toxins like chlorine, lead, and pesticides, which stress the body over time. Checking local water quality through resources like the Environmental Working Group's Tap Water Database and choosing appropriate filtration methods, from simple carbon filters for chlorine and some organic compounds to reverse osmosis systems for heavy metals and fluoride.

These choices may seem small, but they help reduce the quiet, constant stress that environmental toxins place on the body. Creating restorative spaces at home is another way to ease environmental stress. Our surroundings influence how we feel, and cluttered, noisy, or chaotic spaces can increase tension. You can create a sleep haven by ensuring your bedroom is cool, dark, quiet, peaceful, comfortable, and clean. Setting aside a quiet corner for rest, reflection, or prayer can make a powerful difference. It does not have to be elaborate: a chair by a window, a soft blanket, or even a few calming plants. What matters is that it becomes a place where the mind can pause, where the body can release tension, and where peace feels tangible. These spaces serve as daily reminders that rest is allowed, and that calm can be created even in small moments.

Reducing environmental stress is not about achieving perfection. It is about creating little shifts that add up over time. Swapping one product, purifying the air, or carving out a quiet space doesn't just ease stress; it signals to the body that it is safe, supported, and cared for.

Key Takeaways

When we understand how stress affects the body and take intentional steps to manage it, we protect ourselves from the silent damage it can cause. Chronic stress impacts every part of health, from immunity to hormones, mental clarity, and emotional well-being. But it does not have to control us.

As you reflect on this chapter, keep these key takeaways in mind:

Chronic stress is a significant disruptor of health. It weakens the immune system, disrupts hormone balance, clouds mental clarity, and impacts emotional well-being. Stress directly alters gut bacteria composition, increasing inflammatory species while reducing beneficial ones, creating effects throughout the body. Research confirms that even acute psychosocial stress can significantly increase gut permeability in humans, especially in high-cortisol responders.[27]

Stress cannot always be avoided, but it can be managed. Techniques like mindfulness, breathwork, movement, and quiet reflection provide practical ways to ease stress and protect the body. Even short practices, like 60 seconds of deep breathing or 5-10 minutes of mindful movement, can activate the parasympathetic nervous system and begin to reverse the physiological effects of chronic stress.

Emotional resilience is key to handling life's challenges. Building resilience through self-awareness, healthy boundaries, supportive relationships, and intentional rest helps you adapt, recover, and maintain strength even during difficult seasons. Taking control of your stress response changes everything. It reduces inflammation, supports clearer thinking, and helps restore hormonal balance. Managing stress positively influences the gut-brain axis, improving both digestive function and mental clarity through better communication between the enteric nervous system and the central nervous system. Each step you take toward stress management is a step toward greater health and vitality.

Now, take a moment to pause and reflect. These questions are meant to guide you toward deeper insight and more intentional action. Write your answers down or simply consider them thoughtfully.

Questions for Reflection

1. How does stress currently show up in my body and mind?

2. Are there physical symptoms I have been ignoring or emotional patterns that need attention?

3. What stress-management strategies have I tried in the past?

4. Which ones have helped, and which ones have felt ineffective?

5. Where in my life do I need stronger boundaries?

6. Are there people, commitments, or habits that drain my energy and increase stress?

7. What is one small, consistent practice I can begin today to reduce stress? It could be a few moments of reflection, a short walk, or simply taking time to breathe deeply.

8. How might improved stress management support my overall health goals? Consider how reducing stress could enhance energy, sleep, digestion, and emotional well-being.

These reflections offer insight into how stress is showing up and how to better manage it. Each choice you make to ease stress is an act of care and an investment in your health. Learning to manage stress with strength and grace creates a life that feels more balanced and whole. But resilience doesn't stop with a calm mind—it also depends on how we care for the body. One of the most powerful, yet often overlooked, tools for health is movement. The human body was never designed for prolonged sitting, yet modern life encourages it. Without regular activity, metabolism slows, circulation weakens, and mood declines. In the next chapter, we'll explore why movement matters, how it supports every system of the body, and how even small steps each day can restore strength, longevity, and overall health.

CHAPTER 9

Movement Matters

Don't you realize that in a race everyone runs, but only one person gets the prize? So run to win!

— 1 Corinthians 9:24 (NLT)

Most people sit too much, and the body simply wasn't designed for prolonged inactivity. Many of us unknowingly fall into patterns of minimal movement that negatively impact metabolism, blood flow, hormones, and mood. Movement isn't optional. The body requires it for proper function, just as it needs water and sleep. When the body moves, all systems operate more efficiently. Blood circulates freely, delivering oxygen and nutrients to cells. Waste gets cleared through improved lymphatic flow. Muscles pull sugar from the bloodstream without requiring insulin. The brain releases mood-enhancing chemicals that no pill can perfectly replicate. Bones strengthen in response to pressure, and joints receive nourishment through muscle action. Even digestion works more efficiently with regular movement throughout the day.

Without regular activity, bodily systems deteriorate. Metabolism slows, inflammation builds up, stress hormones remain elevated, and natural healing abilities suffer. Joints stiffen, muscles weaken, and bone density decreases. Many symptoms attributed to aging, fatigue, pain, cognitive decline, and reduced mobility are actually signs of movement deficiency.

This chapter explores how regular, everyday movement prevents disease, builds strength, and restores energy. We'll discover practical ways to add more movement to your life, even if you've been inactive for years.

Movement: The Forgotten Medicine

The U.S. Department of Health and Human Services spent years analyzing thousands of studies to create the Physical Activity Guidelines for Americans, and the findings are clear: regular physical activity is one of the most powerful things you can do for your health. Yet nearly 80 percent of adults don't get enough movement, and this inactivity costs us $117 billion annually in healthcare expenses and contributes to 10 percent of premature deaths.[1] Here's what matters for your sleep: physical activity immediately improves sleep quality, reduces anxiety, and stabilizes mood after just one session, and these benefits compound over time to create the deep, restorative rest your body needs to heal. The research shows that some movement is always better than none, and the benefits start right away—not months from now.

Daily physical activity has been systematically removed from modern life. Historically, people stayed active through routine tasks like walking, lifting, and carrying. Modern technology and convenience have eliminated these natural movements. Desks have replaced fields, screens have replaced active play, and machines do the physical work people once did. Washing machines clean clothes, cars transport us door-to-door, and food arrives pre-prepared, often by delivery. This major shift has left the body confused, built for constant motion but forced to stay still for most waking hours. The health problems are clear and widespread. Heart disease, diabetes, obesity, and metabolic disorders have all increased alongside increasingly inactive habits.

The connection between sedentary living and these conditions isn't just correlational; it's causal. When activity levels drop, measurable changes occur in blood vessel function, insulin sensitivity, inflammation markers, and fat metabolism.

Even depression and anxiety are strongly linked to a lack of physical activity, with movement affecting everything from brain structure to neurotransmitter balance. The body needs movement not as some optional health bonus, but as a basic requirement to function properly, just as it needs water, food, and sleep. What's most troubling is how sitting for hours has become so common that many people don't recognize how deeply it affects their health until problems appear. Children sit in classrooms all day, then come home to sit for homework and screen time. Adults commute sitting in cars or public transportation, work sitting at desks, and relax sitting in front of televisions. This results in 10-12 hours daily in seated positions that our bodies weren't designed to maintain. By the time health issues emerge, back pain, fatigue, weight gain, mood disorders, elevated blood sugar, damaged metabolism, muscle loss, and circulation problems have often taken hold and become harder to reverse.

Movement is medicine, a powerful, free therapy that delivers benefits no prescription drug can match. When you move regularly, your body responds with improved circulation, enhanced metabolism, balanced hormones, and better brain function. A simple walk after a meal regulates blood sugar more effectively than diabetes medications. Regular movement throughout the day maintains healthy blood pressure without the side effects of hypertension drugs. The physical act of moving muscles triggers anti-inflammatory responses that no pill can fully replicate. These benefits accrue regardless of fitness level, age, or athletic ability.

Sedentary Lifestyles, Physical Activity, and the Prevention of Chronic Disease

Office jobs, long commutes, and endless screen time have created a genuine health emergency that few people recognize. The average American now spends 6.5 to 8 hours sitting daily, reaching 10 to 12 hours for office workers when you include evening TV time. This unprecedented level of physical inactivity simply didn't exist in previous generations. The body wasn't built for this much stillness, and the effects are serious and wide-ranging.

When you sit for long periods, your muscles become inactive. This directly reduces sugar uptake from your blood, creating insulin resistance even in otherwise healthy people. Blood flow slows dramatically, limiting oxygen and nutrients to tissues while allowing waste to build up. The lymph system, which depends entirely on movement, stagnates, weakening immune function. Even the brain works worse as blood flow decreases during long periods of sitting.

The Physical Activity Guidelines for Americans reveal just how deadly this sedentary lifestyle has become. Strong scientific evidence shows that physical activity delays death from all causes—heart disease, cancer, and other leading killers. The research demonstrates that people who are physically active for approximately 150 minutes per week have a 33 percent lower risk of dying from any cause compared to inactive people. What's remarkable is that only a few lifestyle choices have such a powerful effect on mortality, and you don't need to become a marathon runner to gain these benefits.

What makes sedentary lifestyle so dangerous is how quickly it hurts health. Just two weeks of reduced movement can measurably decrease insulin sensitivity and heart fitness while increasing inflammation.[2] Unlike many health risks that take decades to show symptoms, the effects of sitting too much appear rapidly and get worse if not addressed.

Physical activity includes any bodily movement produced by skeletal muscles that requires energy expenditure. This broad definition includes much more than formal exercise; it includes everyday activities, household tasks, and even fidgeting. When health experts talk about "getting enough physical activity," they mean all the ways the body moves throughout the day. This makes movement accessible to everyone regardless of fitness level, financial resources, or time constraints. It acknowledges that the elderly person tending their garden is engaging in valuable physical activity, as is the parent chasing a toddler. By broadening our understanding beyond structured exercise, we recognize that all movement counts toward health, and small activities accumulate throughout the day to create significant benefits for metabolism, circulation, and well-being.

The truth is that beneficial movement doesn't require any special equipment, gym memberships, or athletic skill. It simply requires breaking up long periods of sitting throughout the day with regular physical activity of *any* kind. This contradicts the fitness industry's campaign that effective movement needs special shoes, technical supplements, costly equipment, or a personal trainer. The body doesn't distinguish between walking on a treadmill and walking through the neighborhood; it simply responds to the movement itself.

The preventive power of movement works through multiple pathways in the body. Regular activity strengthens the heart, improves blood vessel flexibility, and regulates blood pressure and cholesterol, directly countering the main risk factors for heart disease.[3] Each time muscles contract, glucose transporters activate, which pull sugar from the bloodstream without needing insulin, providing natural protection against metabolic disorders and diabetes.

Weight-bearing movement stimulates bone growth, preventing bone loss and maintaining joint health. Muscle contractions pump lymph fluid, improving immune cell circulation and waste removal. Physical activity triggers the release of anti-inflammatory compounds that counter the chronic inflammation underlying most long-term diseases.[4] Perhaps most remarkable are the brain benefits. Movement increases blood flow to the brain, stimulates the production of growth factors, and regulates brain chemicals like serotonin, dopamine, and norepinephrine, providing powerful protection against depression, anxiety, and neurologic disorders.[5] These effects help explain why physically active people report better mental health and maintain sharper thinking as they age.

Movement doesn't just add years to life; it adds life to years by preserving the ability to function and reducing disability as we age. The evidence is clear: no medication, supplement, or treatment comes close to movement in its broad protective power against chronic disease.

Health Benefits Associated With Regular Physical Activity[1]

Adults and Older Adults

- Lower risk of all-cause mortality
- Lower risk of cardiovascular disease mortality
- Lower risk of cardiovascular disease (including heart disease and stroke)
- Lower risk of hypertension
- Lower risk of type 2 diabetes
- Lower risk of adverse blood lipid profile
- Lower risk of cancers of the bladder, breast, colon, endometrium, esophagus, kidney, lung, and stomach
- Improved cognition (executive function, attention, memory, crystallized intelligence, processing speed)
- Reduced risk of dementia (including Alzheimer's disease)
- Improved quality of life
- Reduced anxiety
- Reduced risk of depression
- Improved sleep
- Slowed or reduced weight gain
- Weight loss, particularly when combined with reduced calorie intake
- Prevention of weight regain following initial weight loss
- Improved bone health
- Improved physical function
- Lower risk of falls (older adults)
- Lower risk of fall-related injuries (older adults)

Examples of Different Aerobic Physical Activities and Intensities, Based on Absolute Intensity[1]

Moderate-Intensity Activities

- Walking briskly (2.5 miles per hour or faster)
- Recreational swimming
- Bicycling slower than 10 miles per hour on level terrain
- Tennis (doubles)
- Active forms of yoga (for example, Vinyasa or power yoga)
- Ballroom or line dancing
- General yard work and home repair work
- Exercise classes like water aerobics

Vigorous-Intensity Activities

- Jogging or running
- Swimming laps
- Tennis (singles)
- Vigorous dancing
- Bicycling faster than 10 miles per hour
- Jumping rope
- Heavy yard work (digging or shoveling, with heart rate increases)
- Hiking uphill or with a heavy backpack
- High-intensity interval training (HIIT)
- Exercise classes like vigorous step aerobics or kickboxing

Moving More to Counteract a Sedentary Lifestyle

The most powerful forms of movement are often the simplest: walking, stretching, and everyday activities already part of your routine. No special equipment or skills are needed to benefit. This accessibility removes common barriers that prevent many people from becoming active, making movement possible for everyone regardless of time, budget, or fitness level. According to the Physical Activity Guidelines for Americans, the formula is straightforward: adults should move more and sit less throughout the day, and some physical activity is better than none. For substantial health benefits, you need at least 150 to 300 minutes of moderate-intensity activity per week (like brisk walking), or 75 to 150 minutes of vigorous-intensity activity (like jogging), spread throughout the week. Add muscle-strengthening activities that work all major muscle groups at least 2 days per week, and you'll gain additional benefits.

Walking is perhaps the *most* underrated health intervention available! This basic human movement requires no equipment or special skill, yet delivers remarkable benefits. Brief walks after eating meals significantly lower blood sugar levels, a 10-minute stroll after dinner can reduce how high your blood sugar rises by up to 22%.[6] Walking during phone calls or meetings adds movement without requiring additional time in your schedule. Even short walking breaks every hour significantly improve energy, focus, and metabolic health.

Simple stretching routines integrated into your daily habits maintain flexibility and joint function with minimal time investment. Basic movements like shoulder rolls, gentle spinal twists, and hamstring stretches counteract the muscle tightening and joint stiffness that result from prolonged sitting. Doing these movements for just 2-3 minutes several times daily can preserve mobility and reduce pain. Gardening uses multiple muscle groups through natural, functional movements like squatting, reaching, and lifting. Beyond the physical benefits, connecting with nature while gardening reduces stress hormones and improves mood, creating both physical and mental benefits that support overall health.[7]

Household activities like cleaning, organizing, and yard work all involve reaching, bending, and carrying, movements that maintain functional strength through practical application. Viewing these necessary tasks as opportunities for beneficial movement transforms them from chores into health-promoting activities. Small movements throughout the day, calf raises while brushing teeth, desk stretches during computer work, or balance practice while waiting in line, add significant benefits with minimal disruption to your routine. These small movement "snacks" provide outsized health returns for the time invested. Frequent, brief movement sessions spread throughout the day may deliver greater metabolic benefits than a single workout followed by extended sitting. This movement pattern more closely resembles how humans historically moved, frequent, varied motion throughout waking hours, rather than concentrated exertion followed by prolonged stillness.

Each time you move, even briefly, you trigger beneficial responses: improved circulation, better oxygen delivery, activated metabolism, reduced inflammation, and stimulated brain chemicals. When you spread movement throughout your day, these benefits accumulate and reinforce each other, creating sustained improvements in metabolism, mood, and energy. Walking for just two minutes every half hour significantly improves blood sugar control and energy levels compared to uninterrupted sitting.

This approach provides an accessible strategy for counteracting sedentary patterns, particularly for those with busy schedules, physical limitations, or a dislike of traditional exercise.

The key to success lies in consistency rather than intensity. Regular movement, spread throughout your day, provides greater long-term health benefits than sporadic bursts of vigorous exercise followed by extended periods of inactivity. It's not about pushing your limits occasionally; it's about showing up daily in small, sustainable ways. This shift in mindset removes the pressure to perform and emphasizes steady, ongoing effort. When movement becomes a normal, expected part of your routine, it requires less mental energy and becomes easier to maintain. This principle makes staying active more approachable for everyone, regardless of age, ability, or current fitness level.

Practical Strategies for Overcoming Sedentary Lifestyles

Breaking deeply rooted sedentary habits requires more than good intentions, it demands practical strategies that make movement automatic rather than reliant on willpower. Relying solely on motivation is unsustainable, especially when modern environments are designed for comfort and convenience. Instead, creating systems and environmental cues that prompt regular activity can shift behavior patterns over time. You can set "movement reminders" on your phone, computer, or watch to prompt standing, stretching, or walking every 30-60 minutes. These digital nudges help interrupt the unconscious pattern of prolonged sitting that often takes over during deep work or extended screen time. Without cues, hours can pass unnoticed in a seated position. Timed reminders serve as gentle interruptions, giving your body the signal it needs to reset. Many modern devices and wellness apps now offer customizable movement alerts, making it easier than ever to stay consistent. By building in regular breaks, you create space for movement without needing to rely on memory. Link physical activity to existing habits in your routine. This method leverages the power of behaviors you already perform daily to prompt new ones with minimal resistance. Stand or pace during phone calls, stretch while waiting for the coffee to brew, or do calf raises while brushing your teeth. These movements might seem minor, but their value lies in their consistency. When paired with automatic routines, physical activity becomes just as habitual. These small actions bypass the mental hurdle of making a separate decision, embedding movement seamlessly into your daily flow.

Add movement to current activities instead of trying to carve out extra time for formal exercise. In a busy day, setting aside an hour to work out may feel impossible, but integrating movement into what you're already doing makes it far more achievable. Walk during phone calls, especially long ones, or pace during parent-teacher meetings. Choose stairs over elevators, or park a bit farther from entrances to add effortless walking. Use TV commercial breaks as opportunities to stretch or do quick bodyweight exercises. By blending movement into routine tasks, you remove barriers and reduce the friction that often prevents activity.

Your physical environment *strongly* influences your movement patterns, often more than motivation does. To encourage activity, design your space with movement in mind. Set up a standing or adjustable desk that lets you switch postures throughout the day without interrupting your workflow.

Keep a pair of comfortable walking shoes within easy reach, reducing the steps needed, both literally and mentally, to get moving.

Consider placing frequently used items like your printer, coffee machine, or notebook in separate areas to increase natural movement. These subtle changes promote spontaneous activity and reduce passive behavior, making your environment an active partner in supporting healthier habits.

Adapt your movement goals to accommodate changing energy, motivation, and time constraints. Creating a rigid movement plan often leads to frustration and abandonment at the first disruption. Instead, develop a flexible approach with multiple options for different circumstances. On high-energy days, you might enjoy a longer walk or more challenging activities. During busy periods, brief movement breaks scattered throughout your day might be most realistic.

When fatigue or illness strikes, gentle stretching or simple joint mobility exercises maintain the habit of movement while respecting your body's limitations. Having these flexible options ensures that some activity remains possible even during challenging days. Remember that movement honors the design and function of the body. The human form was not created for sedentary existence; it was intricately designed for motion, with over 600 muscles, 200+ bones, and complex systems that function optimally when regularly activated through movement.

Regular activity maintains these systems and enhances their performance. Physical movement represents more than just an optional health practice; it's fundamental to how the body functions at its best. The body responds to consistent, intentional movement by becoming stronger, more resilient, and better equipped to handle the demands of daily life.

Mental Health Benefits of Physical Activity

The connection between movement and mental health is profound and multifaceted. While many people focus solely on the physical benefits of exercise, the impact on brain function and emotional well-being may be even more significant. Regular movement positively affects multiple aspects of mental health, from mood enhancement to improving symptoms across various conditions. One of the most immediate effects of movement is the release of endorphins, natural opioid compounds that reduce pain perception and trigger positive feelings. These "feel-good" chemicals produce what is often called a "runner's high," though you don't need intense exercise to experience their effects. Movement causes the brain to produce more of these endogenous opioid peptides, which reduce pain and boost mood while decreasing feelings of worry and hopelessness.[8]

Beyond endorphins, moving your body also increases the production of neurotransmitters, including serotonin, dopamine, and norepinephrine.[9] These substances regulate mood, motivation, attention, and energy levels. Low levels are frequently associated with depression and anxiety, which helps explain why regular movement can significantly reduce symptoms of these conditions.

Movement also improves the function of the hypothalamus-pituitary-adrenal (HPA) axis, the body's central stress response system. Regular activity lowers cortisol levels and helps restore balance to other hormones like leptin and ghrelin that regulate appetite and energy. By normalizing these physiological systems, daily movement creates resilience against stress and anxiety.

Activity increases plasma brain-derived neurotrophic factor (BDNF), which plays vital roles in mental health, learning, and cognitive function.[10]

Movement delivers powerful benefits for sleep quality and duration. After regular training, both the quantity and quality of sleep improve. Activity reduces very light sleep and increases REM sleep continuity and performance. Moving moderately and vigorously enhances the overall quality of sleep, which is particularly important for mental health since sleep disturbances are common in many psychological conditions. Moving your body has shown statistically significant effects on the quality of sleep in adults with mental illness, further emphasizing its importance in comprehensive treatment plans.

For those with depression and anxiety, movement provides remarkable benefits. Exercise therapy for depression has shown moderate to large effects compared to no intervention or standard care. While slightly less effective than antidepressant medication in some studies, daily movement remains a crucial adjunctive treatment and may be particularly valuable for those who cannot access or tolerate standard medications.[11] Mind-body practices like yoga have demonstrated positive impacts on depressive symptoms and overall well-being.[12] Movement also shows promise for more complex mental health conditions. For individuals with schizophrenia, staying active helps reduce negative symptoms while addressing medical comorbidities that often accompany psychotic disorders, particularly the metabolic side effects of antipsychotic medications.[13] In substance use recovery, movement helps manage cravings, provides stress relief, and offers a healthy replacement activity. For people with alcohol use disorder, consistent activity has been shown to significantly reduce alcohol intake and binge drinking episodes.

The cognitive benefits of movement extend to everyone. Moving your body can improve attention, focus, memory, cognition, language fluency, and decision-making for up to two hours after activity.[14]

Regular movement enhances overall mood and quality of life, making it one of the most accessible and effective tools for maintaining and improving mental health across the lifespan.

The Immune System and Movement

Regular movement fundamentally transforms how your immune system functions, creating a more balanced defense system that protects against both illness and chronic inflammation.[15] This relationship between moving and immunity has profound implications for overall health, particularly in preventing and managing chronic pain. At its most basic level, moving improves immune cell circulation throughout your body. When you move, muscle contractions help pump lymph fluid, which carries immune cells, through your lymphatic vessels. Unlike the cardiovascular system, the lymphatic system doesn't have its own pump. It relies entirely on bodily movement to function properly. Without regular activity, immune cells stagnate in lymph tissues rather than circulating to locate and address potential threats. Each time you move, you're effectively "stirring the pot" of your immune system, ensuring cells reach the places they're needed most.

Regular moderate activity helps reduce chronic low-grade inflammation, a persistent, subtle inflammatory state that drives numerous chronic diseases, including heart disease, diabetes, and certain types of pain. While intense activity temporarily increases inflammatory markers, regular moderate movement actually decreases baseline inflammation over time. This effect is particularly important because chronic inflammation accelerates tissue aging and significantly increases disease risk. By dampening this inflammatory fire, consistent activity helps protect against the cellular damage that underlies most long-term health conditions.

As your muscles contract when you move, they release special compounds called *myokines*. These are cellular messengers that communicate with other systems throughout your body. Some myokines have direct anti-inflammatory effects, while others stimulate the production of natural antioxidants that protect cells from damage.[16] These muscle-derived substances represent a molecular link between movement and reduced disease risk, demonstrating how activity creates a cascade of protective effects that extend far beyond the muscles themselves.

For people with chronic pain conditions, daily movement helps regulate the immune response that drives symptoms. Regular activity reduces pro-inflammatory substances and increases anti-inflammatory ones at the site of injury and throughout the body. This shift in the inflammatory balance helps reduce pain and support healing. While many pain medications target similar pathways, movement addresses the underlying immune imbalance rather than just masking symptoms. This helps explain why consistent daily movement is now considered essential in managing conditions like arthritis, fibromyalgia, and back pain.

Practical Movement Strategies for Everyone

No matter your current fitness level, age, or health status, adding more beneficial movement into your day goes a long way. Here are some accessible strategies that can work for virtually anyone:

Walking: The Universal Exercise

Walking is the most accessible form of activity available to almost everyone. It requires nothing beyond comfortable shoes and can easily adapt to any fitness level or health status.

For those who have been inactive, starting with just 5-10 minutes of walking makes a significant difference in circulation and energy.

Taking short activity pauses throughout your day provides substantial benefits for both body and mind. Setting a timer to remind yourself to move for just 2-3 minutes every hour during periods of sitting can dramatically improve your health trajectory. These brief interruptions, whether marching in place, stretching gently, or simply walking to refill your water bottle, reset your metabolism and improve blood flow. The cumulative benefit of these brief activity sessions throughout the day often exceeds what a single workout can accomplish, especially when that workout is followed by hours of uninterrupted sitting.

If mobility limitations make standing difficult, chair-based movements provide remarkable benefits. From a seated position, simple exercises like ankle circles, knee lifts, seated marches, arm circles, and gentle torso rotations maintain joint function, improve circulation, and engage core muscles. These seated activities particularly benefit those with arthritis, balance problems, or injury recovery, while still providing meaningful metabolic benefits.

The National Institute on Aging has documented that even people with significant mobility restrictions can improve muscle strength, joint function, and cardiovascular health through consistent chair-based movement.

Your daily routines already contain numerous opportunities for increased activity that require no additional time commitment. Choosing stairs over elevators, when feasible, builds leg strength and cardiovascular fitness in short bursts throughout the day. Parking farther from entrances or carrying groceries in multiple trips might seem insignificant, but these small efforts strengthen your body through functional, practical movements.

These non-exercise physical activities can account for up to 2,000 additional calories of energy used weekly, which is a significant factor in maintaining a healthy metabolism and weight.

Putting Movement Into Your Life

Place visual reminders like colored stickers on doorways in your home as movement triggers. Each time you pass through, do a gentle stretch, five toe raises, or balance briefly on one foot. These small movements might seem insignificant, but they add up throughout the day to create meaningful benefits. While waiting, whether for your coffee to brew, the elevator to arrive, or during TV commercials, practice simple balance exercises, which not only strengthen your muscles but also help prevent falls and maintain independence as you age. Deep breathing paired with gentle arm raises combines oxygen delivery with muscle engagement, making it perfect for anyone, even those with limited mobility who might need to exercise from a seated position or bed.

The social aspect of movement shouldn't be overlooked either. Walking with friends or joining community activities provides both physical benefits and meaningful connections, something research increasingly recognizes as vital for overall health. When possible, take your movement outdoors in natural settings. Parks, gardens, and even your backyard offer mental health benefits beyond the physical activity itself, as time in nature reduces stress hormones and improves mood.[17]

Remember that the most important principle is to begin where you are without comparing yourself to others. Even small increases in daily movement bring significant benefits. If you currently walk zero minutes daily, walking for just two minutes represents an infinite percentage improvement. These small victories accumulate over time, creating sustainable change in both how you feel and how your body functions.

Key Takeaways

Throughout this chapter, we have explored how movement prevents disease, enhances mental health, regulates the immune system, and builds resilience against the effects of aging. The evidence is clear: movement is fundamental to human health, not an optional add-on.

The good news? Moving more is within everyone's reach. By incorporating small, consistent activities throughout your day, you can transform your health trajectory regardless of your starting point. This isn't about intense workouts or athletic performance; it's about honoring your body's basic need for regular movement.

Here's what we know about the power of movement:

- Regular activity is a potent medicine for both preventing and treating chronic disease, from heart conditions and diabetes to depression and cognitive decline.

- Even brief movements, when spread throughout the day, yield significant brain, metabolic and immune benefits that accumulate over time.

- Both the brain and immune system function optimally when regularly activated through movement, creating a powerful foundation for mental clarity and disease resistance.

- Simple, accessible activities can be incorporated into almost *any* lifestyle, regardless of time constraints, physical limitations, or financial resources.

- Consistency matters more than intensity, small, sustainable habits yield greater long-term health benefits than occasional intense exercise.

Questions for Reflection

As we end this chapter, take a moment to reflect on how you move:

1. What does your typical day look like in terms of sitting versus movement? Try to keep a simple log for a few days to see where you might be able to add in some more activity.

2. What three activities, which you already do each day, could be opportunities for more movement? Maybe it's your morning coffee routine, time spent commuting, or free time in the evening.

3. How is your home or workspace set up? Could some simple changes to where you place commonly used items naturally encourage a bit more walking, reaching, or standing?

4. Which forms of movement bring you joy? The activities we enjoy are the ones we'll actually continue doing, so identifying these is key to long-term success.

5. How would having more energy and vitality help you fulfill God's purpose for your life? Consider how being physically stronger might enable you to better serve your family, community, or church. The better you feel, the more you can give!

Movement is not just about fitness or weight, it enhances digestion, clears the mind, lifts mood, and boosts energy. These benefits are available to everyone, regardless of age or fitness level, with each active choice you make. But while movement strengthens the body from within, the environment around us also plays a powerful role in health. Every day, we are exposed to harmful chemicals—pesticides and herbicides such as glyphosate, heavy metals, bisphenols, flame retardants, and even environmental toxins like mold. These exposures can disrupt hormones, weaken immunity, and contribute to chronic disease. In the next chapter, we will look at practical ways to reduce toxic load by limiting exposure, supporting the body's natural detoxification through nutrition, and using supplements strategically to protect and restore health.

CHAPTER 10

Reducing Toxic Load

"They will be able to handle snakes with safety, and if they drink anything poisonous, it won't hurt them. They will be able to place their hands on the sick, and they will be healed."

— Mark 16:18 (NLT)

After months of battling lingering COVID symptoms that conventional medicine couldn't explain, I made a decision that would transform not only my health but my entire approach to healing others. I decided to test myself using the functional medicine principles I was learning. What I discovered shocked me to my core and opened my eyes to an invisible threat that most of us face every single day- toxic burden.

My test results showed dangerously high levels of copper in my tissues. I stared at the numbers in disbelief. How could this be? I was a healthcare professional with over 30 years of experience. I thought I knew everything about health and toxicity. But here I was, poisoned by something I couldn't see, taste, or smell—something that had been accumulating in my body for years while I remained completely unaware. Although copper is not a toxic element, this essential mineral is associated with numerous adverse health effects, including neurodegenerative diseases, adverse reproductive health effects, and increased risk of cardiovascular disease. Additional concerns of gut microbiome disruptions, oxidative stress, liver inflammation, and neurodegenerative diseases like

Alzheimer's and Parkinson's disease [1] increased my risks of adverse effects of copper toxicity. I now had a "root cause" for many of my symptoms: migraines/headaches, fatigue, allergies, brain fog, chronic back pain, and menstrual disorders.[2][3]

As I sat in my kitchen that day, looking at those lab results, a flood of questions overwhelmed me. How had this happened? What were the sources? And most importantly, how many of my patients were suffering from similar imbalances or toxic burdens without anyone, including me, ever investigating this possibility?

This discovery became my wake-up call to the invisible epidemic of toxicity that surrounds us in modern life. From the air we breathe to the food we eat, hidden toxins infiltrate our daily existence, overwhelming our body's natural detoxification systems. Over time, mineral imbalances and toxic burden contribute to oxidative stress, inflammation, hormonal imbalance, immune dysfunction, and chronic disease. But here's what I learned: we don't have to be victims of this toxic world. We can identify these threats, minimize our exposure, and support our body's remarkable ability to heal and detoxify.

Identifying Environmental Toxins

Many sources of toxicity hide in plain sight within our everyday products, creating a steady stream of exposure that gradually overwhelms even the most robust detoxification systems. When I began investigating environmental toxins in my functional medicine practice, I was amazed to discover how pervasive these hidden threats really are. Household cleaners are one of the most significant sources of daily toxic exposure. These products contain harsh chemicals like ammonia, formaldehyde, and chlorine that release volatile organic compounds (VOCs) into our living spaces. What shocked me most was learning from the Environmental Protection Agency that indoor air can be 2-5 times more polluted than outdoor air, largely because of the very products we use to keep our homes clean. This revelation completely changed how I approach home cleaning, both for myself and in recommendations to patients.

Personal care products introduce another layer of chemical burden that most people never consider. Through my research, I discovered that the average woman applies over 168 different chemicals to her body daily through cosmetics, lotions, and personal care items. Parabens, phthalates, and synthetic fragrances act as endocrine disruptors, mimicking estrogen and interfering with our body's delicate hormonal balance. When I share this information with patients, they're often stunned to realize that their daily beauty routine might be contributing to hormonal imbalances they've been struggling to resolve.

The food supply presents its own set of challenges that extend far beyond basic nutrition. Processed foods burden our detoxification organs with additives, preservatives, and pesticide residues that our bodies were never designed to handle. Food colorants, artificial sweeteners, and preservatives have been linked to inflammatory conditions, allergic reactions, and metabolic disruption. Perhaps most concerning is glyphosate, the active ingredient in Roundup herbicide, which disrupts the gut microbiome and has been classified as a *"probably carcinogenic to humans"* (Group 2A), by the International Agency for Research on Cancer (IARC).[4] When patients come to me with unexplained symptoms, we often trace the problem back to these hidden food toxins.

The Six Classes That Changed Everything

My understanding of toxic exposure deepened significantly when I discovered the Green Science Policy Institute's classification of six major chemical classes.[5] This framework revolutionized how I educate patients about environmental toxins—suddenly, the overwhelming world of chemical exposure became manageable and actionable.

1. **Per- and Polyfluoroalkyl Substances, or PFAS**

When I talk with patients about highly fluorinated chemicals, Per- and Polyfluoroalkyl Substances, or PFAS, often called *'forever chemicals,'* I explain that these compounds do not break down in the environment or in our bodies. Over time, they build up and can reach toxic levels. This long-term accumulation has been linked to serious health problems that often show up as chronic diseases, including liver damage, obesity, diabetes, cancer, thyroid disorders, asthma, immune system dysfunction, reduced fertility, low birth weight, and even impacts on children's brain and behavioral development.

PFAS chemicals are found in that water-resistant jacket hanging in your closet, the non-stick pan you use for scrambled eggs, and even the food packaging from your favorite takeout restaurant. I've seen patients make remarkable improvements simply by replacing their non-stick cookware and being more selective about packaged foods. Installing a reliable water-filtration system is one of the most effective ways to protect your home and family from PFAS and other harmful chemicals.

2. Antimicrobials

Antimicrobials are some of the most ironic toxic exposures we encounter. Patients use antibacterial soaps and hand sanitizers, believing they're protecting their health without realizing they're disrupting their beneficial bacteria and contributing to antibiotic resistance. Antimicrobial agents such as triclosan, Quaternary ammonium salts (also known as quats or QACs), and nanosilver are harmful to humans and the ecosystem. Some antimicrobials are *endocrine disruptors,* which are associated with developmental and reproductive harms and allergen sensitivities. Quats like benzalkonium chloride and benzethonium chloride are commonly used in household cleaning products and fabric softeners. Quats have been associated with asthma, dermatitis, and allergies.

When I tell patients that triclosan, which is found in most antibacterial products, has been detected in three-quarters of Americans and nearly all breast milk samples, they're often horrified. On a positive note, in 2016, the FDA stopped the use of triclosan, triclocarban, and 17 other antimicrobials in hand soaps and body washes.

3. Flame Retardants

Flame retardants taught me that even well-intentioned safety regulations can create unintended health consequences. These chemicals are added to furniture, electronics, and children's products to meet flammability standards, but they migrate into household dust that we breathe and ingest daily. I always ask patients about their home furnishings, especially if they have young children who spend time on the floor. Often, replacing fire-retardant clothing, carpeting and furniture embedded with PFAS can significantly reduce exposure.

4. Bisphenols and Phthalates

The bisphenols and phthalates story particularly resonates with patients because plastics are everywhere. These chemicals act as "xenoestrogens"—foreign compounds that mimic estrogen in our bodies.

Early-life exposure to Bisphenol A (BPA) has been linked to asthma and neurodevelopmental concerns, including hyperactivity, anxiety, depression, and aggression. In adults, BPA exposure is associated with obesity, type 2 diabetes, cardiovascular disease, reduced fertility, and cancers of the breast and prostate.

To reduce exposure to harmful chemicals like BPA and phthalates, choose glass, porcelain, or stainless steel containers for hot foods and drinks, and avoid microwaving plastics. Limit the use of plastics labeled with recycle codes 3 or 7, and opt for fresh foods over canned or packaged items. Minimize contact with cash register receipts, and select fragrance-free personal care products to avoid hidden chemicals.

I've learned to look for plastic exposure when patients present with hormonal imbalances, especially when their symptoms don't match their hormone test results. Even products labeled "BPA-free" often contain similar compounds that may be equally harmful—a fact that surprises many health-conscious patients.

5. Some Solvents

Solvents help me explain why some patients feel worse after painting their homes or having carpet installed. These volatile compounds, like toluene, xylene and benzene, easily evaporate at room temperature, making our homes temporary toxic environments. People who work with gasoline, paints, finishes, or dry-cleaning products are at higher risk for harmful solvent exposure. When inhaled or absorbed through the skin, solvents can cause breathing problems, skin irritation, and temporary nervous system effects such as headaches, dizziness, numbness, or confusion. With long-term occupational exposure, certain solvents have been linked to organ damage, increased cancer risk, and neurological harm—especially in infants and young children.

6. **Certain Metals**

The certain metals category encompasses the heavy metals that have become central to my practice. Mercury, lead, arsenic, and cadmium accumulate in our bodies over time, particularly in the brain, kidneys, and bones. These metals help explain why some patients struggle with neurological symptoms, cognitive issues, and organ dysfunction. Understanding heavy metal toxicity completely changed how I approach complex chronic conditions.

Quick Tips to Reduce Heavy Metal Exposure

General Protection

- Control household dust: vacuum with a HEPA filter, wet-mop floors, use door mats, and wash hands often.

- Support your body with nutrition: adequate calcium, iron, and vitamin C help reduce absorption of lead and cadmium.

- Recycle hazardous items properly: dispose of fluorescent lights, batteries, paint, and electronics at approved facilities; choose LED bulbs instead of CFLs.

Mercury

- Avoid high-mercury fish such as shark, swordfish, bluefin tuna, and bigeye tuna.

- Do not use imported skin creams (lightening, acne, or anti-aging) unless confirmed mercury-free.
- Safely clean up broken thermometers or CFL bulbs following EPA guidance.

Arsenic

- For children, limit rice-based foods and offer alternatives when possible.
- Avoid pressure-treated wood manufactured before 2004; seal older decks or playsets every 1–2 years.
- Have children wash their hands after playing on or near older wooden structures.

Cadmium

- Keep children away from inexpensive metal jewelry or charms.
- Do not allow children to handle nickel-cadmium (NiCd/NiCad) rechargeable batteries.

Lead

- In pre-1978 homes, use only lead-safe practices during renovations and repairs.
- Keep children away from chipped or peeling paint.
- Cover bare soil near older homes with grass, bark, or gravel.
- Use cold tap water for drinking and cooking to reduce lead leaching from pipes.

Beyond the Six Classifications

Mold toxicity deserves special mention because it's often the missing piece in complex chronic illness puzzles. I have learned to investigate potential mold exposure whenever patients present with unexplained fatigue, brain fog, or immune dysfunction that doesn't respond to conventional treatments. The mycotoxins produced by certain mold species can trigger inflammatory responses, immune-related reactions, and mitochondrial damage, which are effects that can persist long after the initial exposure.

Agricultural chemicals represent another category that directly impacts every patient I see. The widespread use of glyphosate means virtually everyone has some level of exposure through food and water. When I show patients maps of glyphosate usage across the United States, they begin to understand why gut health issues have become so prevalent. This herbicide doesn't just kill weeds—it disrupts the delicate balance of our gut microbiome.

Understanding How Toxins Impact Our Bodies

Toxins don't target just one organ system; they create widespread dysfunction throughout the body. Neurological symptoms often appear first. Patients complain of headaches, chronic fatigue, and unexplained brain fog that makes them feel like they're living in a mental haze. These are often early indicators that neurotoxins are disrupting normal brain function. The central nervous system is particularly vulnerable because many toxins can cross the blood-brain barrier and accumulate in brain tissue.

Digestive issues are common with toxin exposure. Acid reflux, abdominal pain and irritable bowel syndrome are often manifestations of toxins affecting the gut lining and microbiome.

When toxins disrupt the delicate balance of gut bacteria, compromising intestinal barrier function (i.e., leaky gut) and activating the immune system, patients experience the cascade of symptoms that conventional medicine treats as isolated problems.

Hormonal disruption creates some of the most frustrating symptoms for patients. Low testosterone in men, unexplained weight gain, and reproductive issues often stem from endocrine-disrupting chemicals that interfere with normal hormone production and signaling. These hormone-mimicking substances can trigger effects at extremely low doses, explaining why patients can have "normal" hormone levels but still experience significant symptoms. Additionally, inflammatory conditions throughout the body—joint pain, stiffness, back pain—frequently improve when we address the toxic burden.

Toxins trigger chronic inflammation that manifests differently in each person based on their genetic vulnerabilities and existing health status. What appears as migraines, arthritis, fibromyalgia, or chronic pain, may actually be the body's inflammatory response to ongoing toxic exposure.

Cancer risk increases with cumulative toxic exposure, particularly for hormone-sensitive cancers like breast and thyroid cancer. This doesn't mean toxins directly cause cancer, but they create the inflammatory, hormonally disrupted environment where cancer can more easily develop.

Routes of Toxic Exposure

Understanding how toxins enter our bodies helps us develop strategic protection plans. I use these exposure pathways to help patients identify their highest-risk activities and environments, which allows them to make targeted changes that provide maximum benefit. Contact exposure through the skin represents a significant but often overlooked pathway. Our skin isn't an impermeable barrier; it is designed to absorb beneficial compounds, but this same mechanism allows harmful chemicals to enter our bloodstream. Personal care products, cleaning chemicals, and even clothing treated with flame retardants can introduce toxins through skin contact.

Oral ingestion occurs mainly through sources like contaminated food and water. Pesticide residues on fruits and vegetables accumulate with each meal. Even small amounts of household dust containing flame retardants and other chemicals can be ingested, especially concerning children who frequently touch surfaces and then put their hands in their mouths. Beyond that, inhalation exposure happens continuously as we breathe air containing volatile organic compounds from cleaning products, perfumes, new furniture, scented candles, and building materials. This pathway is particularly concerning because inhaled toxins bypass some of the body's natural filtration systems and can directly access the bloodstream through the lungs. Patients often don't realize that the "new car smell" or freshly cleaned house scent represents chemical exposure that their body must process and eliminate.

Occupational exposure affects millions of workers who encounter higher concentrations of chemicals through their jobs. Healthcare workers exposed to sterilizing chemicals, hairdressers working with dyes and treatments, construction workers around building materials, and office workers in poorly ventilated buildings face elevated exposure risks.

Strategies for Detoxification Through Diet and Lifestyle

The most effective detoxification strategy begins with a simple but powerful principle: stop adding fuel to the fire. When we reduce toxic exposures, we create space for our body's natural elimination processes to address the toxins that have already accumulated. This approach has transformed how I guide patients toward healing: we start by cleaning up their environment, then support their body's innate wisdom to heal itself.

Reducing New Exposures

Food choices are one of our most powerful tools for reducing toxic burden. When I recommend choosing organic produce, I always share the Environmental Working Group's "Dirty Dozen" and "Clean Fifteen" lists with patients. These annual guides identify which fruits and vegetables carry the highest and lowest pesticide residues. I tell patients to prioritize organic options for the Dirty Dozen—strawberries, spinach, kale, nectarines, apples, grapes, cherries, peaches, pears, bell peppers, celery, and potatoes. For the Clean Fifteen—avocados, sweet corn, pineapple, onions, papaya, sweet peas, eggplants, asparagus, kiwi, cabbage, mushrooms, cantaloupe, honeydew, watermelon, and broccoli—conventional versions typically have lower residues and can be budget-friendly alternatives.

Simple swaps in food storage and cooking methods can dramatically reduce chemical exposure. I encourage patients to replace plastic containers with glass, stainless steel, or ceramic alternatives. Canned foods and plastic containers leach chemicals like BPA and phthalates into our food, especially when heated. These compounds disrupt our endocrine system and have been linked to reproductive issues, metabolic disorders, and certain cancers. Water filtration has become non-negotiable in my recommendations. The Environmental Working Group's Tap Water Database reveals concerning levels of contaminants in public water supplies across the United States. I help patients understand their local water quality and choose appropriate filtration methods—from simple carbon filters for chlorine and organic compounds to reverse osmosis systems for heavy metals and fluoride. Clean water is fundamental to every detoxification process in the body.

Indoor air quality improvements can provide immediate relief for many patients. I recommend opening windows for 5-10 minutes daily, even in cold weather, to reduce the concentration of volatile organic compounds and other indoor pollutants. Air purifiers with HEPA and activated carbon filters remove airborne particles, allergens, and gaseous pollutants, creating a cleaner environment for healing.

Personal care and cleaning product swaps often surprise patients with their impact. Our skin absorbs many compounds applied to it, and our lungs take in airborne chemicals released during cleaning. I guide patients to check product safety ratings on the Environmental Working Group's Skin Deep database and introduce them to simple alternatives like vinegar, baking soda, and essential oils for cleaning. These changes often resolve skin issues and respiratory symptoms that patients had accepted as normal.

Supporting Natural Detoxification

While reducing exposures, we simultaneously support the body's innate detoxification systems through targeted dietary and lifestyle practices. Hydration becomes the foundation of every detox protocol I recommend. Water is essential for kidney function, lymphatic movement, and the elimination of water-soluble toxins. I tell patients to consume half their body weight in ounces of filtered water daily, unless they have medical conditions that contraindicate this.

Fiber acts as our internal detox system, and most people don't get nearly enough. Dietary fiber functions like an internal broom, binding toxins in the digestive tract and facilitating their elimination. When patients don't consume adequate fiber, toxins meant for elimination get reabsorbed, creating a cycle of increasing toxic burden. General recommendations for fiber are 30-50 grams per day. Dietary sources from—vegetables, fruits, legumes, and whole grains—support both detoxification and microbiome health. Cruciferous vegetables deserve special attention for their liver-supporting properties. Broccoli, cauliflower, brussels sprouts, and their relatives contain sulfur compounds that activate phase II liver detoxification enzymes. Sulforaphane from broccoli sprouts particularly enhances our body's ability to neutralize and eliminate harmful chemicals. I encourage patients to include these foods regularly rather than occasionally because consistency matters for optimal microbiome and liver support. Sweating provides a powerful elimination pathway that many people underutilize. Our skin is our largest eliminatory organ, and research shows significant elimination of BPA, phthalates, and heavy metals through sweat.[6][7][8]

I recommend regular sauna use when medically appropriate, along with exercise that induces sweating. Patients often report decreased symptoms and improved energy when they incorporate regular sweating into their routine.

Addressing Mold Exposure

Mold toxins, called mycotoxins, are often known as the "Great Masquerader" because they're often the hidden culprit behind persistent health issues. Exposure may cause rashes, coughing, wheezing, stomach upset, headaches, or what seems like repeated infections that never quite go away. In some cases, these toxins have been linked to more serious problems, including certain cancers and birth defects. What makes mycotoxins tricky is that symptoms can come and go, or resemble many different conditions, so the real cause often goes unnoticed. Reducing exposure—whether from indoor air, food contamination, or water-damaged buildings—is a key step in protecting long-term health.[91]

I teach patients that visible mold represents only a fraction of the problem. Most mold growth occurs behind walls, under flooring, or in other hidden spaces where moisture accumulates. Regular inspection of bathrooms, basements, under sinks, and areas around windows can identify problems before they become serious health threats. Food can also be a source of mold exposure. To reduce risk, limit high-mold foods such as peanuts, corn, wheat, dried fruits, coffee, certain aged cheeses, and grain-based alcohol. Whenever possible, choose fresh, high-quality options, store nuts, grains, and coffee in cool airtight containers, and rotate pantry items regularly to minimize mold growth.

For patients with known or suspected mold exposure, air filtration becomes critical. HEPA air purifiers that capture mold spores as small as 0.3 microns can significantly reduce ongoing exposure. I recommend placing these units in bedrooms and frequently used spaces while remediation efforts are underway. Professional assessment may be necessary when patients have unexplained symptoms that worsen in certain environments.

The Role of Supplements in Addressing Toxicity

While diet and lifestyle modifications form the foundation of any detoxification approach, strategic supplementation can provide crucial support for systems overwhelmed by toxic burden. What I've discovered through years of functional medicine practice is that targeted supplements can support detoxification pathways and accelerate healing in patients who have plateaued with lifestyle changes alone. However, supplements work best when approached with wisdom and discernment, not as magic bullets that bypass the foundational work of healing.

Glutathione has become one of the most valuable tools in detoxification medicine, earning its reputation as the body's master antioxidant. This remarkable tripeptide, composed of just three amino acids, is helpful in detoxification, immune function, and cellular protection.[10] What makes glutathione particularly important is that its levels naturally decline with age, stress, and toxic exposure, precisely when we need it most. Various forms offer different benefits: liposomal glutathione provides enhanced absorption, N-acetyl cysteine serves as a precursor, and glutathione-boosting foods like sulfur-rich vegetables and high-quality whey protein support natural production.

N-acetylcysteine (NAC) functions as both a glutathione precursor and a direct antioxidant, making it particularly valuable in detoxification protocols. This modified amino acid demonstrates a remarkable ability to thin mucus and support respiratory health, proving invaluable for addressing air pollution exposure or respiratory symptoms. NAC is best known as the antidote for acetaminophen toxicity, where it protects the liver from severe damage. That same liver-protective capacity also provides an added margin of safety during intensive detoxification protocols, supporting confident implementation while safeguarding vulnerable organ systems. [11] [12] Natural binders like chlorella and spirulina have revolutionized approaches to heavy metal detoxification through their unique binding compounds. [13] [14]

These freshwater algae effectively bind to heavy metals like mercury, lead, and cadmium, facilitating their safe elimination from contaminated water and the body. Beyond their detoxification properties, these superfoods provide complete protein and chlorophyll for blood purification, supporting overall health while addressing toxic burden. [15] [16]

The comprehensive nutrition these algae provide makes them ideal for patients requiring detoxification support without depleting already compromised systems.

Milk thistle is particularly useful at enhancing liver regeneration and detoxification capacity through its active compound silymarin. This powerful herb protects liver cells from damage while increasing glutathione levels and supporting liver tissue regeneration. What's particularly impressive about milk thistle is its ability to enhance both Phase I and Phase II liver detoxification pathways, helping the body process and eliminate both water-soluble and fat-soluble toxins more efficiently. For patients with elevated liver enzymes or those undertaking intensive detoxification, milk thistle provides essential protection during the healing process. [17]

Lastly, activated charcoal serves as nature's emergency binder for acute toxic exposures and digestive tract cleanup. Its highly porous structure can adsorb many times its weight in toxins, making it effective for binding microbial toxins from gastrointestinal infections, environmental chemicals, and certain medications.

The wisdom of effective detoxification supplementation lies in understanding that supplements should support, not replace, the fundamental work of a clean diet, adequate hydration, quality sleep, and stress management. No supplement can compensate for ongoing toxic exposures or poor lifestyle choices—this is a lesson that transforms how we approach healing. The most successful outcomes occur when supplements are built upon a solid foundation of healthy living practices that address root causes rather than simply managing symptoms.

Tools for Detoxification: Diet and Lifestyle

Beyond specific supplements, it's the simple, daily practices that often have the greatest impact on your body's natural ability to detoxify. These foundational habits, when done consistently, support and strengthen the body's own healing systems in a gentle and sustainable way. A meaningful place to start is first thing in the morning, with a glass of warm lemon water. This habit does more than hydrate—it is a good source of vitamin C that provides antioxidant and digestive support.

Throughout the day, make it a point to include antioxidant-rich foods like berries, turmeric, and green tea. These foods help neutralize free radicals produced during detoxification and protect cells from oxidative damage. Their polyphenols not only reduce inflammation but also nourish beneficial gut bacteria. This creates a positive cycle where detoxification and gut health reinforce one another.

Detoxification also relies on physical movement, not just through exercise, but through techniques that support lymphatic flow. The lymphatic system does not have a built-in pump like the heart. It depends on muscle activity and external stimulation. Dry brushing the skin before showering, using a natural bristle brush, can promote lymphatic circulation. Adding contrast showers that alternate between warm and cool water further stimulates blood flow and encourages the movement of lymph.

Breathwork is another powerful yet often overlooked practice. Deep, intentional breathing increases oxygen delivery to tissues and helps remove carbon dioxide and other waste products. It also activates the parasympathetic nervous system, which reduces stress hormone levels. Chronic stress can hinder the detox process, so incorporating daily breathing exercises can ease the load on the body and promote a more relaxed, healing state. Equally important is ensuring regular bowel movements. When waste remains in the colon for too long, toxins that were meant to be eliminated can be reabsorbed into the bloodstream. Supporting regular elimination through hydration, adequate fiber intake, and movement helps complete the detoxification process and prevents further toxic buildup.

Each of these practices may appear small on its own. Yet together, they provide comprehensive support to the liver, lymphatic system, lungs, skin, kidneys, and colon. This creates a full-body approach to reducing toxic burden and restoring balance. Healing does not always come through dramatic interventions. More often, it begins with simple, consistent habits that support the body's natural ability to heal.

Faith and Cleansing the Body

Just as Scripture reminds us that we are protected even in the presence of danger, we are also called to care for the temple that is our body. That care includes minimizing harmful exposures and supporting the body's natural ability to cleanse and renew. The human body is remarkably resilient when given the right conditions. It carries an innate wisdom, a built-in capacity to identify harmful substances, neutralize toxins, and repair what has been damaged. But for that healing to occur, the body must be supported with the proper tools and freed from unnecessary burdens. This means reducing toxic exposures in our environment, food, and personal care products while also nurturing the systems responsible for detoxification.

When you make conscious, consistent choices that align with how the body is designed to function, you are not forcing healing. You are creating space for it. This alignment with the body's natural processes is a powerful act of faith and stewardship. It reflects trust in the body's design and honors its capacity to heal and thrive.

Adopting this approach means moving away from the conventional view of detox as something that happens through a weekend cleanse or short-term regimen. True detoxification is not a singular event. It is a continual process of supporting the organs and systems responsible for keeping the body in balance, most notably the liver, kidneys, gut, skin, lungs, and lymphatic system.

This shift in mindset invites us to see healing not as a temporary fix but as a way of life, one that respects both the physical design of the body and the divine wisdom behind it. When we care for the body in this way, we are walking in alignment with our faith, our biology, and our purpose.

Key Takeaways

Environmental toxins have become one of the most significant yet overlooked contributors to chronic disease, inflammation, and metabolic dysfunction in our modern world. Through my years of working with patients, I have seen how exposure to thousands of synthetic chemicals through food, water, air, and household products creates a perfect storm of health challenges. These compounds accumulate silently in our tissues, disrupting hormones, damaging the cellular powerhouses called mitochondria, and triggering systemic inflammation even at seemingly insignificant doses. What makes this particularly insidious is that most people have no idea this invisible burden is undermining their health until symptoms become severe enough to seek medical attention.

The empowering truth is that reducing toxin exposure through intentional daily choices can dramatically strengthen the body's natural resilience and capacity for healing. Simple yet strategic changes like choosing organic produce for the highest-pesticide foods, installing quality water filtration systems, improving indoor air quality through ventilation and air purifiers, and selecting truly non-toxic personal care products can significantly reduce daily toxic burden.

Supporting the body's natural detoxification pathways becomes equally important as reducing new exposures, creating a comprehensive approach to toxic burden management. Consistent hydration flushes toxins through the kidneys, fiber-rich foods bind harmful compounds in the digestive tract, regular movement promotes lymphatic drainage and sweating, while specific supplements like glutathione and milk thistle enhance the liver's remarkable ability to process and eliminate accumulated toxins. These interventions work synergistically to restore the body's natural capacity for self-cleaning and repair.

True healing requires both protecting the body from cumulative toxic insults and creating an internal environment where optimal health can flourish naturally. What I've learned through years of practice is that effective detoxification isn't about harsh cleanses, extreme purging protocols, or shocking the system into submission. Instead, it's about providing consistent, gentle support for the body's inherent wisdom while systematically minimizing new toxic exposures that interfere with natural healing processes. This balanced approach creates sustainable improvements in health and vitality without overwhelming systems that may already be struggling under a toxic burden.

When we honor the body's remarkable design for self-healing while removing the obstacles that prevent optimal function, we create the conditions for genuine transformation and lasting wellness.

Questions for Reflection

1. Begin by taking a closer look at your home environment. Many household and personal care products contain ingredients that contribute to the body's toxic burden over time. Go room by room and take inventory. Are there cleaning supplies, skincare products, or air fresheners with artificial fragrances or unrecognizable chemicals? As these items run out, consider replacing them with safer, nontoxic alternatives. Change doesn't have to happen all at once. Progress begins with awareness and one intentional choice at a time.

2. Next, consider the hidden exposures in your daily life—heavy metals, mold, and chemical toxins that often go unnoticed. Start by identifying the most meaningful changes you could make based on your personal circumstances. Perhaps it's using a water filter, addressing humidity levels in your home, or replacing non-stick cookware. Ask yourself: What is one practical change I could implement this week to reduce exposure?

3. Now turn to your diet. Are you providing your body with the nutrients it needs to eliminate toxins effectively? Fiber, antioxidants, and hydration play key roles in supporting detoxification pathways. Reflect on your current habits. Could you add more leafy greens, cruciferous vegetables, or brightly colored fruits? Are you drinking enough clean water each day? Even simple shifts can make a noticeable difference in how you feel.

4. As you examine your lifestyle, ask whether you are consistently supporting the body's natural detoxification systems. Movement, hydration, and nutrition are foundational, yet often overlooked. Are there areas where support may be lacking? Sometimes what's missing is not a supplement, but a routine that honors the body's need to move, rest, and replenish.

5. Finally, consider how this understanding shapes your approach to health. Knowing that your body is designed to detoxify can shift the way you view daily choices. It's no longer about chasing perfection. It's about creating an environment—both internally and externally—where your body can thrive. When you see detoxification as an act of alignment rather than force, your health journey becomes more intentional and empowering.

Looking Ahead: The Role of Connection

Supporting detoxification lays an essential foundation for health, but healing is never complete without connection. Social isolation is more than an emotional hardship; it is a biological stressor. It has been shown that loneliness increases inflammation, weakens the immune system, and raises the risk of premature death by nearly 30%. That impact is comparable to smoking fifteen cigarettes a day! In contrast, meaningful relationships protect health in profound ways. Strong social bonds are linked to reduced inflammation, better stress resilience, and improved immune response. They also offer the emotional support that makes healthy habits more sustainable.

The mind-body connection moves in both directions. Supporting detoxification improves mental clarity, emotional balance, and vitality, making it easier to show up fully in relationships. In turn, relationships enhance the body's ability to heal.

In the next chapter, we'll explore The Power of Social Connection, which is how authentic relationships, supportive communities, and intentional networks are not only emotionally enriching but physiologically essential. You'll learn why social connection is not just a wellness bonus. It is a requirement for long-term healing at the deepest level.

CHAPTER 11

Strong Social Connections

And let us not neglect our meeting together, as some people do, but encourage one another, especially now that the day of his return is drawing near.

— Hebrews 10:25 (NLT)

The body, mind, and spirit are deeply intertwined, and so are we. Human beings are designed for relationships. From the very beginning of life, we thrive when we are seen, supported, and surrounded by others. Our nervous system, immune health, hormone regulation, and emotional resilience are all shaped by the presence or absence of meaningful relationships. In fact, strong and supportive connections are among the most powerful predictors of long-term health. It has been shown that people with close, healthy relationships live longer, experience fewer chronic illnesses, and report greater life satisfaction. The impact of connection is comparable to some of the most well-known health interventions.[1] When we feel safe and supported in a relationship, our bodies respond with healing. Oxytocin, serotonin, and other calming neurochemicals are released. Inflammation decreases. Immunity improves. Tissue repair accelerates.

But despite all our modern tools for staying "connected," loneliness is more widespread than ever. We've slowly moved away from the communities that once anchored us—faith gatherings, extended family, neighborhood support systems—and replaced them with digital communication, overbooked schedules, and physical distance. The result is a growing sense of disconnection that impacts not just our mood, but our biology. According to the Centers for Disease Control and Prevention (CDC), social isolation and loneliness are linked to a significantly increased risk of several serious health conditions, including:

- Heart disease and stroke
- Type 2 diabetes
- Depression and anxiety
- Suicidality and self-harm
- Dementia
- Premature death[2]

This chapter will guide you through the essential role of connection in healing. We'll explore the science that explains why relationships are as vital to your well-being as nutrition and movement. We'll also look at the emotional and spiritual nourishment that comes from truly belonging. Most importantly, you'll discover practical ways to cultivate meaningful connections, whether it's rebuilding old ties, creating new ones, or simply learning to open yourself to relationships again.

The Impact of Relationships on Mental and Physical Health

We are created for connection. It's part of our biological design, not just a social preference. From the very beginning of life, relational interaction shapes how the brain develops, how the immune system responds, and how the nervous system learns to regulate itself. Social connection is now recognized as a critical pillar in lifestyle psychiatry and lifestyle medicine, with direct influence on mental, emotional, and physical health. Research shows that meaningful relationships enhance neuroplasticity, support emotional regulation, and reduce chronic stress—factors essential for brain health across the lifespan.[3] In fact, strong social bonds have been associated with improved cognitive function, lower inflammation, and a reduced risk of mental health conditions such as depression and anxiety.

Every time we experience meaningful social engagement, the body releases *oxytocin*, a hormone that quiets the stress response and fosters healing. Oxytocin lowers cortisol, reduces inflammation, improves immune function, and supports cardiovascular health.[4] It's no surprise that people with strong social ties tend to live longer and experience fewer chronic illnesses.

But just as connection heals, disconnection harms. Chronic loneliness—whether due to isolation, loss, or lack of community—disrupts the body's natural rhythms. Elevated cortisol levels, suppressed immunity, and even changes in the gut microbiome all reflect the physiological cost of living without meaningful relational support.

The psychological pain caused by social exclusion is strongly correlated with changes in gut microbiota composition.

These microbial shifts are now being linked to increased inflammation and mood disorders such as anxiety and depression. Targeting microbiome imbalances associated with loneliness may even offer a novel approach to supporting mental health and social reintegration.[5]

Isolation has been linked to higher risks of Alzheimer's disease, high blood pressure, and sleep disturbances. It also alters the microbiome, changing the gut-brain relationship in ways that diminish mood, focus, and cognitive clarity. One analysis found that chronic loneliness carries a health risk comparable to smoking fifteen cigarettes a day.[6] For those already walking through chronic illness, lifestyle change, or recovery from trauma, this additional burden can feel like too much. That's why support matters. Healing is not meant to happen alone.

Relational support, whether through family, friends, a faith community, or a healing partnership, creates an internal environment where restoration becomes possible. When patients feel seen and supported, stress hormones decrease, healing hormones increase, and the nervous system shifts into a state where regeneration can occur. This is more than emotional comfort. It is a measurable, biological response that strengthens outcomes across every chronic condition we see, from cardiovascular disease to autoimmune dysfunction.

We were not designed to do life alone. We certainly were not designed to heal in isolation. True, lasting transformation is most often found in the presence of connection.

Combating Loneliness Through Community

Despite living in what many call a hyperconnected digital world, many patients I see report feeling more isolated and disconnected than ever before. The COVID-19 pandemic only intensified this disconnection, disrupting daily life, weakening community bonds, and leaving many people socially adrift long after restrictions lifted.[7]

The statistics paint a troubling picture: in 2022, nearly 60% of American adults reported experiencing significant loneliness, with the highest rates among young adults aged 18 to 22.[8]

This rising tide of loneliness has drawn national attention. In 2023, the U.S. Surgeon General formally identified loneliness and social isolation as a major public health crisis—on par with smoking and obesity—citing links to increased risks of cardiovascular disease, dementia, depression, and premature death.[9] While digital tools offer the illusion of connection, they often fail to deliver the psychological safety and physiological benefits that come from authentic, face-to-face relationships. The result is an epidemic of disconnection in an age more "connected" than ever.

What I've observed in my practice mirrors broader societal trends: the decline of in-person gatherings, faith-based fellowship, and extended family units has created relational voids that profoundly affect both mental and physical health. Traditional contexts where people naturally formed meaningful connections, such as neighborhood gatherings, community events, regular family meals, and religious services, have diminished in many areas. This growing isolation creates physiological strain that I believe contributes significantly to the rising rates of chronic disease we're seeing across all age groups.

Digital connection, while valuable in certain contexts, simply cannot fully replace the biological benefits of face-to-face interaction. Eye contact, physical proximity, synchronized breathing, and subtle nonverbal cues all trigger regulatory nervous system responses that digital communication fails to replicate.

These physiological differences help explain why virtual connection, while certainly better than complete isolation, does not provide the same health protection and healing benefits as regular in-person gatherings and relationships.

Practical Ways to Rebuild Connection

Faith communities offer one of the most powerful antidotes to modern loneliness that I've witnessed in my practice. Churches, small groups, and prayer meetings provide something our isolated culture desperately needs: regular opportunities for shared experiences, mutual encouragement, and purposeful interaction with a foundation of shared values.

What I find particularly healing about these gatherings is their consistency, which helps establish healthy social rhythms that actively counter isolation's negative effects on both body and spirit. Faith communities also naturally incorporate multiple generations, creating opportunities for the exchange of wisdom and support across age groups, which is something that's become increasingly rare in our age-segregated society. I've seen remarkable transformations when patients join health-focused groups that combine physical wellness with social connection. Walking clubs, fitness classes, and support groups bring people together around shared wellness goals, creating natural bonds through common purpose, faith-based practices and mutual encouragement. What consistently amazes me about these connections is how combining physical activity with social interaction creates synergistic benefits that neither provides alone. Regular movement enhances blood flow, reduces inflammation, and improves mood, and these effects become amplified when experienced within a supportive community that celebrates progress and provides accountability.

Volunteering and service activities address loneliness in ways that naturally overcome many barriers to relationship building. These activities place people in collaborative environments where relationships form organically around shared goals and meaningful contributions to something larger than themselves. I often recommend volunteering to patients struggling with social anxiety because the focus on helping others shifts attention from self-consciousness toward purposeful action. This redirection often allows natural connections to develop without the pressure that can make socializing feel forced or uncomfortable.

Sometimes the most powerful step toward rebuilding connection involves reaching out intentionally to people already in our lives. I encourage patients to reconnect with old friends, initiate coffee dates, or simply check in with someone by phone. What surprises many people is how even brief but genuine interactions generate beneficial physiological responses that counteract isolation's negative effects on health. The frequency of connection often matters more than duration, with regular, brief check-ins providing more consistent biological regulation than occasional, lengthy interactions. Additionally, starting small with everyday interactions can build confidence and capacity for deeper connections over time. Brief, positive interactions with neighbors, local shopkeepers, or even friendly exchanges with strangers create what sociologists call "weak ties"—an important social fabric that contributes significantly to overall well-being. For patients who find social interaction challenging due to anxiety, health limitations, or past relational wounds, I often suggest beginning with these smaller interactions as stepping stones toward more meaningful relationships while still providing immediate benefits for mental and physical health.

Here are some more ways to stay connected:

1. Game night

2. Day trips

3. Bowling

4. Movie night

5. Cooking class

6. Dancing

7. Art night

8. Water-based activities

The wisdom found in Hebrews 10 reminds us that gathering together and encouraging one another isn't merely a social preference but reflects God's spiritual design for endurance and hope. This passage reveals that community isn't optional—it represents a healing force that God specifically intended for our well-being. When we understand social connection as part of divine design rather than simply human preference, it transforms how we approach relationships and community involvement.

We begin to see that investing in meaningful connections is actually an act of stewardship. We are caring for the bodies and spirits we've been given by honoring our fundamental need for relationship and mutual support in our journey toward healing and wholeness.

Health Benefits of Meaningful Social Bonds

1 Corinthians 13:13 (NLT) reminds us that *Three things will last forever—faith, hope, and love—and the greatest of these is love.* Through my years in functional medicine, I've witnessed how this

biblical truth manifests in profound physiological ways that directly impact healing and health outcomes.

What continues to amaze me is how genuine love and support literally activate parasympathetic responses in the body—the "rest-and-digest" functions essential for healing. When patients experience authentic connection and feel truly loved, their nervous system shifts from sympathetic dominance (that constant fight-or-flight state) toward parasympathetic regulation. Heart rate stabilizes, blood pressure decreases, digestion improves, and inflammatory markers decline. These changes create an internal environment conducive to healing and regeneration rather than the stress and deterioration that characterize chronic illness.

It has also been shown that people in loving relationships recover more quickly from illness, demonstrate stronger immune responses, and live significantly longer than their isolated counterparts. The biological mechanisms behind these effects include increased oxytocin production, normalized cortisol rhythms, enhanced immune function, and improved heart rate variability. When I explain these concepts to patients, I emphasize that we're talking about concrete, measurable health benefits: faster gut healing, reduced pain perception, decreased infection risk, and improved treatment response across multiple disease categories. Love isn't just a feeling; it's powerful medicine that activates the body's innate healing capacity.

Relational Safety and the Nervous System

Safe relationships help regulate the vagus nerve, which serves as the primary connection between the brain and many major organs. This remarkable cranial nerve transmits signals that either promote restoration through parasympathetic activation or prepare for threat through sympathetic responses. What I find fascinating is how social connection directly influences which of these signals predominates, creating profound implications for health and healing. When relationships feel supportive and safe, vagal tone improves, supporting numerous aspects of physical health, including better cardiovascular function, improved digestion, and lower inflammation throughout the body. The simple experience of being understood and accepted helps lower anxiety and reduce inflammation in ways that often surprise my patients. When people experience genuine understanding and acceptance, stress hormone levels decrease within minutes, which are measurable with many of the functional labs I use at baseline and for follow-up testing. This hormonal shift triggers a cascade of anti-inflammatory responses throughout the body, creating an internal environment where healing accelerates and disease progression slows. For patients managing chronic conditions, this relational regulation can significantly enhance treatment effectiveness and symptom management in ways that complement medical interventions.

Spiritual and Emotional Resilience Through Relationships

A Christ-centered community offers something truly unique—I've consistently seen it improve healing outcomes. This kind of fellowship brings accountability, shared values, and hope during some of the hardest times in a person's health journey. Faith-based support goes beyond just meeting practical needs, like providing meals during recovery or rides to appointments. It also speaks to the deeper, often unspoken, questions that come with illness. Relationships rooted in love create a strong emotional foundation that makes difficult health changes not just possible, but lasting.

When people feel genuinely cared for and supported, they're more able to take on tough lifestyle changes. In my experience, this kind of connection leads to better treatment follow-through, more lasting dietary improvements, and quicker recoveries.

What I've learned through years of practice is that love truly is the greatest therapeutic force available to us. It costs nothing yet provides benefits that rival the most expensive medical interventions. When we understand relationships as medicine and community as healing, we begin to approach social connection not as a luxury but as a necessity for optimal health and vibrant life.

Key Takeaways

When supportive relationships provide consistent nervous system calibration, the body's regulatory systems function at their optimal capacity. This influence extends far beyond emotional comfort to impact hormone production, immune activity, inflammatory processes, and tissue repair mechanisms—all critical factors that directly determine healing capacity and disease risk.

What I've observed repeatedly is how loneliness dramatically increases the risk for chronic disease while impairing mental clarity, sleep quality, and overall resilience. In physiological terms, social isolation creates a persistent stress state that accelerates tissue damage, compromises immune function, and impairs the cellular repair processes essential for health maintenance. These mechanisms help explain why isolated patients in my practice consistently show higher rates of virtually all chronic diseases, including heart disease, diabetes, autoimmune conditions, and neurodegenerative disorders.

Meaningful relationships provide measurable protection by reducing inflammation, regulating stress responses, and improving long-term outcomes in both physical and emotional health. Through multiple biological pathways, including oxytocin release, cortisol regulation, enhanced vagal tone, and improved immune function, positive social connections create health advantages that I can actually measure in follow-up testing. These physiological benefits translate into reduced disease risk, improved treatment response, and enhanced recovery capacity that often exceeds what medications alone can provide.

Building strong community ties, especially through shared faith, service, and intentional presence, enhances healing and sustains the transformation my patients work so hard to achieve. Regular gathering with others provides the consistency, purpose, and sense of belonging that stabilize physiological processes, improve hormonal balance, and enhance immune function. I've learned that even small steps toward greater connection can produce significant health benefits through these biological pathways, often providing the missing piece that allows other treatments to finally become effective.

Questions for Reflection

1. Do I feel deeply connected to others, or am I experiencing isolation? Take an honest inventory of your current relationships, noting both quantity and quality. Consider how often you engage in meaningful conversation, share authentic emotions, and feel truly understood.

2. What steps can I take this week to build or strengthen my relationships? Identify specific actions, whether reaching out to an old friend, joining a community group, or deepening

existing connections through more vulnerable conversations.

3. How do I show up for others in ways that promote encouragement and hope? Reflect on how you listen, respond, and support those around you. Consider how you might become more present and encouraging in your interactions.

4. What type of community do I long for, and how can I begin creating it? Clarify your vision for meaningful connection. Whether faith-based fellowship, shared interests, or mutual support, defining what you seek helps direct your efforts toward fulfilling relationships.

5. How does God's design for connection inform the way I approach my healing and the healing of others? Consider how the biblical emphasis on community might reshape your understanding of health, recovery, and well-being.

Moving Forward — The Next Healthy Habit

Strong relationships are foundational, but healing also requires a structured approach that addresses the underlying causes of health challenges. While social connection powerfully influences physiological function, many people continue to struggle with persistent symptoms despite having supportive relationships in their lives. The missing piece often lies in identifying and addressing the specific imbalances unique to each patient's biochemistry and health history.

Social connection influences gut bacteria composition, immune function, and stress hormone regulation—all factors that significantly impact health outcomes. Yet these beneficial effects may be limited when underlying dysfunctions remain unaddressed.

Gut dysbiosis, hormone imbalances, nutrient deficiencies, or toxin accumulation can persist even in socially connected people, creating ongoing health challenges that connection alone cannot resolve. What's needed is a comprehensive framework that combines the benefits of social support with personalized, targeted interventions. This approach must recognize both the universal human need for connection and the unique physiological factors that influence each person's health journey. By addressing both relational and biological aspects of health, genuine transformation becomes possible where either approach alone might fall short.

In the next chapter, we will explore the HOPE Method—a structured framework that guides healing through empowerment, testing, and optimization. You will discover how this method identifies the specific factors contributing to your health challenges and creates personalized pathways toward restoration. By combining the healing power of social connection with the precision of functional medicine, this approach offers genuine hope to those who have struggled with chronic health issues despite their best efforts at implementing healthy lifestyle practices.

PART 3

True Transformation
And Your Solution

CHAPTER 12

The HOPE Method

You will be rewarded for this; your hope will not be disappointed.

— Proverbs 23:18 (NLT)

After addressing the six healthy lifestyle habits—nutrition, movement, sleep, stress reduction, toxin elimination, and meaningful connection—the next step in the healing journey is building a personalized path forward. This is where true transformation begins. Not just through generalized wellness advice, but through a tailored approach that honors your body's unique needs and story. That's where HOPE comes in. Not just hope as a feeling, but HOPE as a framework: *H*olistic *O*ptions and *P*ersonal *E*mpowerment. This is the method I created after years of clinical experience, functional medicine training, and personal healing. It is the approach that helped me recover my health when conventional medicine had no more answers. It is the same approach I now offer to others who feel stuck—who've tried to do "everything right," yet still feel unwell.

You've likely made meaningful changes. You've improved your diet, added movement, reduced toxic exposures, worked on sleep, and even begun to foster deeper connections. These are powerful steps, and yet, if symptoms remain, it's not because you've failed. It may simply be because you haven't yet addressed the deeper imbalances unique to your body.

No two bodies are the same. Your biochemistry, genetics, environment, trauma history, and lifestyle patterns all interact in ways that influence how symptoms show up and how healing unfolds. This is why some individuals thrive on a certain eating plan while others feel worse. It explains why a supplement that brings relief to one person may trigger fatigue or inflammation in someone else. Without precision, well-intended efforts can only go so far.

The missing piece is often *personalization.* And the HOPE Method was created to fill that gap. Grounded in functional medicine, HOPE is built on three interconnected pillars: Empower, Test, and Optimize. This is not a quick fix or a temporary protocol. It is a roadmap designed to uncover root causes, apply targeted strategies, and guide you toward sustainable wellness that's aligned with your body's specific needs. This chapter introduces how the HOPE Method works and why it is different from the conventional model of care. If you've ever been told your labs are "normal" but you still feel anything but, or if you've cycled through providers without real answers, this is for you. There *is* a way forward. It begins with the belief that your body is capable of healing when given the right support and the right information. This is the promise of HOPE: not just the return of energy or the relief of symptoms, but the empowerment to understand what's happening in your body and the tools to reclaim your health with clarity, purpose, and confidence.

The HOPE Pillars: Empower, Test, Optimize

While conventional medicine often focuses on diagnosing disease and prescribing medication, lasting transformation requires something more—something deeper. It requires a personalized, comprehensive strategy that moves beyond symptom suppression and engages the whole person in the healing process. That's the foundation of the HOPE Method.

HOPE—Holistic Options and Personal Empowerment—is built on three core pillars: Empower, Test, and Optimize. Each pillar addresses a different aspect of healing. Together, they form a roadmap to restore health by uncovering root causes, applying targeted strategies, and aligning treatment with the body's unique needs.

Empower

True healing begins when you shift from being a passive recipient of care to an active participant in your health journey. The *Empower* pillar equips you with the tools, education, and clarity you need to make informed decisions every day. Rather than simply offering prescriptions, this approach focuses on lifestyle coaching, mindset shifts, and helping you understand how your daily choices shape your health outcomes. When you learn how your digestive system impacts brain health, how hormones affect energy, or how toxins fuel inflammation, you begin to see symptoms not as random events but as signals pointing to deeper imbalances.

Patients who grasp the "why" behind their symptoms and the "how" of healing are more likely to follow through on treatment plans. This isn't about compliance. It's about confidence. When you know what's happening in your body and what to do about it, hope replaces helplessness, and clarity fuels action.

Test

You cannot heal what you cannot see. The *Test* pillar recognizes that precision is essential. Without accurate data, healthcare becomes guesswork. Functional lab testing provides insight into what's actually happening inside your body, often identifying dysfunction long before it becomes diagnosable disease. Testing helps validate symptoms that may have been previously dismissed. It uncovers patterns that explain lingering fatigue, inflammation, or hormone imbalance. It also eliminates the trial-and-error approach that often leaves people discouraged. Areas commonly tested include oxidative stress and inflammatory markers, hormone levels, nutrient deficiencies, gut microbiome composition, food sensitivities, toxic burden, and metabolic function. These data points create a detailed map of your internal environment, guiding the next steps with accuracy and intention. When testing replaces guessing, you stop chasing symptoms and start addressing causes.

Optimize

Once the root causes are uncovered, the focus shifts to *Optimize*—creating a personalized healing plan that restores balance in a way that's sustainable and effective. This is where knowledge becomes action. Optimization may involve nutritional therapy, targeted supplements, detoxification strategies, stress regulation tools, sleep support, and spiritual renewal. These aren't generic recommendations. They're tailored interventions selected based on real-time data from your body. For example, someone with elevated inflammation and microbiome imbalance may benefit from a precision anti-inflammatory protocol rich in fiber and polyphenols known to nourish beneficial gut bacteria.

As healing unfolds in one area, others begin to shift. That's why reassessment and adjustment are essential. This adaptive approach prevents the plateaus common in conventional treatment plans and ensures that your progress continues as your body regains strength and balance. Together, these three pillars—Empower, Test, and Optimize—form the backbone of the HOPE Method. This approach doesn't stop at symptom relief. It guides you into a deeper, more sustainable transformation that honors the complexity of your health, the individuality of your story, and the wisdom of your body. By combining education with advanced testing and targeted interventions, the HOPE Method supports healing at both the physical and emotional levels. It's for anyone who has felt stuck in cycles of frustration, discouraged by "normal" labs, or exhausted by one-size-fits-all answers. This is where things begin to change—not just because you're doing more, but because you're finally doing what's *right* for your body.

Functional vs. Conventional Medicine

Conventional medicine has its strengths. In moments of crisis, when you're facing a heart attack, a broken bone, or a severe infection, it delivers life-saving care that is nothing short of miraculous. The technological advancements, surgical precision, and acute interventions available today have extended and saved countless lives.

But this model often falls short when it comes to chronic conditions that develop slowly over time. These are the fatigue, inflammation, mood changes, gut issues, and hormonal imbalances that don't resolve with a short course of medication or a standard lab panel. Instead of asking *why* these symptoms are occurring, conventional care tends to focus on managing them, usually by assigning a diagnosis and prescribing medication. If you have low energy, joint pain, and digestive discomfort, you might see three different specialists and leave with three different prescriptions. No one is asking what connects these symptoms or what's driving them in the first place.

Far too often, patients are told, "Everything looks normal," even when they know something isn't right. Standard lab ranges are based on population averages, not optimal function. A vitamin D level may fall within the reference range, but that doesn't mean it's ideal for your body. A study has shown how symptoms can arise long before disease is detectable by conventional measures, specifically for cardiometabolic-based chronic diseases like coronary heart disease, heart failure, and atrial fibrillation.[1] That space between "not yet diagnosable" and "definitely not well" is where so many patients are left without answers as symptoms persist and disease develops.

Functional medicine takes a different approach. It begins with the belief that your body is not a collection of individual parts, but an integrated system where everything is connected, such as your gut, hormones, immune function, detox pathways, brain, and energy production. When something is off in one area, it ripples into others. Symptoms like brain fog, joint stiffness, skin rashes, or sleep disturbances are signals that something is not operating normally. Functional medicine evaluates those signals and asks what they're trying to say.

This model also recognizes that healing doesn't begin on a prescription pad. It begins with understanding. You start to see how food, toxins, sleep, stress, and relationships all interact with your biology. You become equipped, not overwhelmed, with knowledge that allows you to take ownership of your healing. Functional care doesn't dismiss your lived experience in favor of numbers on a chart. It honors your symptoms as real, your instincts as valid, and your body as capable of healing when given the right support.

Testing as the Key to Root Cause Discovery

When it comes to chronic symptoms and unresolved health concerns, guessing just isn't enough. You deserve clarity, not assumptions. That's why in the HOPE Method, testing is a foundational pillar. It provides more than just data; it offers direction.

While symptoms are important and often tell us something is off, they rarely tell the whole story. You can have fatigue, headaches, skin issues, or mood swings—but without looking deeper, it's nearly impossible to know what's actually causing them. Functional testing allows us to see beneath the surface. It gives us a window into how your body is functioning at the root level, long before conventional labs would ever detect a problem.

Why Testing Is Foundational

Functional testing shifts us out of the trial-and-error model. It replaces assumptions with answers and turns confusion into clarity. Instead of using general guidelines or hoping that a protocol "might help," we gain real insight into what your body is trying to communicate. I often describe it this way: symptoms are like a compass—they tell us we're heading in the wrong direction. But functional testing gives us a map. It helps us navigate with precision, so we can stop circling the same terrain and finally move forward with purpose.

Common Functional Tests We Use

Every patient is different, and so are the tests we choose. Each one is selected based on your unique symptoms, history, and goals. But there are several foundational tools we often use to get a complete picture of what's going on beneath the surface:

- **Comprehensive Stool Analysis**: This advanced test looks at the gut microbiome, detecting dysbiosis (imbalanced bacteria), pathogens, parasites, and signs of leaky gut. It also evaluates digestion, inflammation, and immune markers—key areas if you're dealing with bloating, brain fog, or immune dysfunction.

- **Hormone Panels**: These tests assess patterns in cortisol (your stress hormone), as well as estrogen, progesterone, DHEA, and testosterone. They help us identify imbalances like estrogen dominance or adrenal fatigue that may be contributing to fatigue, insomnia, anxiety, or weight gain.

- **Minerals and Nutrient Testing**: When you're running low on key nutrients like magnesium, B vitamins, zinc, or vitamin D, your body cannot function optimally. These deficiencies often drive fatigue, mood changes, poor immunity, and even hormone imbalance.

- **Oxidative Stress and Inflammatory Markers**: 8-hydroxy-2' -deoxyguanosine (8-OHdG), a critical biomarker of oxidative stress and carcinogenesis[2] and Quinolinic Acid (QA), a neurotoxic metabolite that contributes to neuronal damage, oxidative stress, and neuroinflammation, playing a key role in Alzheimer's Disease (AD) pathogenesis.[3]

- **Toxin Screens**: Exposure to heavy metals, mold, pesticides, or industrial chemicals can burden your liver, activate immune response, damage mitochondria, and impair brain function. Toxins can cause symptoms that are associated with organ dysfunction, memory impairment, chronic fatigue, and autoimmune diseases. These tests can reveal hidden obstacles to healing.

- **Food Sensitivity Panels:** These are not the same as food allergies. Instead, they identify delayed immune responses (antibodies IgG, IgG4, complement-C3d) to foods that may be silently triggering inflammation, gut disruption, and autoimmune flares.

Too many people spend years trying to figure out what's wrong, cycling through diets, supplements, and protocols with no or partial relief. Functional testing changes that. It brings objectivity into the healing process and helps prevent wasted time, money, and energy on things that aren't actually helping. It also deepens the relationship between patient and provider. When you see the data for yourself, when we sit down together and go over what your body is telling us, you become a true partner in your care. We're no longer guessing. We're working from a place of certainty, and that changes everything.

Testing also allows us to track progress over time. Healing isn't just about feeling better—it's about *knowing* that systems are moving back into balance. That kind of feedback is powerful. It keeps momentum going and reinforces that what you're doing is working. Most importantly, functional testing often reveals hidden dysfunctions, which are those subtle imbalances that don't yet qualify as disease but are already affecting how you feel. This is where functional medicine shines: in the space between "you're fine" and "you're finally thriving."

Key Takeaways

The HOPE Method offers a structured and personalized approach to healing—one that moves beyond symptom management and into true restoration. By focusing on root causes, this method brings clarity, direction, and support to people who've spent too long feeling unheard or stuck. It's built on three pillars: Empower, Test, and Optimize. Together, these pillars guide you through a process that is both data-driven and deeply personal. We begin by equipping you with the knowledge to understand what's happening in your body. We use targeted functional lab testing to uncover what's beneath your symptoms. And we apply interventions that are tailored to your unique needs, not a one-size-fits-all protocol.

Functional medicine stands apart from conventional care in a few key ways. Where traditional models often isolate symptoms and treat each one individually, functional care looks at how everything connects. We recognize that your gut influences your brain and that your hormones shape your immune response. Toxic exposures, even low-grade ones, over time, can reduce your energy and increase your inflammation. These systems don't operate in silos, and neither should your care. Testing is a foundational part of this approach. It gives us insight into how your body is functioning. We look at digestive health, nutrient levels, inflammation, hormone patterns, and toxin load. This allows us to move beyond guesswork. Instead of trying something and hoping it works, we can make informed decisions that are specific to what your body needs right now.

Testing also gives us a way to measure progress. When you can see changes on paper and in how you feel, it builds trust in the process and motivation to keep going. But this is not just about labs and protocols. One of the most important parts of the HOPE Method is the relationship we build together. Healing is more likely to happen when you feel heard, supported, and involved in your own care. When you understand *why* we're doing what we're doing, you're more likely to stay committed. When you see that you're not just reacting to symptoms but actively restoring function, the process becomes much more hopeful and sustainable.

Proverbs 13:12 tells us that *Hope deferred makes the heart sick, but a dream fulfilled is a tree of life (NLT)*. That's what we aim to offer through this work; not false promises or quick fixes, but real, steady progress toward healing. The HOPE Method gives you a framework, a partnership, and a path forward that is grounded in science, built around your body, and rooted in the belief that healing is possible.

Questions for Reflection

1. Have you felt dismissed or discouraged by a conventional care experience? Consider moments when your symptoms were minimized, when you were told "everything looks normal" despite feeling unwell, or when treatments addressed only your symptoms without investigating their causes. How did these experiences affect your health journey and your trust in healthcare?

2. What would it mean for you to participate more actively in your healing process? Reflect on the difference between following instructions passively and engaging as a true partner in your healthcare. How might understanding the "why" behind your symptoms and the "how" of addressing them change your approach to healing?

3. What do you wish you understood more clearly about your symptoms or diagnosis? Identify the gaps in your current understanding—questions about why certain symptoms persist, how different aspects of your health might be connected, or what might be driving your ongoing health challenges.

4. How does "testing, not guessing" offer hope and direction for your next step? Consider how objective data about your specific imbalances could guide more effective interventions and prevent wasted resources on approaches that don't address your unique needs.

5. Which of the HOPE pillars (Empower, Test, Optimize) are you most drawn to right now? Reflect on which aspect of this approach resonates most strongly with your current situation and needs. This attraction often indicates a valuable starting point for your healing journey.

Moving Forward

Once a strong foundation is in place, we can begin to explore the role of supplements. While lifestyle and food remain the cornerstones of healing, supplements can offer focused support when used intentionally and appropriately. Supplementation isn't a shortcut or a replacement for healthy eating. As I often share with my patients, supplements are most effective when they *complement* a nutrient-dense diet, not when they try to substitute for it. Their purpose is to help restore balance, correct deficiencies, support detox pathways, and enhance the body's ability to heal.

In today's world, the need for targeted supplementation has grown. Our soils are more depleted than they were 50 years ago, and with that, the nutrient content of even whole foods has declined. At the same time, we face an unprecedented level of toxic exposure from environmental chemicals to chronic stress, all of which place additional demands on the body's nutrient stores. Stress alone can significantly deplete B vitamins, magnesium, and vitamin C, which are nutrients essential for energy, mood regulation, and immune function. Digestive issues, which are increasingly common, further impair nutrient absorption, meaning that even a healthy diet may not meet all your needs if your gut is compromised.

Having explored the HOPE Method and its three pillars—Empower, Test, and Optimize—we now turn to the cornerstone of lasting health: the gut. Optimizing gut function is not simply one step in the process; it is the foundation upon which overall wellness is built. In the next chapter, we will dive into practical solutions to strengthen and heal the gut: identifying food triggers and reducing inflammation, nourishing with fiber, omega-3s, and polyphenols, managing stress to repair leaky gut, and using targeted probiotics and supplements to restore balance and resilience.

We will also explore what I call Supplementation with Purpose—a strategic, thoughtful approach to choosing foods that heal and selecting supplements that support, rather than overwhelm, the body's healing process. This chapter is designed to take the guesswork out of diet and supplementation. Instead of trial-and-error that leads to frustration, you'll gain the tools to make clear, informed decisions. Building on the insights gathered from testing, symptom tracking, and your unique health history, we will create a plan that truly supports your goals while honoring your body's design. With the HOPE Method as our guide, we are ready to begin where true healing starts—with the GUT!

CHAPTER 13

Solutions for Optimizing Gut Health

He heals the brokenhearted and binds up their wounds.

— Psalm 147:3 (ESV)

Healing the gut isn't just about understanding what's wrong, it's about knowing exactly what to do about it. Basically, gut problems can be remedied with the right treatment. This realization stems from many years of experience treating gut-related illnesses. However, it is important to note that healing is not always linear, and individual timelines can vary. During my health crisis, my gut was a mess, and the conventional approach mainly offered the regular roster of acid blockers and vague advice to "manage stress," but none of that addressed the real dysfunction in my digestive system.

Thankfully, the gut is receptive to proper treatment. This is primarily related to the fact that the cells that line the small intestine replace themselves every three to five days. This reconstructive ability provides part of the framework around which healing can occur. Consequently, targeted gut healing has the potential to produce dramatic improvements when done correctly, especially if proper nutrition is observed.

Understanding Gut-Healing Diet Fundamentals

Gut healing begins with how we eat, beyond just "eating healthy." It means using food as medicine: selecting foods that repair the intestinal lining, removing those that fuel inflammation, and prioritizing eating hygiene habits to ensure the body is in the rest and digest or parasympathetic state. Eating under stress blocks the production of stomach acid, digestive enzymes, and bile flow, leading to undigested food, reduced nutrient absorption, and digestive symptoms such as gas, bloating, and heartburn.

Understanding what foods trigger inflammation or increased permeability ("leaky gut") is also important.[1] Gluten elimination is often the first recommendation. Even without celiac disease, gluten can increase intestinal permeability, allowing harmful substances to pass through the gut lining. During healing, complete gluten removal for three to six months is suggested to allow time for healing while preventing ongoing irritation.

Dairy proteins like casein and whey are also common triggers. While some people tolerate dairy after healing, these proteins may increase gut dysfunction and provoke inflammation, slowing the recovery during the repair phase. Many patients spend months trying to heal their gut while still eating yogurt daily, believing it helps digestion. But true healing requires removing key irritants such as gluten and casein. [2] [3]

Consuming a high-fat diet with processed seed oils like soybean, corn, canola, and safflower doesn't just add excess calories; it interferes with the body's repair process. When heated, these oils oxidize and form compounds that inflame the gut lining. In essence, the oil reacts with oxygen when heated, breaking down and forming harmful, gut-irritating compounds.[4] They're also high in omega-6 fats, which fuel chronic inflammation and endotoxemia (toxins in the bloodstream); a progressive and continuous low-level immune response that, over time, damages tissues and disrupts healing, especially in the gut. A high-fat, high-calorie diet compromises the gut microbiota and the integrity of the intestinal wall, leading to increased permeability.[5] Research also shows a high-fat diet could lead to metabolic endotoxemia resulting from increased lipopolysaccharide (LPS) levels, subsequently triggering low-grade inflammation and metabolic diseases (obesity, diabetes, cardiovascular disease).[6]

However, taking out harmful oils from our diets is only part of the solution. Healing also requires foods that actively repair. For example, bone broth is a key healing food; its collagen, glycine, and glutamine supply the nutrients needed to rebuild the gut lining. Drinking it warm between meals helps these amino acids reach the gut, where they can support repair.

Finally, *when, where,* and *how* we eat also affect gut healing. For example, eating late at night, "on the go" or under stress, can alter the digestive process, impair nutrient absorption, and promote leaky gut, making it difficult for the body to heal. Instead, prioritize mealtimes with mindful eating habits to improve digestion and support healing.

Strategic Probiotic Implementation for Gut Repair

People commonly misunderstand probiotics in two ways: they think all strains are equivalent, and they believe higher doses are always better. When healing serious gut damage, general probiotics from health food stores are often too weak.

Effective gut restoration requires specific strategies for promoting beneficial microbes, increasing helpful metabolites, clearing toxic ones, and reducing inflammatory bacteria. This targeted approach can reduce leaky gut and inflammation while improving metabolic health.[7] Specific bacterial strains have been clinically shown to repair the intestinal barrier, but they need to be the right strains at therapeutic doses.

When choosing a probiotic supplement, it is important to look for the bacterial species contained in the supplement as well as the dose or number of units. Supplements containing probiotics list the number of colony-forming units (CFUs) in a serving. Examples of CFUs that you might see on a label are 1 x 10^9 (1 billion) CFUs and 1 x 10^{10} (10 billion) CFUs. However, higher CFU counts do not necessarily mean that the product has greater health benefits. A product's health benefits, if any, depend more on the specific microorganisms it contains than it does on the number of microorganisms it contains.[8]

Lactobacillus rhamnosus GG (LGG) is one of the most effective strains for gut repair. It produces compounds that strengthen the connections between intestinal cells. LGG-derived products may provide novel approaches for health and disease prevention and treatment, especially for gastrointestinal and respiratory conditions.[9][10][11]

Specific strains like *Bifidobacterium longum* have shown particular promise, as research demonstrates it modulates metabolism, stabilizes gut microbiota, and drives fine-tuned homeostatic balance within the host-microbiome interaction.[12] Additionally, *Saccharomyces boulardii* is a beneficial yeast that supports gut healing. Unlike bacteria, it isn't killed by antibiotics, making it effective for those recovering from antimicrobial treatments. It also produces compounds that strengthen the gut barrier and reduce inflammation.

Dietary sources of prebiotics and probiotics are another option. Fermented foods like sauerkraut, kombucha, yogurt, and kefir help to recolonize the gut with beneficial bacteria, reducing inflammation, supporting the immune system, reducing harmful bacteria, healing the gut lining, as well as providing many other systemic health benefits.[13][14][15][16]

Timing matters with probiotics. Splitting the dose between morning and evening often works better than if taken all at once, especially if taking multiple microbial species. To optimize the benefits of individual microbes, I recommend separating the dosing time of probiotics, as studies on the safety and efficacy of combined administration are lacking. Some probiotics are better absorbed on an empty stomach; others are recommended with food. Generally, it is a good idea to cycle probiotics, taken consistently for four to six weeks, followed by a one- to two-week break. This helps prevent overgrowth of any one strain and allows time to assess how the body is responding. Overall, it's essential to monitor individual responses to probiotics. Increased bloating, digestive upset, or worsening symptoms may signal the wrong strain, too high a dose, or an underlying bacterial overgrowth that needs to be addressed first.

Prebiotic Foods and Fiber for Microbiome Restoration

Prebiotics are a type of non-digestible dietary fiber that selectively stimulates the growth and/or activity of beneficial bacteria in the intestines. They play an important role in maintaining a healthy gut microbiome.

Prebiotics have the potential to:

• Improve digestive function and bowel regularity

• Support the body's immune system

• Improve mineral absorption

• Help regulate your desire to eat, energy balance, and glucose metabolism

Some common prebiotic ingredients include: Galactooligosaccharides (GOS), Fructooligosaccharides (FOS), Oligofructose (OF), Chicory fiber, Inulin, Lactulose, Resistant starch, and Human milk oligosaccharides (HMO).

Most prebiotics for the gut require an oral dose of at least 3 grams per day or more to confer a benefit. Typically, around 5 grams is the target for FOS and GOS in the daily diet—and this includes dietary sources of prebiotics. The recommended daily amount of fiber is 28 g/day, based on a 2000 kcal/day diet.[17]

Introducing specific prebiotic foods strategically is important. Inulin and fructooligosaccharides are types of fiber found in foods like Jerusalem artichokes, chicory root, and garlic. These fibers resist digestion in the small intestine and reach the colon, where they nourish bacteria such as Bifidobacterium and Lactobacillus. For instance, if a patient has severe gut dysbiosis or small intestinal bacterial overgrowth (SIBO), jumping straight into high-prebiotic foods can make them feel worse before they feel better. Harmful bacteria can also feed on these fibers, which may lead to increased bloating and digestive upset.

Resistant starch is a type of fiber that feeds bacteria that produce short-chain fatty acid (SCFA) butyrate, a substance that fuels colon cells and reduces inflammation. Green bananas, cooked and cooled potatoes, and plantains are great sources of resistant starch. The polyphenols in colorful plant foods work as selective prebiotics too. Polyphenols are plant compounds that often survive digestion and make it to the colon, where they help beneficial bacteria thrive while making life difficult for harmful ones. Pomegranate, berries, green tea, and dark leafy greens are packed with these beneficial compounds.

During gut healing, it's often best to begin with gentler fibers. Mucilaginous fibers from plants like slippery elm and marshmallow root coat and soothe inflamed intestinal tissue while also feeding beneficial bacteria. These fibers support healing and provide nutrients needed for repair. Gradually introducing prebiotic foods and monitoring the body's response leads to better outcomes. Starting with small amounts of cooked vegetables and slowly increasing fiber intake as tolerance improves is key.

Essential Nutrients for Gut Lining Regeneration

The intestinal lining is constantly rebuilding itself, but it needs specific nutrients to do this job properly. When these nutrients are missing, healing slows or stops altogether, no matter what else is being done correctly. L-glutamine supports gut healing in two key ways: it nourishes the cells that form the gut lining and strengthens the barrier that prevents harmful substances from entering the bloodstream. This makes it especially useful when the gut barrier is damaged and needs repair.

Zinc is also important for gut healing. However, the form of zinc used during treatment significantly affects results. Some types remain in contact with damaged gut tissue longer, helping repair the connections between cells and rebuild the protective lining more effectively than others. Studies show zinc carnosine promotes gastrointestinal healing and intestinal lining support. [18]

Another important nutrient is Vitamin A. In its active retinol form, vitamin A supports healthy epithelial tissues, including the gut lining. A deficiency increases susceptibility to infections and slows tissue repair.

A study showed that populations at risk for deficiency, especially young children (<5 years old), vitamin A supplementation significantly reduced mortality associated with diarrhea.[19] During gut healing, supplementing vitamin A can be beneficial, but monitoring is essential, as very high doses can be toxic.

The human gut microbiota has the capacity to synthesize vitamins, especially B vitamins[20] and vitamin K.[21] In the presence of dysbiosis or impaired digestive function, these vitamins may be deficient. B vitamins, particularly folate (B9), cobalamin (B12), and pyridoxine (B6), play a crucial role in various bodily functions, primarily acting as coenzymes in many metabolic processes. They are essential for energy production, cell growth and development, nerve function, and the formation of red blood cells. They also support the immune system and may have a role in preventing certain diseases.

Sometimes, sublingual or injectable forms are needed when the digestive system is unable to absorb nutrients (celiac disease) or beneficial microbes are missing (dysbiosis). Vitamin D plays critical roles in gut barrier function and immune regulation throughout the digestive tract. Deficiency has been linked to increased intestinal permeability and inflammatory bowel conditions.[22] Most people need 2,000 to 5,000 IU daily, but the only way to know for sure is to test blood levels. The general finding is that optimal 25(OH)D concentrations to support health and wellbeing are above 30 ng/mL (75 nmol/L).[23]

Collagen peptides provide the specific amino acids, glycine, proline, and hydroxyproline, that are the building blocks of connective tissue in the intestinal wall. Taking 10 to 20 grams of hydrolyzed collagen daily can significantly speed up tissue repair.[24][25]

Polyphenols as Gut Microbiome Medicine

Polyphenols are plant compounds that work like selective antibiotics in the gut; they help beneficial bacteria thrive while making life difficult for harmful ones. These compounds are incredibly powerful for reshaping the microbiome during healing. Quercetin, a flavonoid found in various plants, is being explored for its potential role in supporting gut health, particularly in the context of leaky gut syndrome. It has been shown to influence the gut microbiome, reduce inflammation, provide antioxidant effects and support gut barrier function.[26]

Reducing excessive inflammation creates a more favorable environment for healing. This is why many people see improvements in food sensitivities when they regularly eat quercetin-rich foods like citrus fruits, apples, onions, and berries.

Curcumin from turmeric is a potent anti-inflammatory compound that can significantly reduce intestinal inflammation and improve beneficial gut microbes.[27]

It works by blocking key pathways that trigger inflammation, helping to calm the body's overall inflammatory response. The challenge with curcumin is absorption, most of it gets broken down before it reaches tissues. However, taking it with black pepper or using enhanced formulations helps improve absorption.

Green tea contains compounds called catechins, especially one called EGCG (epigallocatechin-3-gallate) has shown promise in supporting gut health by influencing the gut microbiota and potentially reducing inflammation. EGCG has anti-inflammatory and antioxidant properties that may help alleviate conditions like inflammatory bowel disease (IBD).[28]

Regular green tea drinking has been associated with increased populations of beneficial bacteria. Two to three cups of high-quality green tea daily can provide healing levels of these beneficial compounds. Conversely, Pomegranate polyphenols are transformed by gut bacteria into compounds called urolithins, which are substances that reduce inflammation and protect the gut barrier. Not everyone can produce these beneficial compounds efficiently, which is why direct pomegranate consumption or supplementation can be so helpful.

A striking attribute about polyphenols is that they work better together, combinations of different polyphenols often work better than any single compound alone. This is why eating a variety of colorful plant foods provides benefits that can't be obtained from isolated supplements.

Omega-3 Fatty Acids for Intestinal Inflammation Control

Omega-3 polyunsaturated fatty acids (PUFAs), specifically EPA and DHA, help reduce intestinal inflammation and support the healing process. These fatty acids exert a positive action by improving beneficial microbes that increase the production of anti-inflammatory compounds, like short-chain fatty acids (SCFAs) such a butyrate. Omega-3s have also been shown to help maintain the intestinal wall integrity and host immune response.[29]

EPA, also known as eicosapentaenoic acid and DHA, docosahexaenoic acid, is crucial for maintaining healthy cell membranes and supporting the enteric nervous system (ENS), the network of neurons throughout the gastrointestinal tract. The ENS is often referred to as the "second brain" and can operate independently to control digestion, motility (movement of food), secretion of digestive enzymes, and blood flow to the gut. Studies show that diets rich in polyphenols, omega-3 fatty acids, and probiotics support healthy enteric nervous system (ENS) function, which can help slow or prevent the development of colorectal cancer (CRC). In contrast, diets high in saturated fats and refined sugars promote oxidative stress and inflammation, which can accelerate disease progression.[30]

Adequate EPA and DHA help keep digestion moving properly and support digestive juices while supporting the gut-brain communication that affects mood and cognitive function. The ratio of omega-3 to omega-6 fatty acids in the body significantly affects how much inflammation exists both systemically and within the intestinal tissues. Most people are getting way too many omega-6s from processed foods and vegetable oils, creating a pro-inflammatory environment that fights against gut healing.

While plant sources like flaxseeds and walnuts provide omega-3s, they contain alpha-linolenic acid (ALA), which has to be converted to EPA and DHA, and this conversion is relatively inefficient in most people. For therapeutic gut healing, fish oil or algae-derived omega-3s typically provide more reliable results. For gut healing, 2 to 4 grams of combined EPA and DHA daily is typically recommended, with emphasis on EPA for its anti-inflammatory effects. This is usually more than can be reasonably obtained from food alone, so supplementation becomes necessary. Quality matters enormously with omega-3 supplements! Oxidized fish oils, for instance, promote inflammation rather than reduce it, so look for third-party tested products that guarantee freshness and purity, and keep them refrigerated once opened.

Another promising area of research is pentadecanoic acid (C15:0, PA), an essential odd-chain saturated fatty acid that originates primarily from microbial fermentation, while dietary sources include seafood and dairy products. It has excellent potential for promoting human health.[31]

A study on C:15 supplementation showed an anti-inflammatory effect in mice with chronic ileitis and dextran sodium sulfate (DSS)-induced colitis. The results of this study offer hope for new therapeutic strategies to improve the treatment and management of inflammatory bowel disease (IBD) in humans.[32]

Anti-Inflammatory Foods and Therapeutic Compounds

Creating an anti-inflammatory eating pattern isn't just about avoiding inflammatory foods; it's about actively including foods that reduce inflammation in the gut. For example, ginger is one of the most effective anti-inflammatory foods due to its inhibitory and stimulatory effects on the gut. The gingerols and shogaols in fresh ginger inhibit inflammatory enzymes while stimulating digestive secretions and gut movement. Fresh ginger tea between meals has therapeutic anti-inflammatory effects with additional benefits for overall digestion. Tart cherries also have anti-inflammatory properties. They are packed with anthocyanins, the compounds that give them their deep red color. These compounds significantly reduce inflammatory markers and also support melatonin production, which has beneficial effects on sleep, which in turn is important for tissue repair.

Leafy green vegetables are not just abundant; they also contain multiple anti-inflammatory compounds. Chlorophyll is one such compound. It has direct anti-inflammatory effects on the gut lining and supports the body's detoxification processes. Additionally, leafy greens, beets, and celery are great sources of nitrates that can be converted to nitric oxide by oral microbes. Nitric oxide supports vascular health and provides antimicrobial benefits. Getting two to three servings of varied leafy greens daily helps supply the body with these protective compounds. Cold-water fatty fish like wild salmon, sardines, and anchovies provide omega-3s along with other anti-inflammatory compounds like astaxanthin and selenium. These fish offer the best ratios of beneficial compounds with minimal contamination. Two to three servings weekly provide substantial anti-inflammatory support.

Fermented foods, rich in beneficial bacteria, can positively impact gut health by promoting a diverse and balanced gut microbiome. These foods, like yogurt, kefir, sauerkraut, and kimchi, introduce probiotics that aid digestion, boost immunity, and potentially reduce inflammation.[33][34]

Bone broth, as mentioned earlier, provides collagen peptides, glycine, and proline, amino acids that directly support intestinal barrier repair and offer anti-inflammatory benefits. Its slow cooking process also extracts minerals and compounds not found in regular muscle meats.

Stress Management as Essential Gut Medicine

Even the best gut-healing diet and supplements may fall short if chronic stress isn't addressed. The link between stress and gut function is so strong that managing stress is essential, not optional, for healing. Chronic stress activates the hypothalamic-pituitary-adrenal (HPA) axis, raising cortisol levels that damage the intestinal barrier. Cortisol lowers secretory immunoglobulin A (sIgA), the gut's main immune defense, and disrupts gut movement and digestive enzyme production.

The vagus nerve, which connects the brain to the digestive system, also becomes dysregulated under chronic stress. This affects gut motility, digestive secretions, and inflammation in intestinal tissues. Meditation and mindfulness practices support gut function and reduce inflammation. Regular meditation lowers cortisol and improves heart rate variability, a sign of better nervous system balance. Just ten to twenty minutes a day can have therapeutic effects when done consistently.

Diaphragmatic breathing is an easy, accessible way to manage stress. Deep, slow breaths stimulate the vagus nerve and activate the parasympathetic nervous system, the body's "rest and digest" mode. Making exhales longer than inhales enhances the relaxation response. Additionally, Sleep quality directly impacts gut healing by influencing immune function, hormone levels, and tissue repair. Poor sleep disrupts the body's natural digestive rhythms and raises inflammation, which slows down healing. Finally, social connection and emotional support are also key. Isolation and relationship stress contribute to chronic low-grade inflammation that interferes with repair. In some cases, healing emotional wounds or strengthening relationships can be just as important as dietary changes.

Advanced Gut Healing Protocols and Supplements

Sometimes basic gut healing approaches just aren't enough, especially when dealing with specific conditions like small intestinal bacterial overgrowth (SIBO), candida overgrowth, or severe intestinal permeability. These situations require more targeted interventions. SIBO develops when bacteria that should be in the colon migrate up into the small intestine, where they don't belong. This is often treated with antibiotic medications.

However, newer approaches with high-dose probiotics (fermented yogurt) are showing promise in treating SIBO. Herbal antimicrobials like oregano oil, berberine, and allicin can be effective alternatives to antibiotic therapy. They are comparatively gentler on beneficial bacteria. These natural antimicrobial treatments typically come before probiotic restoration in the protocol sequence.

Candida overgrowth often goes hand-in-hand with bacterial imbalances and requires targeted antifungal interventions. Compounds like caprylic acid, undecylenic acid, and herbs like pau d'arco can help restore balance. But antifungal protocols must be combined with dietary changes that eliminate the sugars and refined carbohydrates that feed fungal overgrowth. For severe intestinal permeability, specific nutrients that support tight junction repair may be necessary. Zinc carnosine, phosphatidylcholine, immunoglobulins and amino acids like glutamine provide targeted support for barrier function restoration.

Also, digestive enzyme supplementation can be helpful if pancreatic function is compromised or when recovering from severe gut damage. Comprehensive enzyme formulations can improve nutrient absorption while reducing the digestive burden on healing tissues. But this should be viewed as temporary support, not permanent replacement. Individuals with very low stomach acid production, a condition called hypochlorhydria, may benefit from betaine hydrochloride with pepsin to restore proper stomach acidity. However, this should never be used if active ulcers or gastritis are present, and it requires careful monitoring. Sometimes, binding agents like bentonite clay or activated charcoal are used during active treatment to help remove bacterial toxins and inflammatory compounds.

They can reduce Herxheimer reactions, temporary symptom flare-ups caused by the release of toxins from dying organisms. Implementing these more intensive protocols should be done under the guidance of a qualified practitioner.

Key Takeaways

Gut healing is absolutely possible, but it requires a comprehensive approach that addresses multiple factors simultaneously. Simply taking a probiotic is rarely sufficient, though that would certainly be more convenient.

The gut responds quickly when given the right support. Intestinal epithelial cells renew every few days, so removing harmful factors and providing targeted repair can lead to noticeable improvements in a short time.

Stress management is not optional in gut healing, it's essential! The gut-brain connection is so strong that ongoing stress can override even the best nutritional strategies.

In some cases, basic steps aren't enough, and targeted interventions are needed for specific conditions. This is when working with a practitioner experienced in advanced gut healing protocols becomes crucial.

The gut is designed to heal; it often just needs the right support and time to do so. Be patient with the process and stay consistent. The transformation that comes from true gut healing can be profound.

Above all, remember that gut healing impacts everything, energy, mood, immunity, and nutrient absorption. A healthy gut lays the foundation for overall health throughout the body.

Questions for Reflection

Take a moment to reflect on these questions:

1. What signs is my body giving me about the current state of my digestion?

2. Take note of recurring symptoms—whether bloating, irregular bowel movements, discomfort after meals, or food reactions—and consider what patterns may be pointing to unresolved gut stress.

3. Have I fully removed the foods and oils that are known to interfere with gut healing? Evaluate your current meals honestly. Consider whether inflammatory ingredients like gluten, processed dairy, or industrial seed oils are still present in your routine, even in small amounts.

4. Am I using targeted nutrients and probiotics with a clear purpose, or just hoping they will help? Think through what you are taking and why. Consider whether your current protocol is based on your actual needs, or if it may be time to reassess what is helping and what may be adding confusion.

5. In what ways could stress or sleep be slowing my digestive repair without me realizing it? Reflect on how your body feels during high-stress periods or poor sleep cycles. Pay attention to how those factors affect your digestion, energy, and ability to follow through with healing routines.

6. What would it mean for my overall health if my gut function were fully restored? Visualize what daily life could feel like if digestion no longer required constant attention. Consider how that shift might impact your energy, mood, immune function, and sense of peace in your body.

Many people start to feel better once their gut begins to heal, but what often surprises them is how quickly that progress can plateau. Bloating may improve, and food sensitivity may decrease, yet fatigue, brain fog, or sleep issues often remain. This isn't because the gut didn't respond. It's because deeper patterns are still active. What I have seen over and over again is that gut healing opens the door, but it doesn't handle every issue. Some people spend months chasing their symptoms without ever identifying the real reasons their gut won't stabilize.

That's where a good strategy becomes essential, not just to keep you moving forward, but for you to know where you are actually going.

By strengthening the gut, we lay the groundwork for whole-body healing. Yet, true prevention requires expanding beyond the gut to embrace the full spectrum of lifestyle practices that sustain health. Prevention begins with simple but profound actions: nourishing the body with real food, prioritizing restorative sleep, moving consistently, creating safer environments, managing stress, and cultivating meaningful connections. Together, these practices care for the whole person—mind, body, and spirit—and create the foundation for lasting wellness.

In the next chapter, we will explore *Food as Medicine* and review clinical practice guidelines for preventing five of the most common chronic diseases: hypertension, cancer, diabetes, stroke, and neurocognitive disorders.

You will notice common themes woven throughout these evidence-based recommendations, principles that reinforce and build upon everything we have discussed so far.

CHAPTER 14

Promoting Health
To Prevent Chronic Disease

*Dear friend, I hope all is well with you and that you are as
healthy in body as you are strong in spirit.*

— 3 John 1:2 (NLT)

Prevention is the most powerful form of medicine, yet most people don't focus on it until their health begins to decline.

Looking back, I now see this pattern everywhere. Patients who were admitted to the hospital with life-threatening or acute exacerbations of their disease, others needing frequent visits to their doctor for evaluation and management of chronic conditions, and many others living with ongoing symptoms due to the progression of their disease. This is the cascade effect of conventional care—one issue leading to another, with more medications added to control symptoms, new conditions developing, and eventually the need for surgeries or hospitalizations. No one got better, they just learned to live with their condition, taking medications, visiting doctors, and having procedures as their quality of life diminished.

Although pharmacists play a vital role in chronic disease and medication management, preventive care and holistic options are not always fully addressed. Our expertise ensures that medications are used safely and effectively, reviewing regimens for interactions, simplifying therapies, improving adherence, and helping patients manage conditions like diabetes, hypertension, COPD, and asthma. Yet, while medications can stabilize symptoms, they often do little to uncover the *why* behind chronic illness. Without addressing underlying imbalances, patients may remain dependent on prescriptions without ever experiencing true wellness.

This is where empowerment and a root-cause approach become essential. Preventive and holistic strategies such as nourishing the body with proper nutrition, restoring quality sleep, reducing toxin exposure, managing stress, strengthening the microbiome, and moving with intention go beyond symptom control to target the sources of disease.

What I've come to understand is that there's a big difference between basic nutrition and using food as medicine. There is a gap between meeting minimum requirements and creating true health. There is a clear difference between generic health advice and personalized strategies that align with your unique body chemistry.

Setting The Foundation for Disease Prevention

We were never meant to simply manage disease. True health is built long before illness begins through the choices we make each day. Yet in today's healthcare system, prevention is often overlooked, and treatment begins only after symptoms appear.

What if the greatest medicine is not found in a prescription bottle, but in how we eat, sleep, move, manage stress, connect with others, and align body, mind, and spirit in faith? These daily practices are not just "healthy habits"; they are essential, evidence-based steps that build resilience and reduce the risk of developing chronic conditions.

Despite this truth, our healthcare system devotes enormous time, resources, and finances to chronic disease management. Insurance often covers medications and procedures, but rarely prioritizes nutrition counseling, lifestyle coaching, or spiritual support. As a result, many patients receive treatments that manage symptoms, while the deeper root causes of disease remain unaddressed.

Chronic illnesses such as heart disease, diabetes, autoimmune disorders, and cancer affect nearly 60% of Americans today. They are the leading drivers of healthcare costs, disability, and reduced quality of life. Yet the majority are influenced not by genetics alone but by lifestyle and environmental factors within our power to change. That reality brings both challenge and hope: while our system may not prioritize prevention, individuals can reclaim health by focusing on daily choices that support long-term wellness.

Prevention begins with simple but profound actions: nourishing our bodies with real food, prioritizing restorative sleep, moving consistently, creating safer environments, managing stress, and cultivating meaningful connections. Adding prayer, meditation, gratitude, and trust in God's design brings strength to sustain these changes and peace to the healing process. Together, these practices address the whole person, mind, body, and spirit, and create the foundation for lasting wellness.

In this chapter, we'll explore the basics of nutrition as medicine and review some examples of clinical practice guidelines on the prevention of 5 common chronic diseases: hypertension, cancer, diabetes, stroke, and neurocognitive diseases. I'm sure you will find some trends in these *evidence-based* recommendations, and I hope they help reinforce what we have previously discussed.

Hypertension

High blood pressure is the most common risk factor for serious health problems like heart disease, stroke, dementia, kidney disease, and even early death. The good news is that it's also one of the most preventable and treatable conditions. For most adults, the goal is to keep blood pressure below 130/80 mmHg. Even in those with a genetic predisposition to hypertension, healthy lifestyle behaviors can *prevent* hypertension.

The 2025 American College of Cardiology/American Heart Association guideline on high blood pressure outlines four stages of blood pressure, providing a clear framework for prevention, detection, and management in adults.

Table 4. Categories of Blood Pressure in Adults [1]

Table 4. Categories of Blood Pressure in Adults*

	SBP		DBP
BP Category			
Normal	<120 mm Hg	and	<80 mm Hg
Elevated	120 to 129 mm Hg	and	<80 mm Hg
Hypertension			
Stage 1	130 to 139 mm Hg	or	80 to 89 mm Hg
Stage 2	≥140 mm Hg	or	≥90 mm Hg

Hypertension results from the combined influence of genetics, lifestyle behaviors, and chronic stress. Importantly, even among those with a genetic predisposition, evidence shows that targeted lifestyle modifications can prevent the onset of high blood pressure. The following strategies are recommended as key preventive measures.

Prevention strategies: [1]

- Includes weight loss for those who are overweight or obese

- A heart-healthy diet such as the DASH (Dietary Approaches to Stop Hypertension) eating plan

- No more than 2300 mg of sodium per day (with the ideal limit of no more than 1500 mg per day for most adults)

- Dietary potassium 3500 to 5000 mg per day

- Aerobic and resistance exercise ($\geq$150 minutes of moderate physical activity per week and resistance exercise $\geq$2 days per week)

- Stress management practices

- Intake of any alcohol is associated with higher SBP in a dose-response manner, including in individuals without hypertension

While lifestyle changes are the foundation for preventing and managing high blood pressure, there are times when additional support is needed. For many people, healthy habits alone may not bring blood pressure down enough to reduce risk. In these cases, combining lifestyle interventions with medication offers the best protection against serious complications.

Cancer

Cancer is the second leading cause of death in the U.S., and while treatment has advanced, prevention remains critical. Many cancers are linked to *modifiable lifestyle factors*, meaning prevention is possible through healthy choices.

The American Cancer Society emphasizes that, beyond tobacco use, the most important factors we can change are body weight, nutrition, physical activity, and alcohol use.[2] Nearly one in five cancers in the U.S. is linked to these areas, showing that prevention is both possible and powerful.

Steps that make a difference include:

- Avoiding tobacco in all forms

- Maintaining a healthy weight

- Staying active through daily movement

- Eating a nourishing diet centered on fruits, vegetables, whole grains, and lean proteins

- Limiting alcohol use

These choices do more than lower cancer risk—they strengthen the body against heart disease, diabetes, and other chronic illnesses. Prevention can also be seen as an act of honoring life: treating the body with care, building resilience, and creating the foundation for living with greater energy, clarity, and purpose.

By combining evidence-based strategies with a spirit of hope, prevention becomes not just a health plan but a pathway to healing and thriving.

Prevention of Diabetes and Prediabetes

The American Diabetes Association (ADA) emphasizes that prevention of type 2 diabetes is possible and highly effective, especially for individuals with prediabetes or those at high risk. The cornerstone of prevention is lifestyle intervention, supported by routine screening and, in some cases, pharmacologic therapy.

Evidence from landmark trials such as the Diabetes Prevention Program (DPP) and the Finnish Diabetes Prevention Study demonstrates that targeted lifestyle changes can reduce diabetes risk by 50–60%.[3][4]

To reduce risk and improve long-term outcomes, the ADA outlines several key steps:

- **Lifestyle Intervention (first-line and most effective):**

  - Aim for ≥150 minutes of moderate physical activity per week (e.g., brisk walking, cycling, swimming).

  - Strive for a 5–7% reduction in baseline body weight for those with overweight or obesity.

  - Emphasize a nutrient-dense, fiber-rich eating pattern, while minimizing refined carbohydrates and excess calories.

- **Screening and Monitoring:**

  - Test for prediabetes and type 2 diabetes in adults beginning at age 35—or earlier if risk factors are present (such as overweight/obesity, family history, hypertension, history of gestational diabetes, or belonging to higher-risk ethnic groups).

  - If results are normal, repeat screening at least every 3 years; if prediabetes is present, monitor annually.

- **Pharmacologic Prevention (when appropriate):**

  - Metformin may be considered in individuals at particularly high risk, such as those with BMI ≥35, age under 60, women with prior gestational diabetes, or those with worsening A1C despite lifestyle efforts.

- o Other agents (e.g., acarbose, GLP-1 receptor agonists) show potential but are not first-line for prevention.

- **Ongoing Support and Education:**

  - o Participation in structured lifestyle change programs (such as CDC's National Diabetes Prevention Program) improves adherence and long-term success.

  - o Counseling on sleep, stress management, and behavioral support enhances outcomes.[5]

Here's another way to think about diabetes prevention—simplified strategies that are easier to follow than dense medical guidelines. Even small, consistent changes can make a big difference in lowering risk. Practical steps include:

- **Maintain a Healthy Weight**: Excess body fat, especially abdominal fat, raises insulin resistance. Even modest weight loss (5–7% of body weight) improves blood sugar control.

- **Choose Nutritious Foods**: Prioritize whole grains, vegetables, fruits, nuts, legumes, and healthy fats while minimizing refined carbohydrates, added sugars, and highly processed foods.

- **Stay Active**: Regular physical activity improves insulin sensitivity, lowers blood sugar, and supports weight management. Aim for at least 30 minutes of moderate activity most days.

- **Limit Sugary Drinks**: Sweetened beverages (soda, fruit drinks, energy drinks) rapidly spike blood glucose and increase diabetes risk. Replace with water, tea, or coffee without added sugar.

- **Avoid Smoking and Excess Alcohol**: Both increase the risk of type 2 diabetes and worsen related health conditions.

- **Get Regular Checkups**: Early detection of elevated blood glucose, blood pressure, or cholesterol allows for timely intervention.

Together, these steps not only help prevent diabetes but also protect against heart disease, stroke, and other chronic illnesses. Regular screening helps identify those at risk, while selective use of medications like metformin may be appropriate when lifestyle alone is insufficient. Prevention is possible—and powerful—when daily habits align with long-term health.

Primary Prevention of Ischemic Stroke (Cerebral Vascular Accident)

The American Heart Association/American Stroke Association guideline [6] provides an overview of the evidence on various established and potential stroke risk factors and largely focuses on an individual patient–oriented approach to stroke prevention.

The first step is to address *modifiable risk factors*, which include: cardiovascular disease, smoking, diabetes, asymptomatic carotid stenosis, atrial fibrillation (nonvalvular), sickle cell disease, dyslipidemia, obesity, physical inactivity, postmenopausal hormone therapy, and dietary factors (sodium intake greater than 2300 mg and potassium intake less than 4700 mg).

Lifestyle modifications are encouraged for all and include (1) weight reduction if overweight, (2) limitation of ethyl alcohol intake, (3) increased aerobic physical activity (30 –45 minutes daily), (4) reduction of sodium intake (<2.34 g), (5) maintenance of adequate dietary potassium (>120 mmol/d), (6) smoking cessation, and (7) DASH diet (Dietary Approaches to Stop Hypertension). This diet is rich in fruit, vegetables, and low-fat dairy products, reduced saturated and total fat, sugar and salt.[7]

Preventing Dementia and Neurocognitive Disease

Alzheimer's, Parkinson's, and other dementias are not simply the result of aging. The greatest opportunities for prevention lie in managing *modifiable risk factors*, especially those tied to vascular health.[8] High blood pressure, diabetes, and obesity damage the brain's blood vessels and accelerate decline. Studies show that controlling blood pressure in midlife lowers the risk of dementia and mild cognitive impairment [9] while managing diabetes and metabolic health also reduces risk.[10]

Diet and lifestyle choices further strengthen protection. Mediterranean and MIND-style diets lower dementia risk while supporting a healthy gut microbiome.[11][12] Regular exercise improves blood flow and cognition,[13] and shows beneficial effects on the severity of motor signs and quality of life (QoL) for most types of physical exercise for people with PD.[14] Restorative sleep is equally important; sleep apnea increases dementia risk and disrupts the gut-brain axis.[15]

Oral and gut health also play a surprising role. Gut dysbiosis, periodontal disease, and tooth loss are linked with higher dementia risk due to inflammation and immune-mediated responses.[16][17][18] Supporting microbial balance through nutrition, oral care, and healthy habits strengthens brain resilience. Avoiding smoking and excess alcohol protects both vascular and microbial health.[19][20] Staying socially and mentally engaged provides additional protection.[21]

Protecting the brain requires caring for the heart, the microbiome, and daily lifestyle habits. Small, consistent steps can build resilience and help preserve memory and cognitive health well into later years.

CDC Key Prevention Steps for Chronic Disease

The CDC identifies four major risk factors that drive most chronic diseases: tobacco use, poor nutrition, physical inactivity, and excessive alcohol consumption. Prevention strategies focus on addressing these risks and strengthening overall health.

Lifestyle Steps:

- Quit smoking

- Eat healthy

- Get regular physical activity

- Limit alcohol

Preventive Care:

- Stay current with recommended vaccinations and health screenings (cancer, diabetes, blood pressure, cholesterol)

- Maintain good oral health with regular dental care

- Prioritize sleep (7+ hours per night) and effective stress management

- Know your family history [22]

Food as Medicine: The Foundation of Disease Prevention

Hippocrates is often credited with the timeless wisdom, "Let food be thy medicine and medicine be thy food." The idea of food as medicine is not new—it has been a guiding principle for health and healing for centuries. Our bodies are designed to respond to the messages that food sends, and these are messages that can either support healing or deepen imbalance. When we begin to look at food as information, not just fuel, we start to understand how our daily choices shape everything from our energy levels to the way we age.

When I work with clients who are exhausted, inflamed, or overwhelmed, one of the first things we look at is *how* they eat—not just what's on their plate, but when and how often they're nourishing themselves. Our bodies crave rhythm. Skipping meals, eating late, or relying on quick fixes throughout the day creates metabolic chaos. Restoring even a basic eating schedule can begin to regulate cortisol, support sleep, and stabilize energy. One traditional eating pattern that continues to stand out in both research and lived experience is the Mediterranean style of eating.[23]

Vegetables, legumes, herbs, olive oil, and fish form the foundation. These foods work together to quiet inflammation, stabilize blood sugar, and nourish the brain and heart. Studies show that this pattern of eating lowers the risk of many chronic conditions, including heart disease, diabetes, cancer, and dementia, especially when it is sustained over time.[24]

What often goes overlooked is how food is prepared and sourced. Avoid processed seed oils, particularly those high in polyunsaturated fats (PUFAs), as they tend to oxidize relatively easily.

Additionally, the refining process used to produce many seed oils can remove natural antioxidants, further contributing to their instability.[25] Wild-caught fish provide anti-inflammatory omega-3s that farmed fish may lack. Even simple choices, like using fresh herbs or cooking at home, influence how our bodies respond to what we eat. Meals prepared in a calm environment, eaten slowly and without distraction, allow for better digestion and absorption.

Our food should nourish and sustain us, yet the reality is far more concerning. In the United States, more than 10,000 chemicals, many with potential toxicity, are permitted in everyday foods, from cereals and snacks to meats. Shockingly, since 2000, nearly 99 percent of these additives were approved not by the FDA, but by the very food and chemical companies that profit from their use. Research has linked many of these substances to cancer, hormone disruption, and developmental harm.

This widespread exposure is made possible by a regulatory loophole known as "generally recognized as safe" (GRAS), which allows manufacturers to decide for themselves if a chemical is safe for consumption. For decades, this loophole has been exploited, leaving consumers vulnerable to hidden risks in the foods they trust. By highlighting some of the worst offenders on the market, the Environmental Working Group's Dirty Dozen Guide to Food Chemicals shows you which chemicals in food to avoid. Some examples are: *potassium bromate, synthetic food dyes (Red 3 & 40, Yellow 5 & 6, Blue 1 & 2, Green 3), titanium dioxide,* and *aspartame.*

Paying attention to environmental toxins from herbicides and pesticides (glyphosate and paraquat) that have been linked to neurologic diseases and cancer. [26] [27] [28]

Choose organic, whole foods when possible to reduce risks of exposure, especially for foods that have the highest level of contamination. This list is updated annually by the Environmental Working Group- Dirty Dozen.[29]

So much of healing begins in the ordinary choices we make—what we buy, how we cook, when we pause to eat. When we choose foods that support rather than stress the body, we begin to transform from coping to restoring.

Vitamin D: The Master Hormone for Disease Prevention

Many patients I've worked with, especially those facing persistent symptoms like fatigue, frequent infections, gut disorders, autoimmune conditions or hormonal imbalance, are unaware that one simple, correctable deficiency may be contributing to their struggles: low vitamin D! In fact, I rarely see someone with chronic health issues whose vitamin D levels are optimal. This deficiency is far more common than most people realize, and correcting it can unlock improvements across many systems of the body.

Vitamin D is not just a "bone health" vitamin. It functions more like a hormone, influencing hundreds of genes involved in immune regulation, inflammation, respiratory health, cardiovascular function, and even cell growth.[30]

Vitamin D also helps in cardiovascular health. It helps regulate blood pressure, improves the function of the endothelial lining of blood vessels, and lowers inflammatory markers associated with heart disease. It has been shown that individuals with low vitamin D levels have a higher risk of heart attack, stroke, and even cardiovascular death.[31]

The presence of vitamin D receptors throughout the body, including in immune cells, muscle tissue, and brain cells, speaks to how fundamental this nutrient is to health. Recent studies have suggested that vitamin D plays a critical role in maintaining overall health, including having a potential impact on gut microbiota composition and efficacy of cancer immunotherapy.[32][33]

Despite all this, deficiency remains widespread, even in people living in sunny climates. That's because several factors affect how efficiently we synthesize vitamin D from sunlight. Sunscreen, while important for skin protection, blocks the UVB rays needed for vitamin D production. People with darker skin tones require longer sun exposure to produce the same amount as someone with lighter skin. Our modern lifestyles that are largely spent indoors often mean we go days or weeks without meaningful sunlight on our skin.

For optimal health and disease prevention, blood levels of 25-hydroxyvitamin D should typically fall between 40 and 60 ng/mL. Achieving that range often requires daily supplementation—anywhere from 2,000 to 4,000 IU of vitamin D3 for most adults.

However, individual needs vary depending on weight, age, skin pigmentation, geographic location, and genetic differences in vitamin D metabolism. That's why regular testing is essential; it's the only reliable way to know whether your dose is sufficient.

Table 5. Optimal 25(OH)D concentrations for various health outcomes.[34]

Nutrients **2022**, *14*, 639

Table 5. Optimal 25(OH)D concentrations for various health outcomes.

Outcome	Type of Evidence	Optimal 25OHD	Reference
All-cause mortality rate	Observational study of 25(OH)D concentration due to vitamin D supplementation	>30 ng/mL	[8]
Alzheimer's disease and dementia	Meta-analysis of observational studies	>25 ng/ml	[93]
Breast cancer	Observational study of 25(OH)D concentration due to vitamin D supplementation	>60 ng/mL	[33]
Colorectal cancer	Meta-analysis of observational studies	30–40 ng/mL	[34]
Cardiovascular disease	Observational study of the CVD mortality rate for CVD patients	>30 ng/mL	[9]
Myocardial infarction	Observational study of 25(OH)D concentration due to vitamin D supplementation'In	>30 ng/mL	[8]
SARS-CoV-2 infection	Retrospective observational study	>50 ng/mL	[75]
COVID-19 mortality	Retrospective cohort study	>60 ng/mL	[82]
Diabetes mellitus type 2	RCT with an analysis of intratrial 25(OH)D for prediabetes patients	>50 ng/mL	[70]
Gene expression	Clinical trial	>40 ng/mL	[45]
Hypertension	Observational study of 25(OH)D concentration due to vitamin D supplementation	>40 ng/mL	[16]
Preterm delivery	Observational study of 25(OH)D concentration due to vitamin D supplementation	>40 ng/mL	[106]

When it comes to supplementation, quality and absorption matter. Research shows that vitamin D3, or cholecalciferol increases serum 25(OH)D levels to a greater extent than vitamin D2 (ergocalciferol) and can maintain those higher levels for longer periods of time.[35] It should always be taken with food, ideally one containing healthy fats, to support absorption. Combining vitamin D with vitamin K2 helps to transport calcium into the bones and teeth, where it is needed for strength. Vitamin K2 also plays a role in maintaining healthy artery function by preventing calcium buildup in blood vessels (calcification). Vitamin K1 (phylloquinone), is used to synthesize clotting factors and is mainly found in green leafy vegetables, while vitamin K2 (menaquinone), is mainly found in fermented dairy and produced by lactic acid bacteria in the intestine.[36][37]

Equally important is ensuring that magnesium status is adequate, as magnesium is required to activate vitamin D in the body. Without it, even high doses may not work as intended.

Magnesium: The Mineral Deficiency Epidemic

Magnesium deficiency may be one of the most overlooked nutritional problems today. This essential mineral is involved in over 300 enzyme reactions in the body, yet most people fall far short of getting enough. It naturally calms the nervous system and is essential in heart health by helping regulate heart rhythm and maintain healthy blood pressure.[38]

For blood sugar balance, magnesium is critical. It improves insulin function and supports glucose metabolism. People with low magnesium levels have a higher risk of blood sugar-related conditions contributing to metabolic syndrome.[39] Increasing magnesium intake often leads to significant improvements.

The nervous system also depends on magnesium for proper brain chemical function and mood regulation. Low levels are commonly found in people dealing with anxiety, sleep disturbances, and mood imbalances. Magnesium depletion has also been associated with cognitive impairment.[40] In many of these cases, increasing magnesium can bring noticeable relief.

Unfortunately, modern food processing and depleted soils have reduced the magnesium content in many foods. Refined grains lose most of their magnesium during processing, and industrial farming practices have lowered mineral levels in the soil. As a result, getting enough from diet alone is difficult.

Ongoing stress and certain medications further reduce magnesium levels. Stress increases magnesium loss through urine, while medications like diuretics, acid blockers, and some antibiotics can impair absorption or increase excretion.

For most people, 300 to 600 mg of elemental magnesium per day is needed for optimal health. Forms like magnesium glycinate and magnesium malate are easily absorbed, yet other forms like magnesium L-threonate may improve cognitive function and magnesium taurate may support heart health and blood pressure. Good food sources include dark leafy greens, nuts, seeds, and beans, but supplementation is often necessary to meet therapeutic needs.

Other Essential Nutrients Most People Are Lacking

Even with more food choices than ever, many people fall short on key nutrients. These are not always full-blown deficiencies with dramatic symptoms. More often, they are subtle imbalances that affect how the body functions and build up slowly over time. One of the most common gaps is omega-3 fatty acids. These essential fats support brain health, heart function, nervous system and help control inflammation. But most diets are heavy in omega-6 fats and very low in omega-3s, creating a ratio that can fuel chronic inflammation and related health problems.

Vitamin K2 is another nutrient often missing. It works with vitamin D to guide calcium into bones and away from soft tissues like arteries. Without enough K2, even high calcium intake can backfire. Since K2 is mostly found in fermented foods and organ meats, many people do not get enough.

Folate, the natural form of vitamin B9 in leafy greens, helps build DNA and supports methylation, a process involved in detoxification, hormone balance, and gene expression. It also helps regulate homocysteine, a compound linked to heart disease when elevated. Many people have genetic differences that make it harder to process synthetic folic acid, so food-based folate is especially important.

Iodine supports thyroid hormone production, which affects metabolism, energy, neurodevelopment and reproductive health. As people move away from iodized salt and eat less seafood, iodine intake has declined. A 2025 study found that when mothers were iodine deficient early in pregnancy, their children had lower mental development scores in the first two years of life, even when the mothers received thyroid treatment. This highlights the importance of getting enough iodine during pregnancy for healthy brain development.[41]

These nutrient gaps develop gradually. People may not notice symptoms at first—just lower energy, poor focus, or more frequent illness. By the time clearer issues appear, the imbalance may have been there for years.

The Power of Personalized Nutrition Approaches

General advice like "eat more vegetables" or "take a multivitamin" is common, but it rarely goes far enough, especially for those dealing with persistent symptoms or chronic discomfort. These blanket recommendations overlook a basic truth: no two bodies are exactly the same. Each of us carries unique genetic patterns, nutrient needs, and metabolic tendencies that shape how we respond to food, supplements, and medication.

For example, some people easily convert beta-carotene from plant foods like carrots or sweet potatoes into retinol, the active form the body uses. But others, due to genetic differences, cannot make that conversion efficiently.

Even with a nutrient-dense diet, they can remain depleted. In those cases, small amounts of retinol from foods like egg yolks or liver may be necessary to support immune function, skin repair, and vision.

Similar variations show up with B vitamins. The MTHFR gene, which affects folate metabolism, can reduce the body's ability to activate certain nutrients. People with this gene variant often need B vitamins in their active or methylated, forms. Without that support, they may struggle with fatigue, low mood, or elevated homocysteine, which is a marker linked to higher cardiovascular risk.

Functional medicine takes these differences seriously. Rather than relying on trial and error, it uses testing to identify what each body actually needs. Blood work, micronutrient evaluations, genetic panels, and stool tests can reveal why conventional strategies fall short and what to do instead. Food sensitivity testing is another layer of insight. Even nutritious foods like eggs, spinach, or almonds can trigger inflammation in some people. When someone says, *"I'm doing everything right, but I still feel awful,"* this is often the missing piece. It is not about adding more rules. It is about understanding what truly supports, rather than stresses, the body.

When nutrition becomes personalized, it stops being about willpower or discipline. It becomes about alignment, specifically by matching what the body needs with what it is actually getting. That is where real healing begins.

Key Takeaways

Preventing chronic disease takes intention and a comprehensive approach. It is not enough to simply avoid what is harmful; the body must be supplied with what it needs to repair and protect itself.

The clinical practice guidelines we've reviewed for hypertension, diabetes, cancer, stroke, and neurocognitive disease all point to the same fundamental truth: lifestyle intervention is our most effective preventive medicine because it addresses root causes rather than merely managing symptoms.

The 6 Healthy Habits we've explored form the cornerstone of chronic disease prevention: nourishing nutrition, restorative sleep, intentional movement, stress management, toxic reduction, and meaningful community connections. Central to all these habits is microbiome health, which influences immune function, inflammation, nutrient absorption, and neurological wellbeing. Supporting beneficial microbes through fermented foods and fiber-rich plants while avoiding processed additives creates the foundation for whole-body healing.

We cannot discuss prevention without acknowledging the toxic burden facing our generation. With over 10,000 chemicals permitted in our food supply—most approved by manufacturers themselves rather than the FDA—our bodies face unprecedented exposure to substances linked to cancer, hormone disruption, and neurological damage. Choosing organic foods when possible and supporting natural detoxification pathways have become essential strategies for long-term health.

Even health-conscious individuals often fall short on critical nutrients like vitamin D, magnesium, omega-3 fatty acids, vitamin K2, folate, and iodine.

Addressing these common deficiencies through personalized nutrition and functional lab testing often unlocks improvements in energy, mood, and resilience that patients had given up hope of experiencing.

This integrative, faith-inspired approach exemplifies the HOPE Method, where we honor both scientific evidence and the body's innate wisdom. When we combine clinical guidelines with personalized functional medicine, support the microbiome, optimize essential nutrients, reduce toxic exposure, and address the whole person, we create conditions for profound healing and lasting wellness.

Questions for Reflection

Now that we've come to the end of this chapter, take a moment to reflect on these questions:

1. What patterns in your family health history could guide your nutrition strategy? Think about conditions that appear often and how targeted nutrient support might lower your risk.

2. Are your vitamin D levels in the optimal range? If not, what steps will you take to correct them, and will you also check your magnesium to ensure vitamin D can be properly activated?

3. If your nutrition plan was designed specifically for your needs, what would you change first? Reflect on what feels out of alignment with your health goals and what adjustments could make the biggest difference right now.

4. What changes can you make to reduce toxic exposure in foods? Consider prioritizing organic options for the Environmental Working Group's Dirty Dozen produce list, avoiding synthetic food dyes and preservatives like those highlighted in EWG's Dirty Dozen Guide to Food Chemicals, and using

EWG.org resources to make informed choices about safer food options.

5. Identify modifiable risk factors in your life. What healthy lifestyle behaviors can you consider for making the greatest impact in preventing chronic disease?

Prevention is not only about avoiding disease—it's about protecting your future quality of life. The choices you make today determine not just how long you live, but how well you live. This brings us to an important distinction: lifespan versus healthspan. Lifespan is the number of years we live; healthspan is how many of those years we remain strong, independent, and well. The gap between the two often represents years of managing chronic illness, losing mobility, or relying on others for care. In the next chapter, we'll explore how to close that gap—shifting the focus from simply adding years to truly living your healthiest life.

CHAPTER 15

Living Your Healthiest Life

"Behold, I will bring to it health and healing, and I will heal them and reveal to them abundance of prosperity and security."

— Jeremiah 33:6 (ESV)

Adding years to our lives means little if those years are filled with pain, fatigue, or the slow loss of independence. What truly matters is our *healthspan,* or the number of years we get to feel strong, clear, and capable, without the burden of chronic illness holding us back.

Too often, the medical system focuses on survival or on preventing death without paying enough attention to how we're actually living. But health is more than the absence of disease. It's the presence of energy, purpose, and freedom in your body.

What many people don't realize is that the breakdowns we feel in midlife or later often begin silently, years earlier. Chronic disease doesn't usually start with a diagnosis, but with subtle imbalances: inflammation, stress overload, hormone shifts, nutrient depletion. These often go unnoticed until symptoms finally speak loud enough to be heard. This is why early, intentional care matters so much. Prevention is about choosing now to support your future self, so that decades from today, you're still living with strength, clarity, and joy.

Healthspan vs. Lifespan:
The Critical Difference

Lifespan is the number of years we live. Healthspan is how many of those years we get to feel strong, independent, and well. The space between them represents the years spent managing chronic illness, losing mobility, or relying on others for basic needs. For many people, that gap has grown wider than they ever expected.

Modern medicine has made it possible for us to live longer. We have advanced treatments for heart disease, diabetes, and cancer. But in the process, something important has been overlooked: we've gotten better at keeping people alive, but not necessarily helping them thrive. In the U.S., the average person now spends the last 12 years of life living with a serious illness or disability.[1] That's more than a decade of decline!

These long periods of poor health take a real toll physically, emotionally, and financially. Medical bills add up, energy fades, and the people around us often become caregivers instead of companions. The vision of retirement as a time of rest and exploration is often replaced with appointments, medications, and limitations.

To change that outcome, we need to change our focus. Instead of waiting until something breaks down and rushing to fix it, we can begin earlier by protecting the parts of our health that matter most: muscle strength, bone density, memory, balanced heart health, and metabolism. These are the foundations of a long, healthy life, and they don't preserve themselves. They require intention and consistency over time.

There's a name for what we're aiming for: *compression of morbidity.* It means shortening the amount of time we spend in poor health at the end of life. This is not to avoid death, but to protect life while we're still living it.

Redefining Aging

Aging is inevitable, but how we age, and how well we feel as the years go by, is more in our hands than most people realize. The number of candles on a birthday cake tells only part of the story. What matters more is how we move, how we think, how we feel, and how much life we still carry in our days. The vitality mindset is understanding that aging doesn't have to mean decline. Too often, we've been told that feeling tired, gaining weight, or losing mental sharpness is just part of getting older. When we believe that's the norm, we stop questioning it. We stop challenging it. But the truth is, those symptoms are often signals of imbalance, not signs that our best years are behind us.

The brain remains adaptable well into later life because of neuroplasticity, or our ability to form new connections and even grow new neurons. Learning something new, staying socially connected, and keeping the body active can all strengthen brain health and protect memory over time. The body, too, responds when we give it what it needs. Sarcopenia, which is the natural loss of muscle mass with age, often begins in our 30s and speeds up after 50. Resistance training, even just a few days a week, has been shown to reverse muscle loss even in people in their 80s.[2]

The vitality mindset also honors what *improves* with age. Emotional clarity, perspective, and the ability to prioritize what truly matters often grow stronger with time.

Biological Age vs. Chronological Age

Biological age reflects how well your body is functioning on the inside—how "old" your cells, tissues, and systems actually are. It often differs from chronological age, which simply counts the years since birth. Two people born on the same day might have vastly different biological ages, depending on how they live, eat, move, and manage stress.

One of the most studied markers of biological age is telomere length, the protective DNA sequences at the ends of chromosomes that shorten with each cell division. While some shortening is natural, accelerated loss of telomeres is linked to chronic stress, poor lifestyle habits, oxidative damage, and inflammation. Importantly, shorter telomeres are associated with a higher risk of age-related diseases, including cardiovascular disease, diabetes, cancer, and neurodegenerative disorders.[3][4][5][6] Thus, telomere length serves not only as a biomarker of biological aging but also as an early signal of disease vulnerability.

Encouragingly, lifestyle choices can protect telomeres. Diets rich in antioxidants, polyphenols, and omega-3s,[7] regular exercise,[8] effective stress management (including mindfulness and prayer)[9][10], and adequate sleep[11] are all associated with slower telomere shortening. These daily habits not only support healthy aging but also reduce the risk of chronic disease.

Another key factor is called advanced glycation end products, or AGEs. These compounds form when sugar binds to proteins (hemoglobin (Hgb A1c%), albumin, insulin, immunoglobulins, low-density lipoproteins (LDL), and collagen) in the body, damaging tissues over time. AGEs stiffen structural proteins like collagen, accelerating aging from the inside out. High sugar intake and poorly managed blood sugar, especially in conditions like diabetes, can drive up AGE formation. Low-grade, chronic inflammation also contributes to biological aging. Biomarkers like C-reactive protein (CRP) and interleukin-6 (IL-6) help reveal how much silent inflammation may be simmering beneath the surface.[12] This slow-burning immune activity often has no obvious symptoms but can gradually damage tissues and increase the risk of many age-related diseases. The term "inflammaging" has been used to describe this pattern.[13] CRP is made by the liver and rises in response to inflammation anywhere in the body. IL-6, a type of signaling molecule called a cytokine, is involved in coordinating the immune response. When IL-6 levels remain high over time, it often signals a state of heightened immune activity tied to chronic disease risk.

Mitochondrial function is another important piece of the puzzle. Mitochondria are the tiny energy factories inside your cells, and their efficiency naturally declines with age. As their performance drops, people may start to notice lower energy, slower recovery, and reduced physical endurance.[14] [15] However, mitochondrial health can be supported through choices like regular movement, intermittent fasting, getting adequate sleep, managing stress, and taking targeted nutrients that boost energy production.[16] Reducing exposure to toxins and supporting the body's natural detoxification processes can help protect mitochondria. Biological age is an empowering concept because it puts more of the aging process into your hands. You cannot change the year you were born, but you can absolutely influence how your body ages on a cellular level through the choices you make every day.

Energy Management Throughout Life Stages

Energy is not just about how awake you feel. It depends on how well your cells create and use fuel. As people get older, energy often changes because of changes in hormones, metabolism, and how well the mitochondria function. Hormones are one of the biggest factors. Thyroid hormones set the pace for your metabolism. Cortisol helps you handle stress and helps in blood sugar regulation. Estrogen and testosterone influence how strong you feel, how well your muscles work, and even how motivated you are. Insulin affects how your body uses sugar for fuel. When these are out of balance, energy drops. But they can be supported through diet, movement, and better sleep and stress routines.

Sleep patterns also matter, especially your circadian rhythm. This internal clock keeps your body running on time. When sleep is irregular, meals are scattered, or you miss out on daylight, the rhythm can change, which often leads to more fatigue. A regular sleep schedule, morning sunlight, and eating meals at consistent times can help reset the rhythm and bring energy levels back up. Another key piece is how flexible your metabolism is. This means how easily your body can switch between burning carbs and fat. As you age, this flexibility can decrease, making you feel more tired or sluggish between meals. But you can train it back. Strength training, daily activity, and occasionally going longer between meals can help your body use stored energy more efficiently.

Energy needs also change based on life stage. In younger adulthood, focus and stamina are usually in high demand. Midlife often brings more stress and responsibility, making recovery just as important as output. In later years, the focus may shift to keeping strength and mobility. But no matter the phase, energy is something you can support, not just something you lose.

Independence and Functional Fitness

Independence, which means being able to take care of yourself and your daily needs, has more to do with functional strength than with how fit you look. The ability to carry groceries, climb stairs, or reach for something on a high shelf makes a bigger difference in everyday life than muscle tone or appearance.

Functional fitness supports this kind of strength. It includes endurance, so you can stay active without getting winded too quickly. It also includes muscle strength to lift, move, and carry things comfortably. Balance and coordination help you stay steady and avoid falls. Flexibility and mobility keep your joints moving well, so it is easier to bend, stretch, or turn without discomfort.

These abilities are what make day-to-day life manageable. Tasks like cooking, getting dressed, cleaning, shopping, or keeping up with grandchildren all rely on this foundation. When strength, balance, or flexibility decline, these everyday actions can become harder or even unsafe. That change often marks the point when people begin needing help with basic needs, which can change their quality of life in significant ways.

Falls are one of the most common and serious risks as we age. Around one in four adults over 65 falls each year, and falls are the leading cause of injury-related death in that age group.[17] Many of those falls are preventable. Regular movement, especially exercises that build strength and improve balance, can greatly reduce the risk.

Mental sharpness also matters. Good executive function, which refers to your ability to plan, organize, and manage details, makes it easier to stay on top of things like finances and medication routines. Memory issues, when they show up, can affect both safety and the ability to live independently. Staying mentally active, socially engaged, and physically mobile all help protect brain function and support continued independence.

The goal of aging well is not just about avoiding illness. It is also about staying capable, connected, and confident in your own body. That kind of outcome is built gradually. The earlier you begin working on functional strength and balance, the more likely you are to stay independent later in life.

Creating a Personal Health Vision

Having a clear and personal vision for your health gives direction to your daily choices. Most people can quickly say what they want to avoid, like chronic illness, fatigue, or losing independence, but have a harder time defining what they actually want for their lives. When health is framed mostly in terms of fear or avoidance, motivation tends to fade. It becomes reactive instead of intentional.

A strong health vision shifts the focus. Instead of saying, *"I don't want to get sick,"* it becomes, *"I want to have the energy to hike with friends,"* or *"I want to stay strong enough to live on my own."* These kinds of goals are specific, personal, and tied to something that matters. They give everyday decisions more meaning.

A meaningful health vision usually includes several dimensions. Physical goals might be about staying active, preserving strength, or having the stamina to keep up with daily life and hobbies. Mental goals often focus on staying sharp, learning new things, and keeping the ability to think clearly and make confident decisions. Emotional goals can involve building stronger relationships, reducing stress, or finding more purpose in day-to-day life. Together, these layers create a fuller picture of what well-being really looks like. What matters most will vary from person to person. Someone who loves gardening might care most about joint mobility. Someone with a strong family history of heart disease may focus more on blood pressure, movement, and nutrition. There is no universal template. A good health vision reflects your own values and the kind of life you want to live.

It should also feel grounded. The goal is not to chase perfection but to create the best possible outcomes from where you are right now. A vision works when it is both realistic and motivating—when it stretches you a little without disconnecting from your current reality. As life changes, so will your priorities. A vision that made sense at 40 may not fit at 60 or 80. That is part of the process. Revisiting it from time to time helps keep your choices aligned with what truly matters to you, whatever chapter you are in.

Legacy Health: Beyond Personal Wellness

Your health choices affect more than just you. They shape the habits, expectations, and well-being of the people around you, especially your children and grandchildren. That is the heart of legacy health. It is not just about genetics or family history. It is about the way routines, behaviors, and priorities are passed down, often without anyone realizing it.

Many people assume that if a disease runs in the family, it is mostly genetic. But in reality, lifestyle tends to matter more. Families often share meals, schedules, stress responses, and sleep habits. These daily patterns influence health just as much as DNA, sometimes more. Children watch what adults eat, how they move, and care for themselves. They learn what is "normal" by what they see every day. If family meals are healthy, if movement is part of the routine, and if rest is valued, those habits tend to stick. The same is true when health is neglected. What starts as one person's routine can quietly become a generational pattern.

There are also practical effects. Chronic illness often brings financial strain, missed work, and caregiving stress. Staying well can ease those burdens. It creates more space to be present, for memory-making, and for daily life to feel manageable. Legacy is also about what gets handed down, such as knowing how to cook real food, how to move regularly, how to manage stress, and how to build a routine that supports energy and calm. These are everyday tools that can make a lasting difference.

When people connect their own health to the people they love, their motivation often deepens. Choices feel less like chores and more like investments in the future—one meal, walk, or bedtime at a time. That is what legacy health really means.

Adapting to Life's Inevitable Changes

Life rarely stays the same for long. Schedules change, roles evolve, and unexpected events come up. When they do, the way we take care of ourselves has to change, too. What worked before might not fit anymore, and that is okay. The key is not to be perfect, but to stay connected to what matters most.

Healthy habits like moving your body, eating well, sleeping enough, and managing stress do not stop being important. But how they show up in daily life might need to change. A new parent might trade long workouts for short walks with the baby. Someone healing from surgery might pause intense exercise in favor of gentle stretching. What matters is staying flexible while keeping your foundation intact, nourishing body, mind, and spirit.

There will be times when energy dips or life feels heavy. Grief, illness, and big transitions can all take a toll. In those moments, showing up for your health may look smaller. That does not mean you have lost your way. It means you are adjusting, and that adjustment is part of staying well. Even aging calls for this kind of flexibility. Maybe certain foods are harder to digest, or high-impact exercise no longer feels good. Maybe sleep patterns will adapt, or your energy levels will vary throughout the day. Instead of fighting those changes, the goal is to listen to them and respond with care. Swap what no longer works for what still does.

Resilience is not about never getting knocked down. It is about knowing how to get back up. One hard week does not erase everything you have built. One detour does not mean the road is gone. Health is not a straight line; it is a process of real life. When you learn to adapt with both wisdom and trust, you make space for growth, healing, and hope at every age.

The Economics of Healthspan

While doctor visits, prescriptions, and hospital stays are easy to track, they are often only a fraction of the true cost. Missed work, lower productivity, and the need for help with daily life can quietly drain far more over time. Choosing to invest in prevention through movement, nutritious food, sleep, and stress support often pays off in ways that are both tangible and long-term. A gym membership, organic produce, or a weekly yoga class might seem like added expenses. But compared to managing diabetes, heart disease, or repeated ER visits, these choices usually cost far less. When health is seen as an investment rather than a cost, spending decisions shift. Groceries, workouts, and therapy become part of a plan to stay independent, energetic, and financially stable. Over time, these small choices add up, often saving far more than they ever cost.

Chronic illness, on the other hand, comes with both visible and hidden costs. There are the obvious expenses, but also the ripple effects: time off work, missed opportunities, and a decline in overall quality of life. In many cases, the indirect costs add up faster than the medical ones. One of the biggest overlooked financial risks is long-term care. The average cost of full-time nursing care now exceeds $100,000 a year.[18] And yet, many people do not plan for it, often assuming they will not need it. Staying strong, mobile, and mentally sharp through daily habits may reduce or even avoid that need entirely.

Being healthy also opens doors. People with more energy, fewer symptoms, and better function can usually work more consistently, travel more freely, and enjoy life without as many limitations. These benefits are not always measured in dollars, but they are deeply valuable.

Building A Longevity Mindset

Longevity thinking means going away from quick fixes and toward what can be sustained for a lifetime. Some choices may give fast results, but they do not always support lasting health. When the focus turns to the long term, everything from how you move your body to how you manage stress begins to change. With a longevity mindset, consistency matters more than intensity. A simple workout routine done regularly over decades is more powerful than bursts of extreme training followed by burnout. The same goes for stress: daily habits like deep breathing, walking, or quiet moments of prayer do far more good than a once-a-year retreat. This kind of thinking also changes how new health trends are viewed. Instead of chasing the latest diet or supplement, the focus shifts to what actually lasts. If something cannot be sustained for the long haul, it probably does not belong in a long-term plan.

It is also about small, steady progress. A little more sleep, a few extra steps each day, or a bit less daily tension might not feel groundbreaking, but over time, these kinds of changes add up. When repeated daily, they create a foundation that gets stronger with age. A longevity mindset accepts that health is never "done." It is not something you check off and walk away from. That idea can feel overwhelming at first, but it can also be freeing. It means every day offers a new chance to make choices that support how you want to live, now and later. Enjoying the process is part of what makes it work. When movement, meals, or rest bring a sense of pleasure or purpose, they become something you want to keep doing, not just something you "should" do. In the end, it is about balance. Good health does not mean giving up everything that brings joy. It means choosing habits that support both how you feel today and how you want to feel in the years ahead. When that balance clicks, the path to longevity begins to feel like something you actually want to walk.

Key Takeaways

Living longer is not the same as living well. Healthspan is about the years you remain strong, clear-minded, and capable, without chronic illness stealing your quality of life. The gap between lifespan and healthspan can be shortened. By protecting strength, mobility, balance, and mental sharpness now, you can reduce the years spent in decline later.

Aging does not have to mean loss. Many symptoms associated with getting older, like fatigue, weight gain, and memory changes, are often signs of imbalance that can be addressed. Biological age matters more than chronological age. Habits that reduce inflammation, protect mitochondria, and maintain healthy blood sugar can slow cellular aging.

Energy changes over time, but it can be supported at every stage. Balanced hormones, a steady circadian rhythm, and metabolic flexibility all contribute to sustained vitality. Your independence depends on functional strength, balance, and cognitive health. These abilities determine how well you manage daily life without assistance.

A clear, personal vision for your health gives purpose to your daily choices. Goals that are specific and meaningful make healthy habits easier to sustain. Your habits influence the health of future generations. Legacy health is built through the example you set and the routines you pass on. Adaptability is essential! Life changes will require adjustments in how you care for yourself, but maintaining your foundation keeps you moving forward.

Investing in prevention is often less costly, financially and physically, than managing chronic illness later in life. A longevity mindset focuses on what can be sustained over decades, prioritizing consistency over quick fixes.

Questions for Reflection

To get more out of what you have learned from this chapter, take a moment to reflect on these questions:

1. How many years of your life do you want to spend in good health, and what would that look like for you?

2. What steps can you take now to protect your strength, balance, and mental sharpness for the future?

3. When you think about aging, which signs of decline do you assume are "normal," and which might be signals you can address?

4. What habits are helping to slow your biological age, and where could you make improvements?

5. How well are your energy levels supported through hormone balance, sleep patterns, and nutrition?

6. Have you clearly defined your vision for health in the years ahead? If not, what would you include?

7. In what ways are you modeling healthy habits for your children, grandchildren, or others who look up to you?

The years ahead can hold strength, clarity, and purpose, but that outcome depends on how you care for yourself today. Every decision, no matter how small, builds the foundation for the health you will carry into the future. By focusing on what is sustainable, you create a life where you are not only living longer, but living well.

In the next chapter, we'll shift from the 'what' of health to the 'how' by exploring *patient empowerment*. True empowerment means more than following instructions; it's about having the knowledge, skills, and confidence to actively shape your care. When you bring your lived experience together with medical insight, healthcare becomes more personal, more precise, and far more effective.

CHAPTER 16

Patient Empowerment

In the same way, wisdom is sweet to your soul. If you find it, you will have a bright future, and your hopes will not be cut short.

— Proverbs 24:14 (NLT)

True empowerment in healthcare goes beyond following instructions or accepting treatments without question. It means developing the confidence, skills, and knowledge to take an active role in your care, even when navigating a system that often feels confusing or impersonal.

If you have ever walked out of a medical appointment with more questions than answers, you are not alone. Many people feel unheard or dismissed, their symptoms reduced to checkboxes or their concerns brushed aside. Over time, this can lead to a sense of powerlessness and frustration, especially when chronic issues remain unresolved.

But the truth is, you are the most important member of your healthcare team. While doctors and specialists bring essential training, no one knows your body, your symptoms, or your quality of life better than you do. When your lived experience is combined with medical insight, care becomes more precise, more meaningful, and more effective.

Empowerment starts with remembering that your voice matters. When you understand your options, ask questions, and speak up about what you notice or feel, you help shape your care in a way that reflects your unique needs.

Developing Health Confidence and Self-Trust

Health confidence comes from learning to listen to your body and trust what it is telling you. But for many people, that trust has been worn down. Maybe you were told your symptoms were all in your head, or that everything looked "normal" even when you felt far from it. Over time, that kind of experience makes it harder to believe what your body is saying.

But your body is always communicating. Whether it is changes in energy, digestion, mood, sleep, or just a sense that something feels off, these signals matter. Learning to notice patterns over time helps you understand when something needs attention. One bad night of sleep is easy to shrug off, but if it keeps happening, that is your body trying to get your attention. The same goes for discomfort that shows up over and over again, even if it seems minor at first.

Building health confidence also means letting go of the idea that "normal" always means healthy. Just because a lab result falls within a reference range does not mean it reflects what is right for you. Additionally, just because something is common does not mean it should be accepted as your baseline. There is a difference between getting by and feeling well.

One of the most effective ways to rebuild trust in your body is by experimenting with small changes and paying attention to how you feel. You might try changing your sleep schedule, eating differently, testing out different ways to manage stress, or incorporating prayer and scripture reading into your daily routine. These low-stakes choices help you notice what helps and what doesn't, without needing anyone else to validate your experience.

Prayer and spending time in God's word can be particularly powerful for rebuilding this connection. Many people find that regular prayer helps them tune into their body's signals, while scripture reading provides wisdom and peace that reduces the stress that often clouds our ability to listen to what our bodies need.

Health confidence is not about handling everything on your own. It is about showing up with more clarity and certainty when you do seek care. The more you know your own patterns and needs, the easier it becomes to have real conversations with your providers, especially when things get complicated. You do not need to know all the answers. You just need to trust that your observations are valid and that your voice belongs in the room.

Becoming a Health Detective

Effective health advocacy means thinking like a detective, watching for patterns, noticing connections, and staying curious about what your body is trying to tell you. It involves observing symptoms over time, tracking lifestyle changes, and piecing together how different factors might be interacting. Instead of seeing symptoms as problems to silence, this approach treats them as clues. Fatigue, pain, bloating, brain fog, and poor sleep do not happen without a reason. They are the body's way of flagging that something is off, even if the cause is not immediately clear.

Timing can be one of the biggest clues. If your energy crashes every afternoon, that might suggest blood sugar swings or hormone dips. If sleep gets worse during times of stress, your nervous system could be staying on high alert. If digestion acts up after certain meals, food sensitivities or enzyme issues may be involved. These are the kinds of patterns that start to show up when you track your symptoms carefully and pay attention to when and how they appear.

The environment also plays a bigger role than most people realize. New skin products, changes in your home or workplace, or even seasonal allergens can trigger subtle changes in how you feel. Sometimes, just looking back at what changed right before symptoms started is enough to spark insight. Family history adds another piece to the puzzle. While genetics are not your destiny, they do shape what might need some attention from you. For example, if digestive issues run in your family, it may make sense to watch for early signs and support gut health more proactively.

Even lab testing becomes more useful with a detective mindset. It is not just about whether a result falls in the "normal" range, but noticing changes and trends over time. A single number might not raise concern, but if it is steadily moving in the wrong direction, it can be an early sign that something needs support. The more you approach your health with curiosity and awareness, the more capable you become of making decisions that actually help. It is not about solving everything on your own. It is about learning to notice what matters, ask the right questions, and stay involved in the process.

Speaking Up in Medical Settings

Communicating clearly with healthcare providers is not always easy, but it makes a big difference. Many people walk into medical appointments feeling rushed, overwhelmed, or unsure of how to explain what they are experiencing. That can lead to misunderstandings, missed information, or treatment plans that do not fully match what someone needs. One of the most helpful ways to make the most of your time is to prepare ahead of the visit. Writing down your main concerns, questions, and goals before you arrive can help you stay focused, especially if the appointment is short. It also helps to bring notes about when symptoms started, what seems to trigger them, and anything that makes them better or worse. This kind of detail can give your provider a much clearer picture.

When you describe what you are feeling, being specific helps more than general statements. Saying something like *"I feel tired all the time"* is a start, but it is even more helpful to say, *"I crash in the afternoon and need another cup of coffee to get through the day."* Adding numbers where possible, like rating your pain or tracking how often something happens, can also make a big difference.

It also helps to ask direct questions. If a provider suggests a medication, asking what it is supposed to do, what the side effects might be, how long it would be taken, and whether there are other options gives you the information you need to decide. The same goes for testing. It is reasonable to ask what a test is meant to show and how it might affect next steps.

Appointments can move quickly, and it is easy to forget details afterward. Taking notes or bringing someone with you can help. If something is unclear, asking for simpler explanations is always okay. Healthcare providers use complex language out of habit, so speaking up when you need more clarity helps everyone.

If you are unsure about a recommendation or it does not feel right to you, it is completely appropriate to say so. You can ask about alternatives, ask for more explanation, or take time to think things through. A good provider will welcome your involvement and work with you to find a plan that fits your needs and values.

Challenging Medical Dismissal

One of the most discouraging experiences in healthcare is feeling dismissed. When symptoms are brushed off, minimized, or explained away without proper evaluation, it can leave people feeling invisible. This happens far too often, especially to women, people with chronic pain, and those dealing with complex or hard-to-categorize symptoms. Dismissal often occurs when test results come back "normal," even though daily life says otherwise. If symptoms don't fit neatly into a diagnosis, they may be attributed to stress, aging, or emotional factors without further investigation. While mental and physical health are certainly connected, assuming symptoms are psychological without exploring physical causes can delay care and block progress. Unfortunately, this often leads providers to prescribe medications to treat the symptoms—anxiety, depression, brain fog, pain—rather than seeking to understand root causes like infections in the microbiome, hormone imbalances, or exposure to toxins.

This symptom-management approach can trap patients in a cycle where medications temporarily mask problems while underlying issues continue to worsen. A patient might receive antidepressants for fatigue and mood changes caused by thyroid dysfunction, or anxiety medication for symptoms actually stemming from gut infections or nutrient deficiencies. While these medications may provide short-term relief, they don't address why the symptoms developed in the first place, leaving the true problem to progress unchecked.

In these situations, staying calm and clear becomes important. Asking directly why symptoms are being linked to psychological causes and what evidence supports that conclusion can bring useful clarity. If you disagree or feel unheard, requesting that your concerns be documented in your medical record can help ensure your experience is acknowledged, even if the provider does not take further action.

If standard lab results do not provide answers, it is reasonable to ask about additional testing or a referral to a specialist. Some root causes only show up with a more detailed investigation. Functional medicine testing or other advanced assessments may uncover patterns that conventional tests overlook. These options are not always covered by insurance, but for some, they offer answers that finally make sense. Getting a second opinion is also a valid step. Different providers bring different perspectives, and a fresh set of eyes may open new possibilities. Just because one provider dismissed your concerns does not mean you are out of options.

Keeping your own record of symptoms can also help move things forward. Notes about when symptoms happen, how intense they are, and how they affect your daily routine create a clear picture of what is going on. This kind of information not only strengthens your case but also gives future providers something specific to work with. In some cases, bringing someone with you to an appointment can change the dynamic. A supportive family member or friend can speak up if needed, offer a second perspective, and reinforce how much the symptoms are affecting your life.

Being heard is essential to getting the care you deserve. If it takes persistence, documentation, or finding a new provider, it is worth it. Your experience is valid, and you are not obligated to accept care that does not acknowledge what you are living with.

Building Accountability Systems

Sustainable health change does not rely on willpower alone. It takes accountability to keep you supported, motivated, and open to adjustment when things do not go as planned. These work best when they fit your life, reflect your values, and offer steady feedback without judgment. It starts with setting clear, specific goals. Vague plans like "eat healthier" or "exercise more" can feel good in the moment, but they rarely lead to lasting change.

Establishing S.M.A.R.T. goals that are *Specific, Measurable, Achievable, Relevant,* and *Time-bound.* This approach helps ensure that goals are well-defined, trackable, and attainable within a specific timeframe.[1] Instead of saying "I want to eat better," a S.M.A.R.T. goal would be "add vegetables to every meal for the next two weeks." Rather than "I need to exercise more," try "walk for 20 minutes each day after dinner for one month." Instead of "I should sleep better," commit to "turn off technology one hour before bedtime every night this week."

These specific, measurable goals give you a clear standard to check in with and help you know whether progress is actually happening. You can track completion, adjust when necessary, and build momentum through small, consistent wins that compound over time.

Regular self-assessment supports this process. Whether you review habits at the end of each week, reflect monthly on what is improving, or do a broader check-in every few months, that consistent reflection helps reveal what is working and what is not. Additionally, accountability from others can make a meaningful difference, too. Friends, family members, or small community groups can help you stay consistent when your motivation dips.

The most helpful relationships are the ones that offer encouragement and understanding, not pressure or guilt. It is about support, not punishment.

In some cases, professional support adds even more structure. Regular check-ins with a healthcare provider, nutritionist, or health coach offer a space for expert insight and guidance. These conversations often provide clarity during slow or frustrating phases and can help adjust your plan to match your real-life challenges.

Technology can also support accountability. Habit-tracking apps, wearable fitness or sleep monitors, and online groups can provide useful tools and extra motivation. Still, even the best tools are no substitute for real human connection and meaningful feedback. They should support the process, not define it. The most effective accountability combines encouragement with the freedom to course correct. Small wins matter because they build momentum and remind you that progress is happening. When setbacks happen, they are not failures. They are part of the process.

Making Difficult Health Decisions

Making complex health decisions is rarely straightforward. There are often several factors to weigh, such as potential benefits, possible risks, personal values, and practical concerns. It can feel even more difficult when the condition is serious, when different professionals offer conflicting advice, or when every option seems to come with a trade-off. The first step is getting clear, reliable information. This means understanding what each option actually involves. What are the expected outcomes? What are the side effects? How likely is it to help? Getting a second or even third opinion can bring a fresh perspective and help clarify the decision.

It can also help to look at both conventional and complementary options. Conventional medicine is often the right choice for urgent or life-threatening problems. But when it comes to long-term or chronic issues, more holistic or integrative approaches might offer support that feels more in line with your values. This is not about choosing one "side" over the other. It is about finding what feels right for your body and your situation. Another part of the process is understanding how much we really know about each option. Some treatments are backed by years of solid research. Others are still being developed or are based on early evidence. Knowing the difference can help you decide what level of uncertainty you are comfortable with.

Personal values also matter. You might care most about minimizing side effects, or you might prioritize keeping your daily routine intact. For someone else, the main goal might be longevity or avoiding certain types of treatment altogether. There is no wrong answer here, because what matters is knowing what matters most to you. It is also worth thinking about how each option might affect your day-to-day life. Will it take a lot of time? Will it interfere with work or caregiving responsibilities? Is it financially realistic?

Finally, try not to let fear or outside pressure drive the decision. Unless something is truly urgent, take time to think things through. Talk to someone you trust. Sleep on it. Write out your thoughts. Pray about it and seek God's guidance through scripture—many find that bringing decisions before God in prayer brings clarity and peace that cuts through confusion. The Bible offers wisdom for decision-making, reminding us that - *If any of you lacks wisdom, you should ask God, who gives generously to all without finding fault, and it will be given to you.* James 1:5 (NIV).

Clarity often comes from giving yourself permission to slow down and think clearly, not from rushing toward a quick answer. When you combine prayer with practical steps like sleeping on decisions and seeking wise counsel, you create space for both divine guidance and human wisdom to work together in pointing you toward the best path forward.

Handling Family and Social Pressure

Making health decisions is hard enough on its own. It gets even harder when those choices go against what your family or close friends expect. Sometimes it shows up as concern, other times as pushback. Either way, it often comes from a good place, but that does not always mean the support feels helpful.

A lot of the time, these reactions are shaped by fear or habit. Maybe a parent had a bad experience and wants to protect you from the same thing. Maybe a sibling is just repeating what they were taught. It helps to keep that in mind, even if you do not agree. You do not have to change your mind to stay kind. Setting boundaries matters. If a conversation starts to feel overwhelming or one-sided, it is okay to step back. A simple *"I've made my decision and I'm not looking to debate it"* can go a long way. You do not need to defend your choices just because someone else is uncomfortable.

It is also completely valid to choose what you share and with whom. Some people will understand and support you without trying to steer the wheel. Others might not, and that is okay, too. You get to decide how much of your health journey is open to others. When someone questions your decision, try to stay grounded. You can say, *"I know this might not make sense to you, but it's something I've thought through."* That keeps the door open without giving away your own clarity. In the long run, doing what feels right for you matters more than avoiding discomfort in the moment. Saying yes to someone else's expectations might keep things smooth for a while, but if it pulls you away from what you believe in, it can create a quiet kind of regret. Standing by your choices is not always easy, but it often brings more peace than trying to please everyone else.

Creating Financial Boundaries for Health

Spending on health often has to compete with other priorities, which makes it critical to be clear about what truly matters and how to sustain it over time. With U.S. healthcare spending projected to grow 7.1% in 2025, reaching an average of $16,570 per person due to increased utilization, an aging population, and rising medical prices, the financial burden highlights the need for a strategic plan.[2] Without one, it's easy to feel overwhelmed or guilty about not doing enough to prioritize health effectively.

A helpful first step is figuring out which choices actually make a difference. Often, the basics like eating real food, staying active, getting rest, and managing stress go further than expensive fixes. These are the things that help prevent problems later, which means they usually save money in the long run. It also helps to be honest about what is essential and what is optional. Some health expenses are non-negotiable. Others might feel helpful but are not urgent. Focusing on what addresses your most immediate needs keeps things manageable.

Thinking about the bigger picture can also change how spending decisions feel. Skipping preventive care may seem like a way to save money now, but it can lead to higher costs down the road. On the other hand, investing a little in things that support your well-being before something goes wrong can spare a lot of stress later.

There are practical ways to keep health spending in check. Cooking at home, finding free or low-cost movement options, and making use of what insurance covers can go a long way. Not everything has to be fancy to be effective. Creating a budget just for health makes those decisions easier. It does not have to be big. What matters is that it fits your life and gives you something steady to build on. Small, regular steps usually do more than big, expensive pushes that are hard to keep up.

Developing Long-Term Health Discipline

Long-term health does not depend on motivation alone. It depends on discipline, which is built through habits, structure, and a clear understanding of what matters. That starts with knowing your goals, specifically the deeper reasons behind them. Maybe it is staying active with your kids, avoiding medications, or feeling clearheaded at work. When your choices are tied to something meaningful, they are easier to stick with.

Small steps are often the most effective because big overhauls tend to burn out quickly. But consistent changes, like adding one extra vegetable to each meal or taking a walk after dinner, can build momentum and create real progress over time. Your environment plays a role, too. When healthy food is easy to reach, when workout clothes are already laid out, and when distractions are reduced, you do not have to rely as much on willpower. Discipline becomes easier when the path is clear.

Daily routines help take the guesswork out of healthy habits. Going to bed and waking up at the same time, scheduling meals, setting aside time to move—all of these reduce the number of choices you have to make and create a reliable rhythm. Flexibility matters too. Life does not always follow a plan, and trying to force rigid routines through every change or disruption often leads to burn-out. A flexible structure that can change with your needs is more sustainable.

When things go off track, which they will at times, the key is not to overreact. Self-criticism does not help. What helps is getting clear on what happened, adjusting, and starting again. Missing a day is not a failure. Letting it stop you completely is. Finally, noticing progress, no matter how small, can help you stay engaged. Maybe you are sleeping better. Maybe your digestion has improved. Maybe you feel more patient or focused. These small signs are proof that your choices are working, and they are worth paying attention to.

Teaching and Mentoring Others

Many people who experience real improvements in their own health feel drawn to help others do the same. Teaching and supporting others can be incredibly meaningful, but it is important to do so with care, respect, and healthy boundaries. One of the most effective ways to begin is by sharing your own experience. Instead of offering advice, simply describe what helped you, what did not, and what you learned along the way. Personal stories can be powerful. They offer insight while still giving others the space to explore what feels right for them.

It also helps to remember that health is deeply personal. What works for one person may not work for another. Differences in biology, background, values, and preferences all shape individual needs. Approaching each conversation with curiosity instead of assumptions keeps it supportive rather than prescriptive. Additionally, listening often goes further than fixing.

Many people just want to feel heard. When you ask honest, open questions about their goals or what they are struggling with, it creates space for reflection. From there, they may be more open to support.

Encouraging others to involve qualified professionals can also make a difference. Your experience might spark ideas or hope, but it should never take the place of professional care, especially when the situation is complex or serious. Clear boundaries matter. Caring about someone's health does not mean taking responsibility for their outcomes. Support is most helpful when it respects autonomy. Letting others own their choices builds confidence and avoids conflict.

Patience is part of the process, too. Change is rarely quick or linear. Even if someone seems uninterested, your example might leave a quiet impression that takes root later on. Respecting their timing helps preserve trust and keeps the relationship strong. Not everyone will be ready, and that is okay. What matters most is offering kindness, perspective, and encouragement, then stepping back and letting people move forward on their own terms.

Empowered Health Through Active Participation

Empowerment in healthcare is not just about following instructions. It is about building the confidence to trust your instincts, the skills to assess your own needs, and the ability to engage with the medical system as an active participant, not a passive recipient. That begins with recognizing that no one knows your body better than you do. Healthcare providers bring expertise, but only you can describe how you feel, what matters most in your daily life, and whether something is truly helping. When that personal insight is taken seriously, healthcare becomes more collaborative, effective, and respectful.

Building accountability systems, setting financial boundaries, and developing consistent discipline around daily habits all contribute to that sense of control.

These tools make it easier to navigate both everyday choices and larger transitions, especially when circumstances are uncertain or challenging.

An empowered person does not reject medical care. They ask questions, express concerns, and participate in decision-making from a place of clarity and self-respect. Outcomes improve not just because the treatments are better, but because the process is rooted in mutual understanding and shared responsibility.

As Proverbs reminds us, wisdom and understanding bring hope. In the context of health, that wisdom comes from learning to listen to your body, to make thoughtful choices, and to advocate for what you need. The goal is not just to live longer, but to live with more agency, more clarity, and more peace of mind. Additionally, offering support doesn't mean becoming responsible for someone else's health outcomes. Letting others take ownership of their choices fosters empowerment and avoids tension.

Being patient is key. Change is difficult and rarely immediate. Even when people seem resistant or uninterested, your example may plant seeds that grow later. Respect for their timing helps maintain trust and keeps communication open.

Ultimately, not everyone will be ready for change, and that's okay. What matters is offering compassion, information, and encouragement—then stepping back and allowing others to move at their own pace.

Key Takeaways

Empowerment in healthcare means more than following instructions. It involves developing the confidence to trust personal instincts, the skills to assess health needs, and the ability to engage actively with the medical system. This empowerment begins by recognizing that each person is the foremost expert on their own body. Healthcare providers contribute knowledge and experience, but only the individual knows how they feel, what matters most, and what's working or not.

By building accountability systems, setting financial boundaries, and developing health discipline, people create the foundation for lasting wellness. These tools help navigate both daily choices and bigger life transitions with resilience.

An empowered person doesn't reject medical care; they collaborate more effectively within it. Better communication, more appropriate decisions, and improved outcomes result when patients are informed, engaged, and confident. As Proverbs reminds us, wisdom and understanding bring hope. In health, this wisdom emerges from learning to make good decisions, advocate for personal needs, and take ownership of long-term well-being. This is not just about living longer, but about living with agency, clarity, and satisfaction. When we align our health choices with our faith, we discover that God desires abundant life for us—not just spiritual abundance, but wholeness in body, mind, and spirit. This abundance includes the energy, clarity, and physical vitality that come from stewarding our bodies well.

Faith-centered health empowerment recognizes that caring for our bodies is both a responsibility and a privilege. We're called to be good stewards of the life we've been given, making choices that honor God and enable us to serve others effectively. When we approach health decisions through prayer and biblical wisdom, we often find the courage to make changes we've been avoiding and the discernment to choose what truly serves our long-term wellbeing rather than what feels easy in the moment.

Questions for Reflection

To reflect on the content of this chapter, please take a moment to think about these questions:

1. When have you felt dismissed or unheard in a medical setting? Consider how that experience influenced your willingness to speak up or return for care, and what you want to do differently next time.

2. What signals has your body been sending that you have ignored or doubted? Decide how you will track those signals and what action you will take when they appear.

3. How would your decisions change if you viewed yourself as the lead detective in your care rather than a passive recipient? Identify one concrete step that puts you in that role.

4. Who or what holds you accountable right now? If support is thin, choose the structure you need—clear goals, regular check-ins, faith-based practice, or a person who will help you stay consistent.

5. What S.M.A.R.T. goal would address your biggest health challenge right now? How will meeting this goal change how you feel in your body day to day?

6. What beliefs about your worth or authority in healthcare are holding you back? Write the words you will use to challenge them, and plan how you will ask questions, set boundaries, or seek a second opinion.

Your answers to these questions are more than just thoughts on a piece of paper. They are the framework for how you will show up in your own care from this point forward! Keep them where you can review them often. As your health needs change, revisit and update your responses so they continue to guide you with accuracy and confidence.

Empowerment means recognizing that your health journey is ultimately in your hands. It's about shifting from being a passive recipient of care to an active participant in your own healing. When you embrace this mindset, every choice—from the food you eat to the way you manage stress—becomes a step toward reclaiming your health and writing a new story for your future.

Up to this point, we've explored how gut health, chronic disease prevention, nutrition, sleep, stress management, and lifestyle choices all shape lasting wellness. You now have the knowledge to transform your health. But knowledge alone isn't enough—what's needed is a clear structure to put it all into practice. That is where the HOPE Blueprint comes in. In this final chapter, I'll share the framework that organizes everything we've covered into four essential pillars: *H*ealthy Nutrition, *O*ptimizing Physical Activity, *P*ositive Mindset, and *E*nvironmental Factors.

Together, these create a practical path toward lasting transformation. Yet the foundation for true resilience reaches even deeper. It comes from faith, trusting that God's design for our bodies is good, that we are wonderfully made, and that healing is possible when we align our choices with His wisdom. With faith at the center, the HOPE Blueprint becomes more than a plan for health, it becomes a path to strength, peace, and long-term success!

CHAPTER 17

The HOPE Blueprint For Success

In everything he did, he had great success,
because the LORD was with him.

— 1 Samuel 18:14 (NIV)

We have now covered many essential factors on gut health, chronic disease, the value of nutrition, the benefit of sleep, and the importance of managing stress. You now have the knowledge to truly transform your health. During my career in pharmacy, when I watched patients accumulate diagnoses and prescriptions without ever truly recovering, I had plenty of knowledge. However, what I was lacking was an understanding centered on health rather than managing conditions, along with a real blueprint for transformation.

This final chapter seeks to provide that blueprint, taking everything we have covered throughout this book and creating a structure that can actually work.

The Four Pillars of Health

During my own health crisis, I discovered that recovery requires a lot more than clinical guidelines, standard protocols, and medications. The HOPE Method framework organizes a path to wellness into four essential pillars that all work together: 1) **H**ealthy nutrition, 2) **O**ptimizing physical activity, 3) **P**ositive Mindset, and 4) **En**vironmental factors.

Healthy Nutrition forms the foundation of all health. As discussed throughout this book, what we eat either fuels healing or feeds disease. For years, I didn't connect my own symptoms to what I was putting in my body.

When functional testing later revealed nutrient deficiencies, mineral imbalances, toxic elements, and food sensitivities, I finally understood that my diet wasn't supporting my health; it was promoting inflammation, fatigue, hormone imbalance, and pain. All this despite following the US Dietary Guidelines for Americans! The eating hygiene tips we have covered remain essential. These simple practices can dramatically improve digestion and nutrient absorption.

Understanding food labels, as we discussed, empowers you to make informed choices about what you are truly eating. Learning the difference between "good" and "bad" fats, why they matter, how to limit saturated fats, and how to ensure you're getting enough essential nutrients like vitamin D, calcium, magnesium, and potassium creates the foundation for lasting health. This knowledge moves you beyond a "fad diet" for quick weight loss toward a way of eating and living that truly supports well-being. Identifying foods that drive inflammation (through food sensitivity testing) and removing them temporarily can accelerate healing and quickly relieve symptoms. Many clients report dramatic improvements, such as freedom from migraines, joint pain, or skin reactions within weeks of eliminating foods that trigger immune reactions. The goal of this pillar is not to strive for perfection, but to develop awareness: to recognize which foods nourish the body and which promote dysfunction, and to practice eating in a mindful, health-supportive way.

Optimizing Physical Activity is done through the benefits of movement or exercise as a powerful foundation for health. Regular physical activity, as mentioned, can help reduce a wide array of risks, from dementia and depression to heart disease. These immediate and long-term benefits explain why movement is so important, and why it is also one of our *Six Healthy Habits*. Combined with the other aspects of health optimization we have covered, movement becomes a key part of a comprehensive approach to preventing and reversing chronic disease.

Positive Mindset does not refer to so-called "toxic positivity" or a sense of pretending that everything is fine when it isn't. Instead, it builds on the definitions of mindfulness, we have covered in this book and rests on the positive aspects of human nature, the strength of social connections, and the depth of spirituality. What matters most is how we respond to the health challenges before us, what we choose to believe, and where we place our faith. Over the years, I have seen many patients accept their diagnoses as if they were a permanent life sentence dictated by fate or genetics. They took their medications without questioning whether improvement was possible or whether other options existed. Today, I encourage my patients to become investigators of their own health. Careful tracking of symptoms often reveals patterns that hold the key to transformation. This mindset of empowerment, combined with the techniques of stress-relieving practices we have discussed, as well as the restoration that comes from quality sleep, creates the resilience needed for lasting change. Ultimately, the way we think shapes the way we heal. A hopeful perspective does not deny reality; it reclaims possibility!

Environmental Factors, of course, relate to the external and internal factors that influence our health. This includes the obvious sources we have covered, such as removing household toxins from our home, testing our drinking water, and avoiding harmful chemicals and agents, like BPA and PFAS, in our products.

The six classes of harmful chemicals covered in this book (highly fluorinated compounds, antimicrobials, flame retardants, bisphenols and phthalates, solvents, and certain metals) all influence our health. However, our environment also includes the social connections, relationships, and sources of support we have in our lives. During my own recovery, I had to examine not just what chemicals were in my home or my body, but also which relationships drained my energy and which ones supported my healing. Some patients end up discovering that their symptoms improve simply by changing their living or working environment, removing mold exposure, or finding a supportive community that understands them and what they are facing.

The four HOPE pillars all work together and are central to any plan for wellness and healing. This book has given you extensive knowledge on what these four pillars are, how to integrate them into your life, and what makes them so essential. Now, it is up to you to use them to empower yourself and begin living a healthier life.

Creating a Personalized Wellness Plan

A successful blueprint always begins with a thorough, systematic assessment of where you are, health-wise, right now. Despite years of medical care, this is something most patients have never experienced. Running general diagnostics is one thing, but an extensive evaluation of your current state of health is another. While there might be a general sense of "not feeling well," without careful documentation, it is nearly impossible to identify the specific triggers, patterns, and connections that reveal what is really going on.

Looking back is just as important as looking at the present. Many patients can pinpoint the onset of their health challenges to a specific event: the loss of a loved one, divorce, an acute illness, financial hardship, trauma, or even childhood adversity. These experiences leave an imprint on the body and can shape how symptoms develop over time. A powerful question to ask yourself is: *When did I last feel well—and what changed before my symptoms began?*

Once you begin reflecting on these questions, the next step is to observe what is happening day to day. Careful tracking allows you to see connections you might otherwise miss, revealing patterns between lifestyle choices, environmental exposures, and symptom flare-ups. This is why it's so important to expand your focus beyond diet, sleep, and stress. Many other factors, often overlooked, can play a critical role in how your body feels and functions.

These additional areas are worth paying attention to, as they often hold the missing pieces of the puzzle. By noticing how each one may be influencing your health, you can begin to connect symptoms to possible triggers and uncover patterns that guide a more personalized wellness plan.

Factors Beyond Diet, Sleep, and Stress

In addition to food, rest, and stress, there are other important influences on health that patients and providers often overlook. Paying attention to these areas can uncover hidden patterns and triggers that may be driving symptoms.

1. Hidden Infections & Immune Triggers

Sometimes, lingering infections, such as recurrent sinus infections, urinary tract infections, yeast overgrowth, or gum disease, create an underlying burden on the immune system. Bacterial or viral reactivations, like chronic Lyme, Epstein-Barr, or herpes viruses, can also flare during times of stress or low immunity. These may show up as unexplained fatigue, brain fog, swollen glands, or flare-ups of joint and muscle pain.

2. Environmental & Toxin Exposure Our bodies are constantly interacting with the environments we live and work in. Mold, heavy metals (mercury, lead, arsenic), pesticides, or chemicals in personal care products and cleaning supplies can add to the body's toxic burden. Patients often notice chronic fatigue, congestion, headaches, dizziness, or increased sensitivity to smells when toxins are a hidden trigger.

3. Food Sensitivities & Intolerances

Beyond obvious allergies, delayed food sensitivities to gluten, dairy, soy, corn, eggs, or histamine-rich foods can quietly fuel inflammation. These reactions may appear hours or even days later and often show up as bloating, rashes, migraines, joint pain, or fatigue.

4. Hormonal Fluctuations

Hormones play a key role in energy, mood, and metabolism. Imbalances in thyroid hormones, adrenal function (cortisol), or sex hormones (estrogen, progesterone, testosterone) can lead to symptoms such as fatigue, weight changes, hot flashes, disrupted sleep, or mood swings.

5. Physical Activity & Movement Patterns

Movement is essential, but too much exercise (overtraining) or too little (sedentary lifestyle) can both disrupt health. Notice if symptoms such as pain, fatigue, or mood shifts worsen after certain types of activity or after long periods of inactivity.

6. Medications & Supplements

Prescription and over-the-counter medications, as well as certain supplements, can sometimes mask or worsen symptoms.

New issues such as digestive upset, headaches, fatigue, or skin changes that appear after starting something new may provide valuable clues.

7. Social & Emotional Environment

Relationships, social support, and emotional well-being deeply affect physical health. Stress from conflict, isolation, or lack of connection may worsen symptoms. Loss and grief can be especially powerful triggers, affecting sleep, mood, and even immune function. Patients may notice flares of pain, anxiety, or fatigue during these times.

8. Environmental Rhythms & Lifestyle Patterns

The body is regulated by daily rhythms. Disruptions from shift work, irregular meal timing, or exposure to artificial light late at night can all disturb the circadian system. This often leads to insomnia, morning fatigue, or mood imbalances.

Connecting Symptoms to Triggers

The goal is not just to document symptoms, but to ask: *What changed right before I felt this way? Did symptoms appear after a specific food, event, or exposure? Do they improve when that trigger is removed?* These questions guide patients to see connections that may otherwise go unnoticed and help create a personalized wellness plan rooted in awareness and empowerment.

Our HOPE Lifestyle 6-Month program is one of the most effective approaches you can take to securing the best blueprint for your health! It provides a comprehensive structure for those who want professional, guided implementation, including a detailed case review that goes far beyond any standard medical history. Included in this program are functional lab testing, personalized nutrition plans based on specific imbalances and preferences, private health coaching sessions, and targeted supplement protocols that can address your unique needs rather than generic recommendations.

Integrating Functional Medicine Insights

Before attempting to address any specific conditions or symptoms, we must first stabilize the basic functions that health depends upon, much like ensuring a house's foundation is solid before renovating the upper floors. Without a stable foundation, even the most sophisticated approaches will fail or potentially cause harm.

Phase 1: Stabilizing the Foundation

The first step in restoring health is not advanced testing or supplements—it is creating balance in the core lifestyle factors that sustain every system of the body. These include:

- **Stress management:** Chronic stress keeps the body in a "fight or flight" state, impairing digestion, hormone balance, immunity, and sleep. Practices such as mindful breathing, journaling, prayer, yoga, or guided imagery help shift the nervous system into "rest and repair," allowing the body to heal.

- **Sleep quality:** Restorative sleep is essential for detoxification, memory consolidation, hormone regulation, and immune function. Addressing sleep hygiene, such as light exposure, bedtime routines, and circadian rhythm alignment, is foundational to all healing.

- **Movement and activity:** Consistent physical activity supports circulation, lymphatic flow, detoxification, and mood regulation.

  Both overtraining and inactivity can create stress on the system; the goal is balanced, sustainable movement.

- **Nutrition basics:** Even before addressing food sensitivities or gut repair, it is critical to establish regular meal timing, whole-food nutrition, adequate hydration, and mindful eating practices. How we eat is as important as what we eat.

Stabilizing these pillars creates the resilience needed for deeper work. Patients who skip this stage often struggle because the body cannot heal if it is constantly fighting stress, exhaustion, or metabolic imbalance.

Phase 2: Targeted Interventions

Once a foundation for health has been stabilized, we can address specific imbalances found through testing or observation. Without proper preparation, these interventions would be useless, or maybe even harmful. Heavy metal toxicity, for instance, is a common factor that often shows up in functional testing. Decades of accumulation from sources people do not usually think about, such as mercury from dental fillings, fish, and lead from old pipes and paint, found in a pre-1978 home, are common factors.

Furthermore, arsenic from our groundwater, aluminum from antiperspirants and cookware, cadmium from cigarette smoke (even secondhand) and other sources.

These metals disrupt cellular energy, mess with our enzyme function, influence the repair of DNA, and create oxidative stress that accelerates aging.

Chelation, the binding of heavy metals or minerals in the body so they can be safely excreted, has to progress slowly. We therefore use gentle agents like modified citrus pectin, chlorella, cilantro, or alpha-lipoic acid, along with binders to prevent redistribution. In addition, supporting the body's natural detoxification pathways is essential. One effective method is sauna therapy, which promotes sweating and the release of toxins through the skin, easing the burden on the liver and kidneys. When combined with proper hydration and mineral support, sauna use can be a powerful complement to nutritional and supplemental detox strategies.

Our hormones also tend to follow a hierarchy you can't skip. Cortisol and insulin, for instance, control many other functions, so they are often addressed first. We might use adaptogens like ashwagandha, rhodiola, or holy basil for cortisol, plus stress management and optimized sleep. Insulin sensitivity, on the other hand, typically requires a change in diet or nutrients like chromium and alpha-lipoic acid. Thyroid hormones come next, as cortisol and insulin affect thyroid production and conversion directly. The sex hormones (estrogen, progesterone, testosterone) usually balance themselves out once the primary hormones normalize, although some cases may benefit from additional support through herbs, bioidentical hormone replacement, or nutrient therapy.

Gut health is foundational to overall wellness, and for many patients, it is the key starting point in their healing journey. Functional medicine often applies the **5R Framework,**[1][2] a stepwise process that addresses the root causes of digestive dysfunction while restoring balance to the microbiome and supporting the entire body.

5R Framework:

1. Remove – Clear Out What Harms

The first step is identifying and removing what is causing harm inside the gut. This may include pathogens such as bacteria, parasites, or yeast overgrowth, as well as food triggers (gluten, dairy, processed foods, or sugar) and environmental toxins.

Removing these obstacles helps reduce inflammation and gives the gut a chance to reset.

2. Replace – Support Digestion

Next, the focus shifts to restoring what may be missing. Digestive support can include stomach acid (HCl), bile salts, or pancreatic enzymes that aid in breaking down food properly. Without these essential factors, nutrients are not absorbed efficiently, and symptoms such as bloating, reflux, or malabsorption can persist.

3. Reinoculate – Rebuild the Microbiome

Once harmful influences are reduced, the gut can be repopulated with beneficial microbes. Probiotics, prebiotics, and fiber-rich foods help cultivate a diverse and resilient microbiome. A balanced microbiome supports immune function, regulates inflammation, and produces key metabolites such as short-chain fatty acids that nourish the intestinal lining.

4. Repair – Heal and Strengthen the Gut Lining

Chronic stress, infections, and toxins can weaken the intestinal barrier, contributing to "leaky gut" and immune reactivity. Repair focuses on supplying nutrients and compounds that support healing—such as L-glutamine, zinc carnosine, omega-3 fatty acids, vitamin D, and botanicals like aloe or slippery elm. This step helps calm the immune system, reduce food sensitivities, and restore resilience.

5. Rebalance – Create a Lasting Foundation

This step is about lifestyle and should be incorporated at the beginning. As true healing requires rebalancing daily habits that support the gut and overall health: restorative sleep, stress management, regular movement, and a nutrient-dense, anti-inflammatory diet. This stage transforms gut healing from a short-term protocol into a sustainable way of living.

Why the 5R Framework Works

The beauty of the 5R approach is that it is both systematic and flexible. While the steps are designed to build upon one another, patients do not always move through them in the same order. For some, especially when symptoms are severe, it may be necessary to begin with **Step 4 (Repair)** to calm inflammation, support the gut–immune system, or ease digestive distress before addressing pathogens. At the same time, I always emphasize the importance of **Step 5 (Rebalance)** from the very beginning of any protocol. Without addressing sleep, stress, and nutrition, symptoms often worsen, particularly during the removal phase, as this can be another form of stress on the body. This adaptability is what makes the 5R framework so effective: it provides both a structure and the flexibility to meet each patient where they are. In doing so, it uncovers what the body truly needs to heal and helps patients move from dysfunction to resilience-restoring not only gut health but also energy, mood, immunity, and long-term wellness.

Case Example: Healing the Gut with the 5R Approach

Maria, a 42-year-old teacher, came to me with years of digestive issues, bloating, constipation, anxiety, and constant fatigue. She also struggled with migraines and frequent urinary tract infections. Despite multiple doctor visits and prescriptions, she was told her labs were "normal" and offered little beyond symptom management.

When we applied the **5R approach**, everything began to shift:

- **Remove:** Stool testing revealed yeast overgrowth, H. Pylori, and significant bacterial overgrowth. She also reacted strongly to gluten. By removing food triggers and addressing the microbial imbalance with targeted herbal antimicrobials, her bloating and migraines began to ease within weeks.

- **Replace:** Maria had low stomach acid and inadequate digestive enzyme function, which explained her discomfort after meals. We supported her digestion with pancreatic enzymes and gall bladder support, which reduced her reflux and improved nutrient absorption.

- **Reinoculate:** Once pathogens were addressed, we introduced probiotics and gradually increased her fiber intake. This helped diversify her gut microbiome and restore healthy bowel movements.

- **Repair:** To strengthen her gut lining, Maria used L-glutamine, zinc carnosine, serum-derived immune globulin, and omega-3 fatty acids. Within months, her digestive symptoms improved, and bowel movements became regular. She even reported more energy and a better mood.

- **Rebalance:** Focusing on lifestyle behaviors was an important first step. Maria committed to a consistent sleep schedule, daily walks, and stress management through journaling and breathwork. These changes gave her the resilience to maintain her improvements long term.

Six months later, Maria's migraines had disappeared, her digestion and bowel movements improved, and she had more energy. Most importantly, she no longer felt defined by her symptoms; she felt empowered by the knowledge of how her body worked and what it needed to thrive.

Steps for Preventing Relapse and Sustaining Results

Phase 3: Maintenance and Optimization

True recovery requires more than simply managing symptoms. Lasting health cannot be achieved if one returns to the very habits and patterns that contributed to illness or dysfunction in the first place.

This is a mistake I repeatedly see: when patients begin to feel better, they often assume they can now go back to their old lifestyle without any concerns. Yet, the practices that restored health must evolve into a sustainable way of healthy *living*. As natural as brushing your teeth, integrated seamlessly into your life, rather than a feeling of being under constant restraint or deprived of things you like.

When we are actively healing, high doses of certain supplements might be needed to correct deficiencies or support a struggling system. However, if we were to continue these doses indefinitely could create new imbalances. The strict elimination diet that successfully reduced inflammation and identified trigger foods can usually be altered once the gut has healed and immune tolerance improves. The intensive protocols for managing stress, which were necessary during acute illness, can be simplified as resilience builds and the nervous system rebalances.

Tracking your process through recurring testing and regularly monitoring your healing can prevent a gradual regression that often occurs when people feel even a bit better and become complacent about their health. I therefore recommend retesting key markers every six to twelve months to adjust your care based on individual needs and current health. After all, the goal is to promote long-lasting health, and not only symptom relief.

Daily Implementation Strategies

Health is built through thousands of continual, small, daily decisions, and not occasional intensive efforts or grand gestures. The key is to consistently nurture daily practices that promote health and well-being.

Your morning routine is one of the key factors of metabolic and hormonal patterns for the entire day, which is why these first hours matter so much. Therefore, getting some bright sunshine within the first thirty minutes of waking up can help establish a healthy circadian rhythm, while suppressing melatonin and allowing cortisol to reach an appropriate level for the morning. Afterward, just *five minutes* of movement—whether that's stretching, going for a short walk, or rebounding—activates your metabolism, improves insulin sensitivity, supports lymphatic flow, and can help keep your mind clear for hours. Furthermore, starting the day with a protein-rich breakfast will help stabilize your blood sugar throughout the morning, which can prevent those energy crashes and cravings that often make us reach for unhealthy snacks before lunch. When you plan and prepare your meals ahead of time, you also avoid making impulsive food choices when hunger hits and there is nothing healthy nearby. Spending a few hours on the weekend, cooking meals in bulk, and preparing healthy grab-and-go snack options like whole fruits or veggies often makes it easier to stay consistent throughout the week. Batch cooking soups, stews, and casseroles can also give you multiple meals to choose from, instead of having to eat the same meal every single day.

A healthy routine in the evening also helps prepare the body for the restorative sleep that is so critical to our health, as poor sleep will sabotage even the most perfect diet and supplement protocol. Not eating late, minimizing screen time, and dimming the lights after sunset tell your pineal gland to start producing melatonin. Taking magnesium glycinate an hour before bed can also help relax muscles and the nervous system, which often improves sleep better than any pharmaceutical sleep aid.

There are plenty of ways to support your health, but the *6 Healthy Habits* covered in this book give you a solid foundation. Putting them into practice can help you build a healthier life, one that is real, lasting, and does not require medication.

From Pain to Purpose

My journey from pain to purpose began with a personal story that evolved into a professional mission that has now transformed hundreds of lives. The conventional system I served so faithfully for thirty years, the system I believed in completely and dedicated my career to, failed me entirely when I needed it the most. However, through functional medicine, I discovered the body possesses a remarkable ability to heal when we stop suppressing its symptoms and start addressing the causes of illness.

This knowledge transformed far more than my personal health; it revolutionized my entire understanding of illness, healing, and the proper role of a healthcare provider in supporting wellness. We should empower patients with knowledge and tools, not create life-long dependence on pharmaceutical treatments. We should investigate why symptoms occur, rather than simply naming and masking them. The HOPE Method framework evolved directly from my own transformation, and I have now organized everything I learned through my own recovery and the insights gained from guiding hundreds of patients through their healing journeys.

Knowledge is one thing, but knowledge without action will never accomplish anything, no matter how profound or comprehensive that knowledge might be. To implement this knowledge into your own life, start with just *one* meaningful change today—not next week, not after the holidays, or when life seems less complicated. Today, right now, make a commitment to yourself. You have the ability to reclaim your health, and you deserve a life lived in wellness.

You now have a complete blueprint, laid out clearly with actionable steps and practical guidance. What happens next depends entirely on your willingness to act, to push through any temporary discomfort, and to maintain faith in the body's ability to heal. The body wants nothing more than to return to balance and vitality; it simply needs the right support and time to restore optimal function. For those who choose action over acceptance, I am here for you.

I believe you can have a future where you can feel energetic again, and where health is an asset you enjoy nurturing, rather than a chore to manage. You do not have to try and change everything all at once, just enough to create momentum.

You will succeed in whatever you choose to do, and light will shine on the road ahead of you.

—Job 22:28 (NLT)

Key Takeaways

This chapter seeks to tie together the main concepts covered in this book. These last key takeaways are meant to reinforce some of the key aspects you can apply to your life, with a direct impact on your health.

- Paying attention to how your body responds is one of the most important tools you have.

- Getting enough sleep, eating real food, and reducing stress support every other aspect of healing.

- Improving your digestion helps with energy, inflammation, mood, and hormonal balance. It is the main foundation for all health.

- Removing processed food, artificial ingredients, and toxins gives your body less to fight against.

- Even without lab testing, you can take simple actions that make a noticeable difference!

- Long-term change comes from routines you can maintain—not fads or trendy protocols or extreme diets or interventions.

- You do not need "perfect days." You need reliable habits you can return to when you fall off track.

- Healing progresses over time, and health is nurtured. What you do most of the time matters more than what you do once in a while.

- Making one change at a time can help you get started, stay focused, and avoid feeling overwhelmed.

- The information in this book is here to be used. Start with what feels doable today and build from there!

Questions for Reflection

The value of this book is not just in what you have learned, but in how you put it into practice. Healing only becomes real when it shows up in the choices we make every day. Use these questions to help you get started—one step at a time.

1. Which of the Six Healthy Habits feels most realistic to begin with right now?

2. What small adjustment could you make this week to improve how you sleep, eat, move, or rest *today?*

3. When do you feel the most grounded and happy, and how can you bring more of that into your life?

4. What part of your environment needs to change for you to better support your health goals?

5. Who in your life encourages you to stay consistent, and how can you stay connected to that person or source of support?

6. How can you make space in your week to reflect, reset, or return to the practices that keep you well?

7. What is *one specific action* you will take this week to begin living by the knowledge you have now gained?

8. What commitment will you make to yourself, from today, to promote a healthier, happier, more energized life?

The journey from chronic illness back to health is one that hundreds of people have now made. The principles covered in this book come from my own experience and the experiences of patients who have successfully used functional medicine to address their health. The HOPE method evolved from the recognition that people need correct knowledge on health, support, and accountability to make a lasting change for themselves. What matters most is taking that first step. The body has a remarkable capacity to heal when given the right support and when the obstacles to healing are removed.

Thank you for taking the time to read this book!

For more information about the HOPE Method or our program, please scan the QR code below or visit our website.

www.drjudym.com

Yours in health,
Dr. Judy Magalhaes, PHARMD, BCGP, CDCES

This poem was given to me by my grandmother when I was young. It helped me to remember that God is always there for us- especially during our most difficult times (and I've had my share of these). I hope this poem gives you peace, knowing you are not alone.

FOOTPRINTS IN THE SAND

One night, I dreamed a dream.
As I was walking along the beach with my Lord.
Across the dark sky flashed scenes from my life.
For each scene, I noticed two sets of footprints in the sand,
One belonging to me and one to my Lord.

After the last scene of my life flashed before me,
I looked back at the footprints in the sand.
I noticed that at many times along the path of my life,
especially at the very lowest and saddest times,
there was only one set of footprints.

This really troubled me, so I asked the Lord about it.
"Lord, you said once I decided to follow you,
You'd walk with me all the way.
But I noticed that during the saddest and most troublesome
times of my life, there was only one set of footprints.
I don't understand why, when I needed You the most, You would
leave me."

He whispered, "My precious child, I love you
and will never leave you
Never, ever, during your trials and testings.
When you saw only one set of footprints,
It was then that I carried you."

Author Unknown.

CONSENT TO CURE

REFERENCE LIST

For readers who wish to dive deeper into the scientific literature behind these concepts, links to the complete reference list is accessible at my website **drjudym.com**

From Chapter 1 – An Introduction To Holistic Health

1] Watson, K. B., Wiltz, J. L., Nhim, K., Kaufmann, R. B., Thomas, C. W., & Greenlund, K. J. (2025). *Trends in multiple chronic conditions among US adults, by life stage, Behavioral Risk Factor Surveillance System*, 2013–2023. Preventing Chronic Disease, 22, E240539. https://doi.org/10.5888/pcd22.240539

https://www.cdc.gov/pcd/issues/2025/24_0539.htm

2] Jokanovic N, Tan EC, Dooley MJ, Kirkpatrick CM, Bell JS. *Prevalence and factors associated with polypharmacy in long-term care facilities: a systematic review.* J Am Med Dir Assoc. 2015 Jun 1;16(6):535.e1-12. doi: 10.1016/j.jamda.2015.03.003. Epub 2015 Apr 11. PMID: 25869992.

https://pubmed.ncbi.nlm.nih.gov/25869992/

3] The Nutrition Source, *Simple Steps to Preventing Diabetes*, no author, no year. Collected 9th Sept. 2025, 5:30 pm. EST.

https://nutritionsource.hsph.harvard.edu/disease-prevention/diabetes-prevention/preventing-diabetes-full-story/

4] Tarakeshwar N, Vanderwerker LC, Paulk E, Pearce MJ, Kasl SV, Prigerson HG. *Religious coping is associated with the quality of life of patients with advanced cancer.* J Palliat Med. 2006 Jun;9(3):646-57. doi: 10.1089/jpm.2006.9.646. PMID: 16752970; PMCID: PMC2504357.

https://pubmed.ncbi.nlm.nih.gov/16752970/

5] Abrignani V, Salvo A, Pacinella G, Tuttolomondo A. *The Mediterranean Diet, Its Microbiome Connections, and Cardiovascular Health: A Narrative Review.* Int J Mol Sci. 2024 Apr 30;25(9):4942. doi: 10.3390/ijms25094942. PMID: 38732161; PMCID: PMC11084172.

https://pubmed.ncbi.nlm.nih.gov/38732161/

From Chapter 2 – The Chronic Disease Epidemic

1] World Health Organization. (n.d.). *Noncommunicable diseases.* Retrieved September 8, 2025, from

https://www.who.int/health-topics/noncommunicable-diseases#tab=tab_1

2] National Cancer Institute. (n.d.). *Disease.* In Dictionary of Cancer Terms. Retrieved September 8, 2025, from

https://www.cancer.gov/publications/dictionaries/cancer-terms/def/disease

3] Quagliani D, Felt-Gunderson P. *Closing America's Fiber Intake Gap: Communication Strategies From a Food and Fiber Summit.* Am J Lifestyle Med. 2016 Jul 7;11(1):80-85. doi: 10.1177/1559827615588079. PMID: 30202317; PMCID: PMC6124841.

https://pubmed.ncbi.nlm.nih.gov/30202317/

4] Tristan Asensi M, Napoletano A, Sofi F, Dinu M. *Low-Grade Inflammation and Ultra-Processed Foods Consumption: A Review.* Nutrients. 2023 Mar 22;15(6):1546. doi: 10.3390/nu15061546. PMID: 36986276; PMCID: PMC10058108.

https://pubmed.ncbi.nlm.nih.gov/36986276/

5] Wiertsema SP, van Bergenhenegouwen J, Garssen J, Knippels LMJ. *The Interplay between the Gut Microbiome and the Immune System in the Context of Infectious Diseases throughout Life and the Role of Nutrition in Optimizing Treatment Strategies.* Nutrients. 2021 Mar 9;13(3):886. doi: 10.3390/nu13030886. PMID: 33803407; PMCID: PMC8001875.

https://pubmed.ncbi.nlm.nih.gov/33803407/

6] El-Zawawy HT, Farag HF, Tolba MM, Abdalsamea HA. *Improving Hashimoto's thyroiditis by eradicating Blastocystis hominis: Relation to IL-17. Therapeutic Advances in Endocrinology and Metabolism.* 2020;11. doi:10.1177/2042018820907013

https://pmc.ncbi.nlm.nih.gov/articles/PMC7036484/

7] Bertalot, G., Montresor, G., Tampieri, M., Spasiano, A., Pedroni, M., Milanesi, B., Fa-vret, M., Manca, N., & Negrini, R. (2004). *Decrease in thyroid autoantibodies after eradication of Helicobacter pylori infection.* Clinical Endocrinology, 61(6), 649–653. https://doi.org/10.1111/j.1365-2265.2004.02137.x

https://pubmed.ncbi.nlm.nih.gov/15521972/

8] Blue Cross, Blue Shield, *Early-Onset Dementia and Alzheimer's Rates Grow for Younger American Adults*

https://www.bcbs.com/news-and-insights/report/early-onset-dementia-alzheimers-disease-affecting-younger-american-adults

9] Alzheimer's Association, 2019 *Alzheimer's Disease and Facts And Figures*, 2019 Alzheimer's Disease Facts and Figures Report

https://www.alz.org/getmedia/4be8a3fe-b60d-4349-b167-8db03b16e272/alzheimers-facts-and-figures-2019-r.pdf

10] Gibbs T, Sabine N. *Chronic Disease Management and the Healthcare Workforce.* Dela J Public Health. 2022 Dec 31;8(5):176-196. doi: 10.32481/djph.2022.12.043. PMID: 36751614; PMCID: PMC9894075.

https://pmc.ncbi.nlm.nih.gov/articles/PMC9894075/

From Chapter 3 – All Disease Begins In The Gut

1] Human Microbiome Project Data Coordination Center. (n.d.). *Overview.* Retrieved August 14, 2025, from

https://www.hmpdacc.org/overview/

https://commonfund.nih.gov/hmp

2] Ursell LK, Metcalf JL, Parfrey LW, Knight R. *Defining the human microbiome.* Nutr Rev. 2012 Aug;70 Suppl 1(Suppl 1):S38-44. doi: 10.1111/j.1753-4887.2012.00493.x. PMID: 22861806; PMCID: PMC3426293.

https://pubmed.ncbi.nlm.nih.gov/22861806/

3] Jean Guy LeBlanc, Christian Milani, Graciela Savoy de Giori, Fernando Sesma, Douwe van Sinderen, Marco Ventura, *Bacteria as vitamin suppliers to their host: a gut microbiota perspective*, Current Opinion in Biotechnology, Volume 24, Issue 2, 2013, Pages 160-

168, ISSN 0958-1669, https://doi.org/10.1016/j.copbio.2012.08.005.

https://www.sciencedirect.com/science/article/pii/S095816691200119X

4] Mousa WK, Chehadeh F, Husband S. *Microbial dysbiosis in the gut drives systemic autoimmune diseases.* Front Immunol. 2022 Oct 20;13:906258. doi: 10.3389/fimmu.2022.906258. PMID: 36341463; PMCID: PMC9632986.

https://pmc.ncbi.nlm.nih.gov/articles/PMC9632986/

5] Gao Fangfang, Cheng Canyu, Li Runwei, Chen Zongcun, Tang Ke, Du Guankui, *The role of Akkermansia muciniphila in maintaining health: a bibliometric study*, Frontiers in Medicine, Volume 12 – 2025. DOI=10.3389/fmed.2025.1484656 ISSN=2296-858X

https://www.frontiersin.org/journals/medicine/articles/10.3389/fmed.2025.1484656

6] Pasta A, Formisano E, Calabrese F, Plaz Torres MC, Bodini G, Marabotto E, Pisciotta L, Giannini EG, Furnari M. *Food Intolerances, Food Allergies, and IBS: Lights and Shadows.* Nutrients. 2024 Jan 16;16(2):265. doi: 10.3390/nu16020265. PMID: 38257158; PMCID: PMC10821155.

https://pmc.ncbi.nlm.nih.gov/articles/PMC10821155/

7] Yoon SJ, Yu JS, Min BH, Gupta H, Won SM, Park HJ, Han SH, Kim BY, Kim KH, Kim BK, Joung HC, Park TS, Ham YL, Lee DY, Suk KT. *Bifidobacterium-derived short-chain fatty acids and indole compounds attenuate nonalcoholic fatty liver disease by modulating the gut-liver axis.* Front Microbiol. 2023 Mar 1;14:1129904. doi: 10.3389/fmicb.2023.1129904. PMID: 36937300; PMCID: PMC10014915.

https://pubmed.ncbi.nlm.nih.gov/36937300/

8] Stuivenberg GA, Burton JP, Bron PA, Reid G. *Why Are Bifidobacteria Important for Infants?* Microorganisms. 2022 Jan 25;10(2):278. doi: 10.3390/microorganisms10020278. PMID: 35208736; PMCID: PMC8880231.

https://pubmed.ncbi.nlm.nih.gov/35208736/

9] Brenner DM, Chey WD. Bifidobacterium infantis 35624: *a novel probiotic for the treatment of irritable bowel syndrome.* Rev Gastroenterol Disord. 2009 Winter;9(1):7-15. PMID: 19367213.

https://pubmed.ncbi.nlm.nih.gov/19367213/

10] Ahmad SR, AlShahrani AM, Kumari A. *Effects of Probiotic Supplementation on Depressive Symptoms, Sleep Quality, and Modulation of Gut Microbiota and Inflammatory Biomarkers: A Randomized Controlled Trial.* Brain Sci. 2025 Jul 18;15(7):761. doi: 10.3390/brainsci15070761. PMID: 40722352; PMCID: PMC12293967.

https://pubmed.ncbi.nlm.nih.gov/40722352/

11] Muguerza-Rodríguez L, Mier A, Ponce-González JG, Casals C, Corral-Pérez J. *Systematic Review on the Importance of Gut Microbiota in the Regulation of Type 2 Diabetes Through Physical Activity and Exercise.* Curr Issues Mol Biol. 2025 Jul 1;47(7):505. doi: 10.3390/cimb47070505. PMID: 40728974; PMCID: PMC12293346.

https://pubmed.ncbi.nlm.nih.gov/40728974/

12] Wexler HM. *Bacteroides: the good, the bad, and the nitty-gritty. Clin Microbiol* Rev. 2007 Oct;20(4):593-621. doi: 10.1128/CMR.00008-07. PMID: 17934076; PMCID: PMC2176045.

https://pubmed.ncbi.nlm.nih.gov/17934076/

13] Augustynowicz G, Lasocka M, Szyller HP, Dziedziak M, Mytych A, Braksator J, Pytrus T. *The Role of Gut Microbiota in the Development and Treatment of Obesity and Overweight: A Literature Review.* J Clin Med. 2025 Jul 11;14(14):4933. doi: 10.3390/jcm14144933. PMID: 40725626; PMCID: PMC12295081.

https://pubmed.ncbi.nlm.nih.gov/40725626/

14] El-Kholy O, Nichols L, Elsayed AAR, Basson MD. *The Correlation Between Carbohydrate Loading Diet and Gut Microbiome: A Systematic Review. Microbiologyopen.* 2025 Aug;14(4):e70045. doi: 10.1002/mbo3.70045. PMID: 40765268; PMCID: PMC12326083:

https://pubmed.ncbi.nlm.nih.gov/40765268/

15] Diagnostic Solutions Lab. (n.d.). *GI-MAP interpretive guide.* Retrieved August 14, 2025, from https://www.diagnosticsolutionslab.com/assets/documents/gi-map-interpretive-guide.pdf

16] Ju T, Bourrie BCT, Forgie AJ, Pepin DM, Tollenaar S, Sergi CM, Willing BP. *The Gut Commensal Escherichia coli Aggravates High-Fat-Diet-Induced Obesity and Insulin Resistance in Mice.* Appl Environ Microbiol. 2023 Mar 29;89(3):e0162822. doi: 10.1128/aem.01628-22. Epub 2023 Feb 21. PMID: 36809030; PMCID: PMC10057047.

https://pubmed.ncbi.nlm.nih.gov/36809030/

17] Seto T, Grondin JA, Khan WI. *Food Additives: Emerging Detrimental Roles on Gut Health.* FASEB J. 2025 Jul 15;39(13):e70810. doi: 10.1096/fj.202500737R. PMID: 40622070; PMCID: PMC12232514.

https://pubmed.ncbi.nlm.nih.gov/40622070/

18] Kidangathazhe A, Amponsah T, Maji A, Adams S, Chettoor M, Wang X, Scaria J. *Synthetic vs. non-synthetic sweeteners: their differential effects on gut microbiome diversity and function.* Front Microbiol. 2025 May 15;16:1531131. doi: 10.3389/fmicb.2025.1531131. PMID: 40443994; PMCID: PMC12119465.

https://pubmed.ncbi.nlm.nih.gov/40443994/

19] Foster DM, Kellum JA. *Endotoxic Septic Shock: Diagnosis and Treatment.* Int J Mol Sci. 2023 Nov 10;24(22):16185. doi: 10.3390/ijms242216185. PMID: 38003374; PMCID: PMC10671446.

https://pubmed.ncbi.nlm.nih.gov/38003374/

20] Kalyan M, Tousif AH, Sonali S, Vichitra C, Sunanda T, Praveenraj SS, Ray B, Gorantla VR, Rungratanawanich W, Mahalakshmi AM, Qoronfleh MW, Monaghan TM, Song BJ, Essa MM, Chidambaram SB. *Role of Endogenous Lipopolysaccharides in Neurological Disorders.* Cells. 2022 Dec 14;11(24):4038. doi: 10.3390/cells11244038. PMID: 36552802; PMCID: PMC9777235.

https://pubmed.ncbi.nlm.nih.gov/36552802/

21] *Proton pump inhibitors affect the gut microbiome Floris Imhann,* Marc Jan Bonder, Arnau Vich Vila, Jingyuan Fu, Zlatan Mujagic, Lisa Vork, Ettje F Tigchelaar, Soesma A Jankipersadsing, Maria

Carmen Cenit,2 Hermie J M Harmsen, Gerard Dijkstra, Lude Franke, Ramnik J Xavier, Daisy Jonkers, Cisca Wijmenga, Rinse K Weersma, Alexandra Zhernakova, Received 16 July 2015 Revised 28 October 2015 Accepted 30 October 2015 Published Online First 9 December 2015.

https://gut.bmj.com/content/gutjnl/65/5/740.full.pdf

22] Ray H, Khatum J, Haldar S, Bhowmik P. *Second brain: reviewing the gut microbiome's role in lifestyle diseases.* BioTechnologia (Pozn). 2025 Mar 31;106(1):103-122. doi: 10.5114/bta/195495. PMID: 40401130; PMCID: PMC12089934.

https://pubmed.ncbi.nlm.nih.gov/40401130/

23] Christine Fülling, Timothy G. Dinan, John F. Cryan, *Gut Microbe to Brain Signaling: What Happens in Vagus...,* Neuron, Volume 101, Issue 6, 2019, Pages 998-1002, ISSN 0896-6273, https://doi.org/10.1016/j.neuron.2019.02.008

https://www.sciencedirect.com/science/article/pii/S0896627319301175

24] Carabotti M, Scirocco A, Maselli MA, Severi C. *The gut-brain axis: interactions between enteric microbiota, central and enteric nervous systems.* Ann Gastroenterol. 2015 Apr-Jun;28(2):203-209. PMID: 25830558; PMCID: PMC4367209.

https://pubmed.ncbi.nlm.nih.gov/25830558/

25] Fatima SN, Arif F, Khalid R, Khan M, Naseem K. *Immunomodulatory role of gut microbiota in autoimmune disorders and the advancement of gut microbiota-based therapeutic strategies.* Microb Pathog. 2025 Oct;207:107882. doi: 10.1016/j.micpath.2025.107882. Epub 2025 Jul 9. PMID: 40645350.

https://pubmed.ncbi.nlm.nih.gov/40645350/

26] Zhang T, Guo F, Zhang C, Xiang Y. *Decoding the role of gut mycobiota in immune regulation and disease.* Virulence. 2025 Dec;16(1):2541704. doi: 10.1080/21505594.2025.2541704. Epub 2025 Aug 17. PMID: 40820365; PMCID: PMC12363511.

https://pubmed.ncbi.nlm.nih.gov/40820365/

27] Jawamis A, Al-Domi H, Al Sarayreh N. *Effect of dietary fat intake on metabolic endotoxemia: Mechanisms and clinical insights.*

Clin Nutr ESPEN. 2025 Jul 28;69:415-420. doi: 10.1016/j.clnesp.2025.07.1124. Epub ahead of print. PMID: 40738208.

https://pubmed.ncbi.nlm.nih.gov/40738208/

28] Baddam S, Burns B. *Systemic Inflammatory Response Syndrome.* 2025 Jun 20. In: StatPearls [Internet]. Treasure Island (FL): StatPearls Publishing; 2025 Jan–. PMID: 31613449.

https://pubmed.ncbi.nlm.nih.gov/31613449/

29] Gogesch P, Ortega Iannazzo S, Rupp N, Rom J, Kreuz M, Reiche K, Anzaghe M, Waibler Z; imSAVAR Consortium. *Immune cells play a critical role in cytokine- and endotoxin-mediated endothelial permeability.* PLoS One. 2025 Aug 14;20(8):e0329700. doi: 10.1371/journal.pone.0329700. PMID: 40811745; PMCID: PMC12352842.

https://pubmed.ncbi.nlm.nih.gov/40811745/

30] Parantainen J, Barreto G, Strandberg TE, Mars N, Nurmi K, Eklund KK. *Increased intestinal mucosal permeability and metabolic endotoxemia predict the risk of cardiovascular mortality.* Atherosclerosis. 2025 Jun;405:119220. doi: 10.1016/j.atherosclerosis.2025.119220. Epub 2025 Apr 26. PMID: 40319651.

https://pubmed.ncbi.nlm.nih.gov/40319651/

31] Pouramir A, Nosratiyan N, Askari H, Ghasemi-Kasman M, Shirzad M, Pouramir M. *Arbutin improves spatial learning and memory in a lipopolysaccharide-induced neuroinflammation model via attenuating of astrocytes activation and oxidative stress.* Neurosci Lett. 2025 Aug 11;865:138356. doi: 10.1016/j.neulet.2025.138356. Epub ahead of print. PMID: 40803547.

https://pubmed.ncbi.nlm.nih.gov/40803547/

32] Elbehiry A, Marzouk E, Aldubaib M, Abalkhail A, Anagreyyah S, Anajirih N, Almuzaini AM, Rawway M, Alfadhel A, Draz A, Abu-Okail A. *Helicobacter pylori Infection: Current Status and Future Prospects on Diagnostic, Therapeutic and Control Challenges.* Antibiotics (Basel). 2023 Jan 17;12(2):191. doi: 10.3390/antibiotics12020191. PMID: 36830102; PMCID: PMC9952126.

https://pmc.ncbi.nlm.nih.gov/articles/PMC9952126/

33] Carabotti M, Annibale B, Lahner E. *Common Pitfalls in the Management of Patients with Micronutrient Deficiency: Keep in Mind the*

Stomach. Nutrients. 2021 Jan 13;13(1):208. doi: 10.3390/nu13010208. PMID: 33450823; PMCID: PMC7828248.

https://pubmed.ncbi.nlm.nih.gov/33450823/

34] Sun LJ, Li JN, Nie YZ. *Gut hormones in microbiota-gut-brain cross-talk. Chin Med J (Engl).* 2020 Apr 5;133(7):826-833. doi: 10.1097/CM9.0000000000000706. PMID: 32132364; PMCID: PMC7147657.

https://pubmed.ncbi.nlm.nih.gov/32132364/

35] Magne F, Gotteland M, Gauthier L, Zazueta A, Pesoa S, Navarrete P, Balamurugan R. *The Firmicutes/Bacteroidetes Ratio: A Relevant Marker of Gut Dysbiosis in Obese Patients*? Nutrients. 2020 May 19;12(5):1474. doi: 10.3390/nu12051474. PMID: 32438689; PMCID: PMC7285218.

https://pubmed.ncbi.nlm.nih.gov/32438689/

From Chapter 4 – Gut Imbalances And Chronic Disease

1] Hou K, Wu Z-X, Chen X-Y, Wang J-Q, Zhang D, Xiao C, Zhu D, Koya JB, Wei L, Li J, Chen Z-S. *Microbiota in health and diseases.* Signal Transduction and Targeted Therapy. 2022;7(1):135. doi:10.1038/s41392-022-00974-4

https://www.nature.com/articles/s41392-022-00974-4#Bib1

2] Stecher B. *The Roles of Inflammation, Nutrient Availability and the Commensal Microbiota in Enteric Pathogen Infection.* Microbiology Spectrum. 2015;3(3):MBP-0008-2014. doi:10.1128/microbiolspec.MBP-0008-2014

https://journals.asm.org/doi/10.1128/microbiolspec.mbp-0008-2014

3] Martel J, Chang S-H, Ko Y-F, Hwang T-L, Young JD, Ojcius DM. *Gut barrier disruption and chronic disease.* Trends in Endocrinology & Metabolism. 2022;33(4):247-265. doi:10.1016/j.tem.2022.01.002

https://pubmed.ncbi.nlm.nih.gov/35151560/

4] Magne F, Gotteland M, Gauthier L, Zazueta A, Pesoa S, Navarrete P, Balamurugan R. The Firmicutes/Bacteroidetes Ratio: *A Relevant Marker of Gut Dysbiosis in Obese Patients?* Nutrients. 2020

May 19;12(5):1474. doi: 10.3390/nu12051474. PMID: 32438689; PMCID: PMC7285218.

https://pubmed.ncbi.nlm.nih.gov/32438689/

5] Määttä AM, Salminen A, Pietiäinen M, Leskelä J, Palviainen T, Sattler W, Sinisalo J, Salomaa V, Kaprio J, Pussinen PJ. *Endotoxemia is associated with an adverse metabolic profile.* Innate Immun. 2021 Jan;27(1):3-14. doi: 10.1177/1753425920971702. Epub 2020 Nov 27. PMID: 33243051; PMCID: PMC7780360.

https://pmc.ncbi.nlm.nih.gov/articles/PMC7780360/

6] Moreira AP, Texeira TF, Ferreira AB, Peluzio Mdo C, Alfenas Rde C. *Influence of a high-fat diet on gut microbiota, intestinal permeability and metabolic endotoxaemia.* Br J Nutr. 2012 Sep;108(5):801-9. doi: 10.1017/S0007114512001213. Epub 2012 Apr 16. PMID: 22717075.

https://pubmed.ncbi.nlm.nih.gov/22717075/

7] Lassenius MI, Pietiläinen KH, Kaartinen K, Pussinen PJ, Syrjänen J, Forsblom C, Pörsti I, Rissanen A, Kaprio J, *Mustonen J, Groop PH, Lehto M; FinnDiane Study Group. Bacterial endotoxin activity in human serum is associated with dyslipidemia, insulin resistance, obesity, and chronic inflammation.* Diabetes Care. 2011 Aug;34(8):1809-15. doi: 10.2337/dc10-2197. Epub 2011 Jun 2. PMID: 21636801; PMCID: PMC3142060.

https://pubmed.ncbi.nlm.nih.gov/21636801/

8] Augustynowicz G, Lasocka M, Szyller HP, Dziedziak M, Mytych A, Braksator J, Pytrus T. *The Role of Gut Microbiota in the Development and Treatment of Obesity and Overweight: A Literature Review.* J Clin Med. 2025 Jul 11;14(14):4933. doi: 10.3390/jcm14144933. PMID: 40725626; PMCID: PMC12295081.

https://pubmed.ncbi.nlm.nih.gov/40725626/

9] Arukha AP, Nayak S, Swain DM. *Effect of Akkermansia muciniphila on GLP-1 and Insulin Secretion.* Nutrients. 2025 Jul 31;17(15):2516. doi: 10.3390/nu17152516. PMID: 40806100; PMCID: PMC12348610.

https://pubmed.ncbi.nlm.nih.gov/40806100/

10] Ke Z, Ma Q, Ye X, Jin Y, Wang Y, Zhao X, Su Z. *Oral delivery of GLP-1 peptide using recombinant Lactobacillus gasseri for the treatment of type 2 diabetes mellitus.* Microbiol Spectr. 2025 Aug 5;13(8):e0282824. doi: 10.1128/spectrum.02828-24. Epub 2025 Jun 18. PMID: 40530879; PMCID: PMC12323307.

https://pubmed.ncbi.nlm.nih.gov/40530879/

11] Jardon KM, Umanets A, Gijbels A, Trouwborst I, Hul GB, Siebelink E, Vliex LMM, Bastings JJAJ, Argamasilla R, Chenal E, Venema K, Afman LA, Goossens GH, Blaak EE. *Distinct gut microbiota and metabolome features of tissue-specific insulin resistance in overweight and obesity.* Gut Microbes. 2025 Dec;17(1):2501185. doi: 10.1080/19490976.2025.2501185. Epub 2025 May 7. PMID: 40336254; PMCID: PMC12064058.

https://pubmed.ncbi.nlm.nih.gov/40336254/

12] Alang N, Kelly CR. *Weight gain after fecal microbiota transplantation.* Open Forum Infect Dis. 2015 Feb 4;2(1):ofv004. doi: 10.1093/ofid/ofv004. PMID: 26034755; PMCID: PMC4438885.

https://pubmed.ncbi.nlm.nih.gov/26034755/

13] Ribeiro G, Schellekens H, Cuesta-Marti C, Maneschy I, Ismael S, Cuevas-Sierra A, Martínez JA, Silvestre MP, Marques C, Moreira-Rosário A, Faria A, Moreno LA, Calhau C. *A menu for microbes: unraveling appetite regulation and weight dynamics through the microbiota-brain connection across the lifespan.* Am J Physiol Gastrointest Liver Physiol. 2025 Mar 1;328(3):G206-G228. doi: 10.1152/ajpgi.00227.2024. Epub 2025 Jan 15. PMID: 39811913.

https://pubmed.ncbi.nlm.nih.gov/39811913/.

14] Cani, Patrice D., Emilie Moens de Hase, and Matthias Van Hul. 2021. *"Gut Microbiota and Host Metabolism: From Proof of Concept to Therapeutic Intervention"* Microorganisms 9, no. 6: 1302. *https://doi.org/10.3390/microorganisms9061302*

https://www.mdpi.com/2076-2607/9/6/1302.

15] Heaney RP. *"Vitamin D in health and disease."* Clinical Journal of the American Society of Nephrology 3, no. 5 (2008): 1535–1541. https://doi.org/10.2215/CJN.01160308.

https://pmc.ncbi.nlm.nih.gov/articles/PMC4571146/

16] Vigna L, Speciani MC, Tirelli AS, Bravi F, La Vecchia C, Conte C, Gori F. *"Vitamin D and metabolic syndrome in working age subjects from an obesity clinic." Nutrients* 15, no. 18 (2023): 4048. https://doi.org/10.3390/nu15184048.

https://www.mdpi.com/2072-6643/15/20/4354

17] Almetwazi MS, Noor AO, Almasri DM, Popovici I, Alhawassi T, Alburikan KA, Harrington CA. *The association of vitamin D deficiency and glucose control among diabetic patients.* Saudi Pharm J. 2017 Dec;25(8):1179-1183. doi: 10.1016/j.jsps.2017.09.001. Epub 2017 Sep 12. PMID: 30166907; PMCID: PMC6111131.

https://pubmed.ncbi.nlm.nih.gov/30166907/

18] Kazemian N, Mahmoudi M, Halperin F, Wu JC, Pakpour S. *Gut microbiota and cardiovascular disease: opportunities and challenges.* Microbiome. 2020 Mar 14;8(1):36. doi: 10.1186/s40168-020-00821-0. PMID: 32169105; PMCID: PMC7071638.

https://pubmed.ncbi.nlm.nih.gov/32169105/

19] Liu H, Chen X, Hu X, Niu H, Tian R, Wang H, Pang H, Jiang L, Qiu B, Chen X, Zhang Y, Ma Y, Tang S, Li H, Feng S, Zhang S, Zhang C. *Alterations in the gut microbiome and metabolism with coronary artery disease severity.* Microbiome. 2019 Apr 26;7(1):68. doi: 10.1186/s40168-019-0683-9. PMID: 31027508; PMCID: PMC6486680.

https://pubmed.ncbi.nlm.nih.gov/31027508/

20] Hemmati M, Kashanipoor S, Mazaheri P, Alibabaei F, Babaeizad A, Asli S, Mohammadi S, Gorgin AH, Ghods K, Yousefi B, Eslami M. *Importance of gut microbiota metabolites in the development of cardiovascular diseases (CVD).* Life Sci. 2023 Sep 15;329:121947. doi: 10.1016/j.lfs.2023.121947. Epub 2023 Jul 16. PMID: 37463653.

https://pubmed.ncbi.nlm.nih.gov/37463653/

21] Witkowski M, Weeks TL, Hazen SL. *Gut Microbiota and Cardiovascular Disease.* Circ Res. 2020 Jul 31;127(4):553-570. doi: 10.1161/CIRCRESAHA.120.316242. Epub 2020 Jul 30. PMID: 32762536; PMCID: PMC7416843.

https://pubmed.ncbi.nlm.nih.gov/32762536/

22] Łuc, M., Misiak, B., Pawłowski, M., Stańczykiewicz, B., Zabłocka, A., Szcześniak, D., Pałęga, A., & Rymaszewska, J. (2021). *Gut microbiota in dementia: Critical review of novel findings and*

their potential application. *Progress in Neuro-Psychopharmacology and Biological Psychiatry, 104*,
110039. https://doi.org/10.1016/j.pnpbp.2020.110039

https://www.sciencedirect.com/science/article/pii/S0278584620303559?via%3Dihub

23] Sepúlveda-Rivera V, Olivieri-Henry G, Morales-González H, Ruiz-Adames J, Herrero-Rivera C, Rentas-Echeverria A, Cardona-Berdecia V, Soler-Llompart C, Sala-Morales AC, Pérez-Montero G, Blanco-Ruiz E, Godoy-Vitorino F. *Gut microbiota distinguishes aging hispanics with Alzheimer's disease: associations with cognitive impairment and severity.* Sci Rep. 2025 Aug 5;15(1):28505. doi: 10.1038/s41598-025-13262-2. PMID: 40764790; PMCID: PMC12325907.

https://pubmed.ncbi.nlm.nih.gov/40764790/

24] Chen Y, Xu J, Chen Y. *Regulation of Neurotransmitters by the Gut Microbiota and Effects on Cognition in Neurological Disorders.* Nutrients. 2021 Jun 19;13(6):2099. doi: 10.3390/nu13062099. PMID: 34205336; PMCID: PMC8234057.

https://pubmed.ncbi.nlm.nih.gov/34205336/

25] Zhang, Yuan, Wanpeng Yu, Lei Zhang, Man Wang, and Wenguang Chang. 2022.*"The Interaction of Polyphenols and the Gut Microbiota in Neurodegenerative Diseases" Nutrients* 14, no. 24: 5373. https://doi.org/10.3390/nu14245373

https://www.mdpi.com/2072-6643/14/24/5373

26] Cheng LH, Liu YW, Wu CC, Wang S, Tsai YC. *Psychobiotics in mental health, neurodegenerative and neurodevelopmental disorders.* J Food Drug Anal. 2019 Jul;27(3):632-648. doi: 10.1016/j.jfda.2019.01.002. Epub 2019 Feb 10. PMID: 31324280; PMCID: PMC9307042.

https://pubmed.ncbi.nlm.nih.gov/31324280/

27] Cardona F, Andrés-Lacueva C, Tulipani S, Tinahones FJ, Queipo-Ortuño MI. *Benefits of polyphenols on gut microbiota and implications in human health.* J Nutr Biochem. 2013 Aug;24(8):1415-22. doi: 10.1016/j.jnutbio.2013.05.001. PMID: 23849454.

https://pubmed.ncbi.nlm.nih.gov/23849454/

28] Chattopadhyay I, Shankar EM. *SARS-CoV-2-Indigenous Microbiota Nexus: Does Gut Microbiota Contribute to Inflammation and Disease Severity in COVID-19?* Front Cell Infect Microbiol. 2021 Mar 11;11:590874. doi: 10.3389/fcimb.2021.590874. PMID: 33791231; PMCID: PMC8006403.

https://pubmed.ncbi.nlm.nih.gov/33791231/

29] Battaglini D, Robba C, Fedele A, Trancă S, Sukkar SG, Di Pilato V, Bassetti M, Giacobbe DR, Vena A, Patroniti N, Ball L, Brunetti I, Torres Martí A, Rocco PRM, Pelosi P. *The Role of Dysbiosis in Critically Ill Patients With COVID-19 and Acute Respiratory Distress Syndrome.* Front Med (Lausanne). 2021 Jun 4;8:671714. doi: 10.3389/fmed.2021.671714. PMID: 34150807; PMCID: PMC8211890.

https://pubmed.ncbi.nlm.nih.gov/34150807/

30] Rampelotto PH, Taufer CR, da Silva J. *The Role of Beneficial Microbiota in COVID-19: Insights from Key Bacterial Genera.* Microorganisms. 2025 Apr 29;13(5):1029. doi: 10.3390/microorganisms13051029. PMID: 40431202; PMCID: PMC12113938.

https://pubmed.ncbi.nlm.nih.gov/40431202/

31] Paray BA, Albeshr MF, Jan AT, Rather IA. *Leaky Gut and Autoimmunity: An Intricate Balance in Individuals Health and the Diseased State.* Int J Mol Sci. 2020 Dec 21;21(24):9770. doi: 10.3390/ijms21249770. PMID: 33371435; PMCID: PMC7767453.

https://pubmed.ncbi.nlm.nih.gov/33371435/

32] El-Zawawy HT, Farag HF, Tolba MM, Abdalsamea HA. *Improving Hashimoto's thyroiditis by eradicating Blastocystis hominis: Relation to IL-17.* Ther Adv Endocrinol Metab. 2020 Feb 21;11:2042018820907013. doi: 10.1177/2042018820907013. PMID: 32128107; PMCID: PMC7036484.

https://pubmed.ncbi.nlm.nih.gov/32128107/

33] Bertalot G, Montresor G, Tampieri M, Spasiano A, Pedroni M, Milanesi B, Favret M, Manca N, Negrini R. *Decrease in thyroid autoantibodies after eradication of Helicobacter pylori infection.* Clin Endocrinol (Oxf). 2004 Nov;61(5):650-2. doi: 10.1111/j.1365-2265.2004.02137.x. PMID: 15521972.

https://pubmed.ncbi.nlm.nih.gov/15521972/

34] Wang H, Zhang J, Yang M, Chen J, Yang X, Yang N, Zhao B. *Causal relationship between gut microbiome, immune cell, and systemic lupus erythematosus: A Mendelian randomization analysis. Medicine (Baltimore).* 2025 Aug 1;104(31):e43703. doi: 10.1097/MD.0000000000043703. PMID: 40760547; PMCID: PMC12323915.

https://pubmed.ncbi.nlm.nih.gov/40760547/

35] De Luca F, Shoenfeld Y. *The microbiome in autoimmune diseases.* Clin Exp Immunol. 2019 Jan;195(1):74-85. doi: 10.1111/cei.13158. PMID: 29920643; PMCID: PMC6300652.

https://pubmed.ncbi.nlm.nih.gov/29920643/

36] Zhang J, Wang T, Mao X, Hu X, Lv L, Qi H, Zheng L. *Biomarkers in body fluids and their detection techniques for human intestinal permeability assessment.* Clin Chem Lab Med. 2025 Aug 13;63(11):2115-2129. doi: 10.1515/cclm-2025-0318. PMID: 40793775.

https://pubmed.ncbi.nlm.nih.gov/40793775/

37] Inoue R, Suzuki K, Takaoka M, Narumi M, Naito Y. *Effects of Dietary Fiber Supplementation on Gut Microbiota and Bowel Function in Healthy Adults: A Randomized Controlled Trial.* Microorganisms. 2025 Sep 5;13(9):2068. doi: 10.3390/microorganisms13092068. PMID: 41011400; PMCID: PMC12471990.

https://pubmed.ncbi.nlm.nih.gov/41011400/

38] Fu Y, Wang Y, Gao H, Li D, Jiang R, Ge L, Tong C, Xu K. *Associations among Dietary Omega-3 Polyunsaturated Fatty Acids, the Gut Microbiota, and Intestinal Immunity.* Mediators Inflamm. 2021 Jan 2;2021:8879227. doi: 10.1155/2021/8879227. PMID: 33488295; PMCID: PMC7801035.

https://pubmed.ncbi.nlm.nih.gov/33488295/

39] Zeng Q, Zhu J, Hu Y, Su S, Chen J. *The critical role of diet, exercise, and sleep in shaping the gut microbiota of children with idiopathic short stature: a Retrospective study.* Front Immunol. 2025 Aug 1;16:1566722. doi: 10.3389/fimmu.2025.1566722. PMID: 40821812; PMCID: PMC12353712.

https://pubmed.ncbi.nlm.nih.gov/40821812/

40] Mohr AE, Mach N, Pugh J, Grosicki GJ, Allen JM, Karl JP, Whisner CM. *Mechanisms underlying alterations of the gut microbiota by exercise and their role in shaping ecological resilience.* FEMS Microbiol Rev. 2025 Jan 14;49:fuaf037. doi: 10.1093/femsre/fuaf037. PMID: 40796291; PMCID: PMC12366553.

https://pubmed.ncbi.nlm.nih.gov/40796291/

41] Shi S, Liu D, Baranova A, Cao H, Zhang F. *Investigating bidirectional causal relationships between gut microbiota and insomnia.* Gen Psychiatr. 2025 Aug 12;38(4):e101855. doi: 10.1136/gpsych-2024-101855. PMID: 40822499; PMCID: PMC12352136.

https://pubmed.ncbi.nlm.nih.gov/40822499/

From Chapter 5 – Finding Your Why

1] Wiertsema, S.P., van Bergenhenegouwen, J., Garssen, J., & Knippels, L.M.J. (2021). *The Interplay between the Gut Microbiome and the Immune System in the Context of Infectious Diseases throughout Life and the Role of Nutrition in Optimizing Treatment Strategies.* Nutrients, 13(3), 886. doi:10.3390/nu13030886

https://pubmed.ncbi.nlm.nih.gov/33803407/

2] Mahdavifar B, Hosseinzadeh M, Salehi-Abargouei A, Mirzaei M, Vafa M. *Dietary intake of B vitamins and their association with depression, anxiety, and stress symptoms: A cross-sectional, population-based survey.* J Affect Disord. 2021 Jun 1;288:92-98. doi: 10.1016/j.jad.2021.03.055. Epub 2021 Mar 26. PMID: 33848753.

https://pubmed.ncbi.nlm.nih.gov/33848753/

3] Grant, W.B., Al Anouti, F., Boucher, B.J., et al. *A Narrative Review of the Evidence for Variations in Serum 25-Hydroxyvitamin D Concentration Thresholds for Optimal Health. Nutrients.* 2022;14(3):639. doi:10.3390/nu14030639

https://pubmed.ncbi.nlm.nih.gov/35276999/

4] Al-khalidi, B., Kimball, S.M., Rotondi, M.A., Ardern, C.I. *Standardized serum 25-hydroxyvitamin D concentrations are inversely associated with cardiometabolic disease in U.S. adults: a cross-sectional analysis of NHANES, 2001–2010. Nutrition Journal.* 2017;16:16. doi:10.1186/s12937-017-0237-6

https://pubmed.ncbi.nlm.nih.gov/28241878/

5] Pludowski, P., Takacs, I., Boyanov, M., et al. *Clinical Practice in the Prevention, Diagnosis and Treatment of Vitamin D Deficiency: A Central and Eastern European Expert Consensus Statement.* Nutrients. 2022;14(7):1483. doi:10.3390/nu14071483

https://pubmed.ncbi.nlm.nih.gov/35406098/

From Chapter 6 – Food As Medicine

1] National Research Council (US) Committee on Nutrition in Medical Education. *Nutrition Education in U.S. Medical Schools.* Washington (DC): National Academies Press (US); 1985. 4, Current Programs. Available from:

https://www.ncbi.nlm.nih.gov/books/NBK216788/

2] Bhardwaj RL, Parashar A, Parewa HP, Vyas L. *An Alarming Decline in the Nutritional Quality of Foods: The Biggest Challenge for Future Generations' Health.* Foods. 2024 Mar 14;13(6):877. doi: 10.3390/foods13060877. PMID: 38540869; PMCID: PMC10969708.

https://pmc.ncbi.nlm.nih.gov/articles/PMC10969708/#abstract1

3] Grant, W.B., Al Anouti, F., Boucher, B.J., et al. *A Narrative Review of the Evidence for Variations in Serum 25-Hydroxyvitamin D Concentration Thresholds for Optimal Health.* Nutrients. 2022;14(3):639.

https://www.mdpi.com/2072-6643/14/3/639

4] Holick MF, Chen TC. *Vitamin D deficiency: a worldwide problem with health consequences.* Am J Clin Nutr. 2008 Apr;87(4):1080S-6S. doi: 10.1093/ajcn/87.4.1080S. PMID: 18400738.

https://pubmed.ncbi.nlm.nih.gov/18400738/

5] Al-khalidi, B., Kimball, S.M., Rotondi, M.A., Ardern, C.I. *Standardized serum 25-hydroxyvitamin D concentrations are inversely associated with cardiometabolic disease in U.S. adults.* Nutrition Journal. 2017;16:16.

https://pubmed.ncbi.nlm.nih.gov/28241878/

6] Pludowski P, Takacs I, Boyanov M, Belaya Z, Diaconu CC, Mokhort T, Zherdova N, Rasa I, Payer J, Pilz S. *Clinical Practice in the Prevention, Diagnosis and Treatment of Vitamin D Deficiency: A Central and Eastern European Expert Consensus Statement.* Nutrients. 2022 Apr 2;14(7):1483. doi: 10.3390/nu14071483. PMID: 35406098; PMCID: PMC9002638.

https://pubmed.ncbi.nlm.nih.gov/35406098/

7] Fan, L., et al. Magnesium *Depletion Score and Metabolic Syndrome in US Adults: Analysis of NHANES* 2003 to 2018.

https://pubmed.ncbi.nlm.nih.gov/38366015/

8] Zhang, H., Kuang, L., Wan, Q. *Higher magnesium depletion score increases the risk of all-cause and cardiovascular mortality in US adults with diabetes.* PLoS ONE. 2025.

https://pubmed.ncbi.nlm.nih.gov/38831178/

9] Nestle, Marion. (1993). *Food Lobbies, the Food Pyramid, and U.S. Nutrition Policy.* International journal of health services: planning, administration, evaluation. 23. 483-96. 10.2190/32F2-2PFB-MEG7-8HPU.

https://www.researchgate.net/publication/14823257_Food_Lobbies_the_Food_Pyramid_and_US_Nutrition_Policy

10] Ojeda-Belokon C, González-Palacios S, Compañ-Gabucio LM, Oncina-Cánovas A, García-de-la-Hera M, Vioque J, Torres-Collado L. *Adherence to Three Mediterranean Dietary Indexes and All-Cause, Cardiovascular, and Cancer Mortality in an Older Mediterranean Population.* Nutrients. 2025 Sep 13;17(18):2956. doi: 10.3390/nu17182956. PMID: 41010481; PMCID: PMC12472705.

https://pubmed.ncbi.nlm.nih.gov/41010481/

11] Kearns, C. E., Schmidt, L. A., & Glantz, S. A. (2016). *Sugar industry and coronary heart disease research: a historical analysis of internal industry documents. JAMA Internal Medicine,* 176(11), 1680-1685.

https://pubmed.ncbi.nlm.nih.gov/27617709/

12] The Washington Post, *Eating Lab, Many of today's unhealthy foods were brought to you by Big Tobacco,* September 19, 2023, by Anahad O'Connor.

https://www.washingtonpost.com/wellness/2023/09/19/addiction-foods-hyperpalatable-tobacco/

13] Environmental Working Group. Available at:

https://www.ewg.org

14] Stavropoulou, E., Bezirtzoglou, E., Papadaki, A., & Dimitriou, M. (2024). *Autoimmune protocol diet: A personalized elimination diet for patients with autoimmune diseases.* Clinical Nutrition ESPEN, 62, 124-134.

https://www.sciencedirect.com/science/article/pii/S2589936824000744

From Chapter 7 – The Transformative Power Of Sleep

1] Patel AK, Reddy V, Shumway KR, et al. Physiology, *Sleep Stages*. [Updated 2024 Jan 26]. In: StatPearls [Internet]. Treasure Island (FL): StatPearls Publishing; 2025 Jan-. Available from:

https://www.ncbi.nlm.nih.gov/books/NBK526132/

2] Centers for Disease Control and Prevention. (n.d.). *About sleep.*

https://www.cdc.gov/sleep/about/?CDC_AAref_Val=https://www.cdc.gov/sleep/about_sleep/how_much_sleep.html

3] Centers for Disease Control and Prevention. (n.d.). *FastStats: Sleep in adults.*

https://www.cdc.gov/sleep/data-research/facts-stats/adults-sleep-facts-and-stats.html

4] Office of Disease Prevention and Health Promotion. (n.d.). *Sleep. Healthy People 2030.*

https://odphp.health.gov/healthypeople/objectives-and-data/browse-objectives/sleep

5] Centers for Disease Control and Prevention. (n.d.). *BRFSS Prevalence & Trends Data.*

https://www.cdc.gov/brfss/brfssprevalence/index.html

6] Liu Y, Wheaton AG, Chapman DP, Cunningham TJ, Lu H, Croft JB. *Prevalence of Healthy Sleep Duration among Adults*--United States, 2014. MMWR Morb Mortal Wkly Rep. 2016 Feb 19;65(6):137-41. doi: 10.15585/mmwr.mm6506a1. PMID: 26890214.

https://pubmed.ncbi.nlm.nih.gov/26890214/

7] Grandner MA, Patel NP. *From sleep duration to mortality: implications of meta-analysis and future directions.* J Sleep Res. 2009 Jun;18(2):145-7. doi: 10.1111/j.1365-2869.2009.00753.x. PMID: 19645959; PMCID: PMC3685145.

https://pmc.ncbi.nlm.nih.gov/articles/PMC3685145/

8] Rahelić V, Perković T, Romić L, Perković P, Klobučar S, Pavić E, Rahelić D. *The Role of Behavioral Factors on Chronic Diseases-Practice and Knowledge Gaps.* Healthcare (Ba-sel). 2024 Dec 12;12(24):2520. doi: 10.3390/healthcare12242520. PMID: 39765947; PMCID: PMC11675894. The Role of Behavioral Factors on Chronic Diseases—Practice and Knowledge Gaps - PMC

https://pubmed.ncbi.nlm.nih.gov/39765947/

9] Alfikany M, Sakhr K, Kremers S, El Khatib S, Adam T, Meertens R. *The Role of Sex in the Impact of Sleep Restriction on Appetite- and Weight-Regulating Hormones in Healthy Adults: A Systematic Review of Human Studies.* Clocks Sleep. 2025 Jul 29;7(3):39. doi: 10.3390/clockssleep7030039. PMID: 40843663; PMCID: PMC12372055.

https://pubmed.ncbi.nlm.nih.gov/40843663/

10] Schüssler P, Uhr M, Ising M, Weikel JC, Schmid DA, Held K, Mathias S, Steiger A. *Nocturnal ghrelin, ACTH, GH and cortisol secretion after sleep deprivation in humans.* Psychoneuroendocrinology. 2006 Sep;31(8):915-23. doi: 10.1016/j.psyneuen.2006.05.002. Epub 2006 Jun 30. PMID: 16814473.

https://pubmed.ncbi.nlm.nih.gov/16814473/

11] Spiegel K, Tasali E, Penev P, Van Cauter E. *Brief communication: Sleep curtailment in healthy young men is associated with decreased leptin levels, elevated ghrelin levels, and increased hunger and appetite.* Ann Intern Med. 2004 Dec 7;141(11):846-50. doi: 10.7326/0003-4819-141-11-200412070-00008. PMID: 15583226.

https://pubmed.ncbi.nlm.nih.gov/15583226/

12] Nedeltcheva AV, Kilkus JM, Imperial J, Kasza K, Schoeller DA, Penev PD. *Sleep curtailment is accompanied by increased intake of calories from snacks.* Am J Clin Nutr. 2009 Jan;89(1):126-33. doi:

10.3945/ajcn.2008.26574. Epub 2008 Dec 3. PMID: 19056602; PMCID: PMC2615460.

https://pubmed.ncbi.nlm.nih.gov/19056602/

13] Schmid SM, Hallschmid M, Jauch-Chara K, Born J, Schultes B. *A single night of sleep deprivation increases ghrelin levels and feelings of hunger in normal-weight healthy men.* J Sleep Res. 2008 Sep;17(3):331-4. doi: 10.1111/j.1365-2869.2008.00662.x. Epub 2008 Jun 28. PMID: 18564298.

https://pubmed.ncbi.nlm.nih.gov/18564298/

14] Rogers EM, Banks NF, Jenkins NDM. *The effects of sleep disruption on metabolism, hunger, and satiety, and the influence of psychosocial stress and exercise: A narrative review.* Diabetes Metab Res Rev. 2024 Feb;40(2):e3667. doi: 10.1002/dmrr.3667. Epub 2023 Jun 2. PMID: 37269143.

https://pubmed.ncbi.nlm.nih.gov/37269143/

15] Maybrier HR, Jackson JJ, Toedebusch CD, Lucey BP, Head D. *Influence of sleep and cardiovascular health on cognitive trajectories in older adults.* Neurobiol Aging. 2025 Aug;152:34-42. doi: 10.1016/j.neurobiolaging.2025.04.008. Epub 2025 Apr 19. PMID: 40318496.

https://pubmed.ncbi.nlm.nih.gov/40318496/

16] Winer JR, Deters KD, Kennedy G, Jin M, Goldstein-Piekarski A, Poston KL, Mormino EC. *Association of Short and Long Sleep Duration With Amyloid-β Burden and Cognition in Aging.* JAMA Neurol. 2021 Oct 1;78(10):1187-1196. doi: 10.1001/jamaneurol.2021.2876. PMID: 34459862; PMCID: PMC8406215.

https://pubmed.ncbi.nlm.nih.gov/34459862/

17] Liu J, Yuan Q, Zhang Y, Wang X, Zhai L, Wang R, Zheng C, Hong Z. *Sleep health: an unappreciated key player in colorectal cancer.* J Cancer. 2025 Mar 3;16(6):1934-1943. doi: 10.7150/jca.107117. PMID: 40092705; PMCID: PMC11905398.

https://pubmed.ncbi.nlm.nih.gov/40092705/

18] Al-Farsi HY, Al-Fahdi EY, Al-Balushi MA, Al-Jahwari AN, Al-Maskari AM, Das S. *Sleep Disturbances Associated with Different Systems of the Body: Underlying Mechanisms Involved and Consequences.* Curr Med Chem. 2025 Apr 23. doi:

10.2174/0109298673350476250331181123. Epub ahead of print. PMID: 40277067.

https://pubmed.ncbi.nlm.nih.gov/40277067/

19] Carissa Gardiner, Jonathon Weakley, Louise M. Burke, Gregory D. Roach, Charli Sargent, Nirav Maniar, Minh Huynh, Dean J. Miller, Andrew Townshend, Shona L. Halson, *The effect of alcohol on subsequent sleep in healthy adults: A systematic review and meta-analysis*, Sleep Medicine Reviews, Volume 80, 2025, 102030, ISSN 1087-0792, https://doi.org/10.1016/j.smrv.2024.102030.

https://www.sciencedirect.com/science/article/pii/S1087079224001345

20] Lie JD, Tu KN, Shen DD, Wong BM. *Pharmacological Treatment of Insomnia.* P T. 2015 Nov;40(11):759-71. PMID: 26609210; PMCID: PMC4634348.

https://pubmed.ncbi.nlm.nih.gov/26609210/

21] Caballero-Gallardo K, Quintero-Rincón P, Olivero-Verbel J. *Aromatherapy and Essential Oils: Holistic Strategies in Complementary and Alternative Medicine for Integral Wellbeing.* Plants (Basel). 2025 Jan 29;14(3):400. doi: 10.3390/plants14030400. PMID: 39942962; PMCID: PMC11821193.

https://pubmed.ncbi.nlm.nih.gov/39942962/

22] Yu Y, Wang H, Li W, Guo H, Chen Y. *Non-pharmacological interventions for sleep in older adults: an umbrella review and evidence map of randomized controlled trials.* Front Neurol. 2025 Sep 2;16:1655192. doi: 10.3389/fneur.2025.1655192. PMID: 40963939; PMCID: PMC12439529.

https://pubmed.ncbi.nlm.nih.gov/40963939/

From Chapter 8 – Managing Stress For Resilience

1] Liu YZ, Wang YX, Jiang CL. Inflammation: *The Common Pathway of Stress-Related Diseases.* Front Hum Neurosci. 2017 Jun 20;11:316. doi: 10.3389/fnhum.2017.00316. PMID: 28676747; PMCID: PMC5476783.

https://pubmed.ncbi.nlm.nih.gov/28676747/

2] Lei AA, Phang VWX, Lee YZ, Kow ASF, Tham CL, Ho YC, Lee MT. *Chronic Stress-Associated Depressive Disorders: The Impact of HPA Axis Dysregulation and Neuroinflammation on the Hippocampus-A Mini Review.* Int J Mol Sci. 2025 Mar 24;26(7):2940. doi: 10.3390/ijms26072940. PMID: 40243556; PMCID: PMC11988747.

https://pubmed.ncbi.nlm.nih.gov/40243556/

3] Madison, A.A., & Bailey, M.T. *Stressed to the Core: Inflammation and Intestinal Permeability Link Stress-Related Gut Microbiota Shifts to Mental Health Outcomes. Biological Psychiatry*, 2024.

https://pubmed.ncbi.nlm.nih.gov/38353184/

4] Madison A, Kiecolt-Glaser JK. *Stress, depression, diet, and the gut microbiota: human-bacteria interactions at the core of psychoneuroimmunology and nutrition.* Curr Opin Behav Sci. 2019 Aug;28:105-110. doi: 10.1016/j.cobeha.2019.01.011. Epub 2019 Mar 25. PMID: 32395568; PMCID: PMC7213601.

https://pmc.ncbi.nlm.nih.gov/articles/PMC7213601/

5} Cryan JF, O'Riordan KJ, Cowan CSM, Sandhu KV, Bastiaanssen TFS, Boehme M, Codagnone MG, Cussotto S, Fulling C, Golubeva AV, Guzzetta KE, Jaggar M, Long-Smith CM, Lyte JM, Martin JA, Molinero-Perez A, Moloney G, Morelli E, Morillas E, O'Connor R, Cruz-Pereira JS, Peterson VL, Rea K, Ritz NL, Sherwin E, Spichak S, Teichman EM, van de Wouw M, Ventura-Silva AP, Wallace-Fitzsimons SE, Hyland N, Clarke G, Dinan TG. *The Microbiota-Gut-Brain Axis.* Physiol Rev. 2019 Oct 1;99(4):1877-2013. doi: 10.1152/physrev.00018.2018. PMID: 31460832.

https://pubmed.ncbi.nlm.nih.gov/31460832/

6] Guzzetta KE, Cryan JF, O'Leary OF. *Microbiota-Gut-Brain Axis Regulation of Adult Hippocampal Neurogenesis.* Brain Plast. 2022 Oct 21;8(1):97-119. doi: 10.3233/BPL-220141. PMID: 36448039; PMCID: PMC9661352.

https://pubmed.ncbi.nlm.nih.gov/36448039/

7] Roberts BL, Karatsoreos IN. *Brain-body responses to chronic stress: a brief review.* Fac Rev. 2021 Dec 16;10:83. doi: 10.12703/r/10-83. PMID: 35028648; PMCID: PMC8725649.

https://pmc.ncbi.nlm.nih.gov/articles/PMC8725649/

8] Silva YP, Bernardi A, Frozza RL. *The Role of Short-Chain Fatty Acids From Gut Microbiota in Gut-Brain Communication.* Front Endocrinol (Lausanne). 2020 Jan 31;11:25. doi: 10.3389/fendo.2020.00025. PMID: 32082260; PMCID: PMC7005631.

https://pmc.ncbi.nlm.nih.gov/articles/PMC7005631/

9] De Cillis F, Petrillo G, D'Aprile I, Marizzoni M, Saleri S, Mazzelli M, Zonca V, Di Benedetto MG, Riva MA, Cattaneo A. *Prenatal Stress Rewires the Gut-Brain Axis: Long-Term, Sex-Specific Effects on Microbiota, Intestinal Barrier, and Hippocampal Inflammation.* Nutrients. 2025 Aug 29;17(17):2812. doi: 10.3390/nu17172812. PMID: 40944198; PMCID: PMC12429922.

https://pubmed.ncbi.nlm.nih.gov/40944198/

10] Du D, Yuan Y, Guan X, Xie Q, Sun X, Dong Z. *Gut microbiota, circadian rhythms and their interactions: implications for the pathogenesis and treatment of depression.* Ann Med. 2025 Dec;57(1):2561222. doi: 10.1080/07853890.2025.2561222. Epub 2025 Sep 18. PMID: 40963403; PMCID: PMC12447470.

https://pubmed.ncbi.nlm.nih.gov/40963403/

11] National Center for Complementary and Integrative Health. (2024). *Mind and body approaches for stress and anxiety.*

https://www.nccih.nih.gov/health/providers/digest/mind-and-body-approaches-for-stress

12] Gherardi-Donato ECDS, Gimenez LBH, Fernandes MNF, Lacchini R, Camargo Júnior EB, Díaz-Serrano KV, Melchior M, Pérez RG, Riquelme-Galindo J, Reisdorfer E. *Mindfulness Practice Reduces Hair Cortisol, Anxiety and Perceived Stress in University Workers: Randomized Clinical Trial.* Healthcare (Basel). 2023 Oct 31;11(21):2875. doi: 10.3390/healthcare11212875. PMID: 37958019; PMCID: PMC10648523.

https://pmc.ncbi.nlm.nih.gov/articles/PMC10648523/

13] Song C, Ikei H, Park BJ, Lee J, Kagawa T, Miyazaki Y. *Psychological Benefits of Walking through Forest Areas.* Int J Environ Res Public Health. 2018 Dec 10;15(12):2804. doi: 10.3390/ijerph15122804. Erratum in: Int J Environ Res Public Health. 2020 Feb 18;17(4):E1316. doi: 10.3390/ijerph17041316. PMID: 30544682; PMCID: PMC6313311.

https://pubmed.ncbi.nlm.nih.gov/30544682/

14] Niles AN, Haltom KE, Mulvenna CM, Lieberman MD, Stanton AL. *Randomized controlled trial of expressive writing for psychological and physical health: the moderating role of emotional expressivity.* Anxiety Stress Coping. 2014 Jan;27(1):1-17. doi: 10.1080/10615806.2013.802308. Epub 2013 Jun 6. Erratum in: Anxiety Stress Coping. 2014 Jan;27(1):I. PMID: 23742666; PMCID: PMC3830620.

https://pmc.ncbi.nlm.nih.gov/articles/PMC3830620/

15] Bear T, Dalziel J, Coad J, Roy N, Butts C, Gopal P. *The Microbiome-Gut-Brain Axis and Resilience to Developing Anxiety or Depression under Stress.* Microorganisms. 2021 Mar 31;9(4):723. doi: 10.3390/microorganisms9040723. PMID: 33807290; PMCID: PMC8065970.

https://pubmed.ncbi.nlm.nih.gov/33807290/

16] Kim TW, Jeong JH, Hong SC. *The impact of sleep and circadian disturbance on hormones and metabolism.* Int J Endocrinol. 2015;2015:591729. doi: 10.1155/2015/591729. Epub 2015 Mar 11. PMID: 25861266; PMCID: PMC4377487.

https://pubmed.ncbi.nlm.nih.gov/25861266/

17] Madison A, Kiecolt-Glaser JK. *Stress, depression, diet, and the gut microbiota: human-bacteria interactions at the core of psychoneuroimmunology and nutrition.* Curr Opin Behav Sci. 2019 Aug;28:105-110. doi: 10.1016/j.cobeha.2019.01.011. Epub 2019 Mar 25. PMID: 32395568; PMCID: PMC7213601.

https://pubmed.ncbi.nlm.nih.gov/32395568/

18] Reilly CB, Bernier SG, Shahriar S, Horvath V, Lewandowski M, Javorsky E, Budnik B, Ingber DE. *Dietary flavonoids form supramolecular assemblies, alter biochemistry, and enhance cell resilience.* Front Nutr. 2025 Sep 2;12:1649867. doi: 10.3389/fnut.2025.1649867. PMID: 40964684; PMCID: PMC12439166.

https://pubmed.ncbi.nlm.nih.gov/40964684/

19] Johns Hopkins Medicine. *"Anti-Inflammatory Diet."* Johns Hopkins Medicine, https://www.hopkinsmedicine.org/health/wellness-and-prevention/anti-inflammatory-diet

20] Office of Dietary Supplements. (n.d.). *Magnesium.* National Institutes of Health.

https://ods.od.nih.gov/factsheets/Magnesium-HealthProfessional/

21] Office of Dietary Supplements. (2024). *Omega-3 fatty acids.* National Institutes of Health.

https://ods.od.nih.gov/factsheets/Omega3FattyAcids-HealthProfessional/

22] Zhou P, Chen C, Patil S, Dong S. *Unveiling the therapeutic symphony of probiotics, prebiotics, and postbiotics in gut-immune harmony.* Front Nutr. 2024 Feb 8;11:1355542. doi: 10.3389/fnut.2024.1355542. PMID: 38389798; PMCID: PMC10881654.

https://pmc.ncbi.nlm.nih.gov/articles/PMC10881654/

23] Sarkar A, Lehto SM, Harty S, Dinan TG, Cryan JF, Burnet PWJ. *Psychobiotics and the Manipulation of Bacteria-Gut-Brain Signals.* Trends Neurosci. 2016 Nov;39(11):763-781. doi: 10.1016/j.tins.2016.09.002. Epub 2016 Oct 25. PMID: 27793434; PMCID: PMC5102282.

https://pmc.ncbi.nlm.nih.gov/articles/PMC5102282/

24] Sears ME, Genuis SJ. *Environmental determinants of chronic disease and medical approaches: recognition, avoidance, supportive therapy, and detoxification.* J Environ Public Health. 2012;2012:356798. doi: 10.1155/2012/356798. Epub 2012 Jan 19. PMID: 22315626; PMCID: PMC3270432.

https://pmc.ncbi.nlm.nih.gov/articles/PMC3270432/

25] Green Science Policy Institute. (n.d.). *Six classes of harmful chemicals.*

https://greensciencepolicy.org/harmful-chemicals/

26] Warren, A., et al. *Dangers of the Chronic Stress Response in the Context of the Microbiota-Gut-Immune-Brain Axis and Mental Health: A Narrative Review. Frontiers in Immunology,* 2024.

https://pubmed.ncbi.nlm.nih.gov/38756771/

27] La Torre, D., et al. *Psychosocial Stress-Induced Intestinal Permeability in Healthy Humans: What Is the Evidence?* Neurobiology of Stress, 2023.

https://pubmed.ncbi.nlm.nih.gov/37842017/

From Chapter 9 – Movement Matters

1] U.S. Department of Health and Human Services. (2018). *Physical Activity Guidelines for Americans* (2nd ed.).

https://health.gov/sites/default/files/2019-09/Physical_Activity_Guidelines_2nd_edition.pdf

2] Yaribeygi H, Maleki M, Sathyapalan T, Jamialahmadi T, Sahebkar A. *Pathophysiology of Physical Inactivity-Dependent Insulin Resistance: A Theoretical Mechanistic Review Emphasizing Clinical Evidence.* J Diabetes Res. 2021 Oct 7;2021:7796727. doi: 10.1155/2021/7796727. PMID: 34660812; PMCID: PMC8516544.

https://pmc.ncbi.nlm.nih.gov/articles/PMC8516544/

3] Tian D, Meng J. *Exercise for Prevention and Relief of Cardiovascular Disease: Prognoses, Mechanisms, and Approaches.* Oxid Med Cell Longev. 2019 Apr 9;2019:3756750. doi: 10.1155/2019/3756750. PMID: 31093312; PMCID: PMC6481017.

https://pmc.ncbi.nlm.nih.gov/articles/PMC6481017/

4] Rusu L, Mihai TA, Schenker RA, Marin MI, Schenker M, Streba CT, Gheonea DI, Piele D. *The effect of physical exercises on TNF-a, IL-6, and IL-8 cytokines expression and NK cells in cancer.* Rom J Morphol Embryol. 2025 Jan-Mar;66(1):89-98. doi: 10.47162/RJME.66.1.08. PMID: 40384195; PMCID: PMC12236277.

https://pubmed.ncbi.nlm.nih.gov/40384195/

5] Lin TW, Kuo YM. *Exercise benefits brain function: the monoamine connection.* Brain Sci. 2013 Jan 11;3(1):39-53. doi: 10.3390/brainsci3010039. PMID: 24961306; PMCID: PMC4061837.

https://pubmed.ncbi.nlm.nih.gov/24961306/

6] Reynolds, A.N., Mann, J.I., Williams, S. *et al. Advice to walk after meals is more effective for lowering postprandial glycaemia in type 2 diabetes mellitus than advice that does not specify timing: a random-ised crossover study. Diabetologia* 59, 2572–2578 (2016). https://doi.org/10.1007/s00125-016-4085-2

https://link.springer.com/article/10.1007/s00125-016-4085-2#citeas

7] Van den Dungen P, Maas J. Natuur op recept *Nature prescriptions: is it time to bring more nature into healthcare?* Ned Tijdschr Geneeskd. 2025 Apr 10;169:D8444. Dutch. PMID: 40223755.

https://pubmed.ncbi.nlm.nih.gov/40223755/

8] Boecker H, Sprenger T, Spilker ME, Henriksen G, Koppenhoefer M, Wagner KJ, Valet M, Berthele A, Tolle TR. *The runner's high: opioidergic mechanisms in the human brain.* Cereb Cortex. 2008 Nov;18(11):2523-31. doi: 10.1093/cercor/bhn013. Epub 2008 Feb 21. PMID: 18296435.

https://pubmed.ncbi.nlm.nih.gov/18296435/

9] Meeusen R, De Meirleir K. *Exercise and brain neurotransmission. Sports Med.* 1995 Sep;20(3):160-88. doi: 10.2165/00007256-199520030-00004. PMID: 8571000.

https://pubmed.ncbi.nlm.nih.gov/8571000/

10] K.I. Erickson,M.W. Voss,R.S. Prakash,C. Basak,A. Szabo,L. Chaddock,J.S. Kim,S. Heo,H. Alves,S.M. White,T.R. Wojcicki,E. Mailey,V.J. Vieira,S.A. Martin,B.D. Pence,J.A. Woods,E. McAuley, & A.F. Kramer, *Exercise training increases size of hippocampus and improves memory, Proc.* Natl. Acad. Sci. U.S.A. 108 (7) 3017-3022, https://doi.org/10.1073/pnas.1015950108 (2011).

https://pubmed.ncbi.nlm.nih.gov/21282661/

11] Cooney GM, Dwan K, Greig CA, Lawlor DA, Rimer J, Waugh FR, McMurdo M, *Mead GE. Exercise for depression. Cochrane Database of Systematic Reviews 2013*, Issue 9. Art. No.: CD004366. DOI: 10.1002/14651858.CD004366.pub6.

https://www.cochranelibrary.com/cdsr/doi/10.1002/14651858.CD004366.pub6/full

12] Burnett-Zeigler I, Schuette S, Victorson D, Wisner KL. Mind-*Body Approaches to Treating Mental Health Symptoms Among Disadvantaged Populations: A Comprehensive Review.* J Altern Complement Med. 2016 Feb;22(2):115-24. doi:

10.1089/acm.2015.0038. Epub 2015 Nov 5. PMID: 26540645; PMCID: PMC4761814.

https://pubmed.ncbi.nlm.nih.gov/26540645/

13] Vancampfort D, Firth J, Stubbs B, Schuch F, Rosenbaum S, Hallgren M, Deenik J, Ward PB, Mugisha J, Van Damme T, Werneck AO. *The efficacy, mechanisms and implementation of physical activity as an adjunctive treatment in mental disorders: a meta-review of outcomes, neurobiology and key determinants.* World Psychiatry. 2025 Jun;24(2):227-239. doi: 10.1002/wps.21314. PMID: 40371806; PMCID: PMC12079350.

https://pubmed.ncbi.nlm.nih.gov/40371806/

14] Mahindru A, Patil P, Agrawal V. *Role of Physical Activity on Mental Health and Well-Being: A Review.* Cureus. 2023 Jan 7;15(1):e33475. doi: 10.7759/cureus.33475. PMID: 36756008; PMCID: PMC9902068.

https://pubmed.ncbi.nlm.nih.gov/36756008/

15] Sever E, Yılmaz S, Koz M. *Acute and Chronic Immunological Responses to Different Exercise Modalities: A Narrative Review.* Healthcare (Basel). 2025 Sep 8;13(17):2244. doi: 10.3390/healthcare13172244. PMID: 40941596; PMCID: PMC12428347.

https://pubmed.ncbi.nlm.nih.gov/40941596/

16] Brandt C, Pedersen BK. *The role of exercise-induced myokines in muscle homeostasis and the defense against chronic diseases.* J Biomed Biotechnol. 2010;2010:520258. doi: 10.1155/2010/520258. Epub 2010 Mar 9. PMID: 20224659; PMCID: PMC2836182.

https://pmc.ncbi.nlm.nih.gov/articles/PMC2836182

17] Hand MD, Ihara ES, Moore M, Shaw M. *Integrating music and nature: a scoping review of research on interventions involving both music- and nature-based strategies for mental health and wellbeing.* Front Hum Neurosci. 2025 Aug 26;19:1664304. doi: 10.3389/fnhum.2025.1664304. PMID: 40932877; PMCID: PMC12418201.

https://pubmed.ncbi.nlm.nih.gov/40932877/

Chapter 10 – Reducing Toxic Load

1] Li L, Lv L, Wang Z, Liu X, Wang Q, Zhu H, Jiang B, Han Y, Pan X, Zhou X, Ren L, Chang Z. *From copper homeostasis to cuproptosis: a new perspective on CNS immune regulation and neurodegenerative diseases.* Front Neurol. 2025 May 29;16:1581045. doi: 10.3389/fneur.2025.1581045. Erratum in: Front Neurol. 2025 Jul 29;16:1664184. doi: 10.3389/fneur.2025.1664184. PMID: 40510202; PMCID: PMC12158703.

https://pubmed.ncbi.nlm.nih.gov/40510202/

2] Wu D, Lin Q, Hou S, Cui X, Shou N, Yuan X, Xu W, Fu K, Wang Q, Shi Z. *Gut Microbiota and Its Metabolite Taurine-β-Muricholic Acid Contribute to Antimony- and/or Copper-Induced Liver Inflammation.* Int J Mol Sci. 2025 Apr 3;26(7):3332. doi: 10.3390/ijms26073332. PMID: 40244173; PMCID: PMC11989503.

https://pubmed.ncbi.nlm.nih.gov/40244173/

3] Sharma M, Rajawat NK. *Neurotoxicity study of copper oxide nanoparticles and the protective role of a probiotic (Lactobacillus acidophilus) in Swiss albino mice.* Toxicol Ind Health. 2025 Jul;41(7):398-408. doi: 10.1177/07482337251350165. Epub 2025 Jun 10. PMID: 40492926.

https://pubmed.ncbi.nlm.nih.gov/40492926/

4] International Agency for Research on Cancer. (2018, July 19). *IARC monograph on glyphosate.* World Health Organization. https://www.iarc.who.int/featured-news/media-centre-iarc-news-glyphosate/

5] Green Science Policy Institute. (n.d.). *Six classes of harmful chemicals.* Green Science Policy Institute.

https://greensciencepolicy.org/harmful-chemicals/

6] Genuis SJ, Beesoon S, Birkholz D, Lobo RA. *Human excretion of bisphenol A: blood, urine, and sweat (BUS) study.* J Environ Public Health. 2012;2012:185731. doi: 10.1155/2012/185731. Epub 2011 Dec 27. PMID: 22253637; PMCID: PMC3255175.

https://pubmed.ncbi.nlm.nih.gov/22253637/

7] Genuis SJ, Beesoon S, Lobo RA, Birkholz D. *Human elimination of phthalate compounds: blood, urine, and sweat (BUS) study.* ScientificWorldJournal. 2012;2012:615068. doi: 10.1100/2012/615068. Epub 2012 Oct 31. PMID: 23213291; PMCID: PMC3504417.

https://pubmed.ncbi.nlm.nih.gov/23213291/

8] Sears ME, Kerr KJ, Bray RI. *Arsenic, cadmium, lead, and mercury in sweat: a systematic review.* J Environ Public Health. 2012;2012:184745. doi: 10.1155/2012/184745. Epub 2012 Feb 22. PMID: 22505948; PMCID: PMC3312275.

https://pmc.ncbi.nlm.nih.gov/articles/PMC3312275/

9] Etzel RA. *What the primary care pediatrician should know about syndromes associated with exposures to mycotoxins.* Curr Probl Pediatr Adolesc Health Care. 2006 Sep;36(8):282-305. doi: 10.1016/j.cppeds.2006.05.003. PMID: 16935759.

https://pubmed.ncbi.nlm.nih.gov/16935759/

10] Hope J. *A review of the mechanism of injury and treatment approaches for illness resulting from exposure to water-damaged buildings, mold, and mycotoxins.* ScientificWorldJournal. 2013 Apr 18;2013:767482. doi: 10.1155/2013/767482. PMID: 23710148; PMCID: PMC3654247.

https://pubmed.ncbi.nlm.nih.gov/23710148/

11] Tenório MCDS, Graciliano NG, Moura FA, Oliveira ACM, *Goulart MOF. N-Acetylcysteine (NAC): Impacts on Human Health.* Antioxidants (Basel). 2021 Jun 16;10(6):967. doi: 10.3390/antiox10060967. PMID: 34208683; PMCID: PMC8234027.

https://pubmed.ncbi.nlm.nih.gov/34208683/

12] Atkuri KR, Mantovani JJ, Herzenberg LA, Herzenberg LA. *N-Acetylcysteine--a safe antidote for cysteine/glutathione deficiency.* Curr Opin Pharmacol. 2007 Aug;7(4):355-9. doi: 10.1016/j.coph.2007.04.005. Epub 2007 Jun 29. PMID: 17602868; PMCID: PMC4540061.

https://pubmed.ncbi.nlm.nih.gov/17602868/

13] Zhang B, Zhang L, Fu H, Li C, Mao B. *Combining Chlorella vulgaris and metal-organic framework for enhanced Pb^{2+} removal.* Bioresour Technol. 2025 Sep 29;440:133414. doi: 10.1016/j.biortech.2025.133414. Epub ahead of print. PMID: 41033500.

https://pubmed.ncbi.nlm.nih.gov/41033500/

14] Bhattacharya S. *The Role of Spirulina (Arthrospira) in the Mitigation of Heavy-Metal Toxicity: An Appraisal.* J Environ Pathol Toxicol

Oncol. 2020;39(2):149-157. doi: 10.1615/JEnvironPatholToxi-colOncol.2020034375. PMID: 32749124.

https://pubmed.ncbi.nlm.nih.gov/32749124/

15] Bito T, Okumura E, Fujishima M, Watanabe F. *Potential of Chlorella as a Dietary Supplement to Promote Human Health.* Nutrients. 2020 Aug 20;12(9):2524. doi: 10.3390/nu12092524. PMID: 32825362; PMCID: PMC7551956.

https://pubmed.ncbi.nlm.nih.gov/32825362/

16] Alves JLB, Costa PCTD, Sales LCS, Silva Luis CC, Bezerra TPT, Souza MLA, Costa BA, de Souza EL. *Shedding light on the impacts of Spirulina platensis on gut microbiota and related health benefits.* Crit Rev Food Sci Nutr. 2025;65(11):2062-2075. doi: 10.1080/10408398.2024.2323112. Epub 2024 Feb 29. PMID: 38420934.

https://pubmed.ncbi.nlm.nih.gov/38420934/

17] Abenavoli L, Capasso R, Milic N, Capasso F. *Milk thistle in liver diseases: past, present, future.* Phytother Res. 2010 Oct;24(10):1423-32. doi: 10.1002/ptr.3207. PMID: 20564545.

https://pubmed.ncbi.nlm.nih.gov/20564545/

From Chapter 11 – Strong Social Connections

1] Martino J, Pegg J, Frates EP. *The Connection Prescription: Using the Power of Social Interactions and the Deep Desire for Connectedness to Empower Health and Wellness.* Am J Lifestyle Med. 2015 Oct 7;11(6):466-475. doi: 10.1177/1559827615608788. PMID: 30202372; PMCID: PMC6125010.

https://www.ncbi.nlm.nih.gov/pmc/articles/PMC6125010/

2] CDC, *Social Connections, Health Effects of Social Isolation and Loneliness,* No author, May 2024.

https://www.cdc.gov/social-connectedness/risk-factors/index.html

3] Merlo G, Snellman L, Sugden SG. Connectedness: *The Updated and Expanded Pillar of Lifestyle Psychiatry and Lifestyle Medicine.* Am J Lifestyle Med. 2025 Jun 2:15598276251345455. doi:

10.1177/15598276251345455. Epub ahead of print. PMID: 40469950; PMCID: PMC12129969.

https://pubmed.ncbi.nlm.nih.gov/40469950

4] Itskovich E, Bowling DL, Garner JP, Parker KJ. *Oxytocin and the social facilitation of placebo effects.* Mol Psychiatry. 2022 Jun;27(6):2640-2649. doi: 10.1038/s41380-022-01515-9. Epub 2022 Mar 25. PMID: 35338314; PMCID: PMC9167259.

https://pubmed.ncbi.nlm.nih.gov/35338314/

5] Kim CS, Shin GE, Cheong Y, Shin JH, Shin DM, Chun WY. *Experiencing social exclusion changes gut microbiota composition.* Transl Psychiatry. 2022 Jun 17;12(1):254. doi: 10.1038/s41398-022-02023-8. PMID: 35715396; PMCID: PMC9205890.

https://pubmed.ncbi.nlm.nih.gov/35715396/

6] Kidambi N, Lee EE. *Insight into Potential Mechanisms Linking Loneliness and Cognitive Decline: Commentary on "Health Factors as Potential Mediator the Longitudinal Effect of Loneliness on General Cognitive Ability".* Am J Geriatr Psychiatry. 2020 Dec;28(12):1284-1286. doi: 10.1016/j.jagp.2020.08.015. Epub 2020 Aug 28. PMID: 32950365; PMCID: PMC7452903.

https://pubmed.ncbi.nlm.nih.gov/32950365/

7] Atshan S, Ayer L, Parker AM, Strough J, Ghosh-Dastidar B. *Disrupted and Dis-connected Post Disaster: Associations Between the Social and Built Environ-ment and Loneliness During COVID-19 in a U.S. Gulf Coast Sample.* Int J Envi-ron Res Public Health. 2025 Jan 31;22(2):203. doi: 10.3390/ijerph22020203. PMID: 40003429; PMCID: PMC11855155.

https://pubmed.ncbi.nlm.nih.gov/40003429/

8] Demarinis S. *Loneliness at epidemic levels in America. Explore (NY).* 2020 Sep-Oct;16(5):278-279. doi: 10.1016/j.explore.2020.06.008. Epub 2020 Jun 28. PMID: 32674944; PMCID: PMC7321652.

https://pubmed.ncbi.nlm.nih.gov/32674944/

9] Albertorio-Diaz JR, Wheldon CW. *Prevalence of loneliness states among the US adult population: Findings from the 2022 HINTS-6.* Am J Prev Med. 2025 Jun 11:107935. doi: 10.1016/j.amepre.2025.107935. Epub ahead of print. PMID: 40513912.

https://pubmed.ncbi.nlm.nih.gov/40513912/

Chapter 12 – The HOPE Method

1] Mechanick JI, Farkouh ME, Newman JD, Garvey WT. *Cardiometabolic-Based Chronic Disease, Addressing Knowledge and Clinical Practice Gaps*: JACC State-of-the-Art Review. J Am Coll Cardiol. 2020 Feb 11;75(5):539-555. doi: 10.1016/j.jacc.2019.11.046. PMID: 32029137; PMCID: PMC8168371.

https://pubmed.ncbi.nlm.nih.gov/32029137/

2] Valavanidis A, Vlachogianni T, Fiotakis C. *8-hydroxy-2' -deoxyguanosine (8-OHdG): A critical biomarker of oxidative stress and carcinogenesis.* J Environ Sci Health C Environ Carcinog Ecotoxicol Rev. 2009 Apr;27(2):120-39. doi: 10.1080/10590500902885684. PMID: 19412858.

https://pubmed.ncbi.nlm.nih.gov/19412858/

3] Liang Y, Xie S, He Y, Xu M, Qiao X, Zhu Y, Wu W. *Kynurenine Pathway Metabolites as Biomarkers in Alzheimer's Disease.* Dis Markers. 2022 Jan 19;2022:9484217. doi: 10.1155/2022/9484217. PMID: 35096208; PMCID: PMC8791723.

https://pubmed.ncbi.nlm.nih.gov/35096208/

Chapter 13 – Solutions for Optimizing Gut Health

1] Camilleri M. *Review: Human Intestinal Barrier-Optimal Measurement and Effects of Diet in the Absence of Overt Inflammation or Ulceration.* Aliment Pharmacol Ther. 2025 Jul;62(2):128-145. doi: 10.1111/apt.70225. Epub 2025 Jun 13. PMID: 40515459.

https://pubmed.ncbi.nlm.nih.gov/40515459/

2] Al Dera H, Alrafaei B, Al Tamimi MI, Alfawaz HA, Bhat RS, Soliman DA, Abuaish S, El-Ansary A. *Leaky gut biomarkers in casein- and gluten-rich diet fed rat model of autism.* Transl Neurosci. 2021 Dec 31;12(1):601-610. doi: 10.1515/tnsci-2020-0207. PMID: 35070443; PMCID: PMC8724359.

https://pubmed.ncbi.nlm.nih.gov/35070443/

3] Robinson SR, Greenway FL, Deth RC, Fayet-Moore F. *Effects of Different Cow-Milk Beta-Caseins on the Gut-Brain Axis: A Narrative Review of Preclinical, Animal, and Human Studies.* Nutr Rev. 2025 Mar 1;83(3):e1259-e1269. doi: 10.1093/nutrit/nuae099. PMID: 39024213; PMCID: PMC11819488.

https://pubmed.ncbi.nlm.nih.gov/39024213/

4] Martínez-Augustin O, Tena-Garitaonaindia M, Ceacero-Heras D, Jiménez-Ortas Á, Enguix-Huete JJ, Álvarez-Mercado AI, Ruiz-Henares G, Aranda CJ, Gámez-Belmonte R, Sánchez de Medina F. *Macronutrients as Regulators of Intestinal Epithelial Permeability: Where Do We Stand?* Compr Rev Food Sci Food Saf. 2025 May;24(3):e70178. doi: 10.1111/1541-4337.70178. PMID: 40421830; PMCID: PMC12108046.

https://pubmed.ncbi.nlm.nih.gov/40421830/

5] Dimba NR, Mzimela N, Mosili P, Ngubane PS, Khathi A. *Investigating the Association Between Diet-Induced "Leaky Gut" and the Development of Prediabetes.* Exp Clin Endocrinol Diabetes. 2023 Nov;131(11):569-576. doi: 10.1055/a-2181-6664. Epub 2023 Sep 26. PMID: 37751850.

https://pubmed.ncbi.nlm.nih.gov/37751850/

6] Jawamis A, Al-Domi H, Al Sarayreh N. *Effect of dietary fat intake on metabolic endotoxemia: Mechanisms and clinical insights.* Clin Nutr ESPEN. 2025 Jul 28;69:415-420. doi: 10.1016/j.clnesp.2025.07.1124. Epub ahead of print. PMID: 40738208.

https://pubmed.ncbi.nlm.nih.gov/40738208/

7] Mishra S, Jain S, Agadzi B, Yadav H. *A Cascade of Microbiota-Leaky Gut-Inflammation- Is it a Key Player in Metabolic Disorders?* Curr Obes Rep. 2025 Apr 10;14(1):32. doi: 10.1007/s13679-025-00624-0. PMID: 40208464.

https://pubmed.ncbi.nlm.nih.gov/40208464/

8] National Institutes of Health, Office of Dietary Supplements. (2023, November 3). *Probiotics: Fact sheet for consumers.*

https://ods.od.nih.gov/factsheets/Probiotics-Consumer/

9] Yan F, Polk DB. Lactobacillus rhamnosus GG*: An Updated Strategy to Use Microbial Products to Promote Health.* Funct Food Rev. 2012 Jun;4(2):77-84. PMID: 24795791; PMCID: PMC4006995.

https://pmc.ncbi.nlm.nih.gov/articles/PMC4006995/

10] Hidayat K, Zhang L, Wei H, Zhang W, Qin L, Ou Y, Li N. *The effects of Lacticaseibacillus rhamnosus GG supplementation on gastrointestinal and respiratory outcomes: a systematic review and meta-analysis of randomized controlled trials.* Food Funct. 2025 Aug 11;16(16):6275-6292. doi: 10.1039/d5fo01780g. PMID: 40702885.

https://pubmed.ncbi.nlm.nih.gov/40702885/

11] Ahmadi-Khorram M, Hatami A, Asghari P, Jafarzadeh Esfehani A, Afshari A, Javdan F, Nematy M. *Probiotics mitigate stress and inflammation in malnourished adults via gut microbiota modulation: a randomized controlled trial.* Front Nutr. 2025 Jul 16;12:1615607. doi: 10.3389/fnut.2025.1615607. PMID: 40740643; PMCID: PMC12307372.

https://pubmed.ncbi.nlm.nih.gov/40740643/

12] Chyn Boon Wong, Toshitaka Odamaki, Jin-zhong Xiao, *Beneficial effects of Bifidobacterium longum subsp. longum BB536 on human health: Modulation of gut microbiome as the principal action,* Journal of Functional Foods, Volume 54, 2019, Pages 506-519, ISSN 1756-4646, https://doi.org/10.1016/j.jff.2019.02.002. https://www.sciencedirect.com/science/article/pii/S1756464619300684

13] Leeuwendaal NK, Stanton C, O'Toole PW, Beresford TP. *Fermented Foods, Health and the Gut Microbiome.* Nutrients. 2022 Apr 6;14(7):1527. doi: 10.3390/nu14071527. PMID: 35406140; PMCID: PMC9003261.

https://pubmed.ncbi.nlm.nih.gov/35406140/

14] Pihelgas S, Ehala-Aleksejev K, Kutti ML, Kuldjärv R, Kazantseva J. *Impact of fresh and fermented vegetable consumption on gut microbiota and body composition: insights from diverse data analysis approaches.* Front Nutr. 2025 Jul 15;12:1623710. doi: 10.3389/fnut.2025.1623710. PMID: 40735240; PMCID: PMC12306187.

https://pubmed.ncbi.nlm.nih.gov/40735240/

15] Dimidi E, Cox SR, Rossi M, Whelan K. Fermented Foods: *Definitions and Characteristics, Impact on the Gut Microbiota and Effects on Gastrointestinal Health and Disease.* Nutrients. 2019 Aug 5;11(8):1806. doi: 10.3390/nu11081806. PMID: 31387262; PMCID: PMC6723656.

https://pubmed.ncbi.nlm.nih.gov/31387262/

16] Borresen EC, Henderson AJ, Kumar A, Weir TL, Ryan EP. *Fermented foods: patented approaches and formulations for nutritional supplementation and health promotion*. Recent Pat Food Nutr Agric. 2012 Aug;4(2):134-40. doi: 10.2174/2212798411204020134. PMID: 22702745; PMCID: PMC5175401.

https://pubmed.ncbi.nlm.nih.gov/22702745/

17] International Science Applications. (n.d.). Home. https://isapp-science.org/

18] Mahmood A, FitzGerald AJ, Marchbank T, Ntatsaki E, Murray D, Ghosh S, Playford RJ. *Zinc carnosine, a health food supplement that stabilises small bowel integrity and stimulates gut repair processes*. Gut. 2007 Feb;56(2):168-75. doi: 10.1136/gut.2006.099929. Epub 2006 Jun 15. PMID: 16777920; PMCID: PMC1856764. https://pmc.ncbi.nlm.nih.gov/articles/PMC1856764/

19] Iyer N, Vaishnava S. *Vitamin A at the interface of host-commensal-pathogen interactions*. PLoS Pathog. 2019 Jun 6;15(6):e1007750. doi: 10.1371/journal.ppat.1007750. PMID: 31170262; PMCID: PMC6553882.

https://pubmed.ncbi.nlm.nih.gov/31170262/

20] LeBlanc JG, Milani C, de Giori GS, Sesma F, van Sinderen D, Ventura M. *Bacteria as vitamin suppliers to their host: a gut microbiota perspective*. Curr Opin Biotechnol. 2013 Apr;24(2):160-8. doi: 10.1016/j.copbio.2012.08.005. Epub 2012 Aug 30. PMID: 22940212.

https://pubmed.ncbi.nlm.nih.gov/22940212/

21] Tarracchini C, Lugli GA, Mancabelli L, van Sinderen D, Turroni F, Ventura M, Milani C. *Exploring the vitamin biosynthesis landscape of the human gut microbiota*. mSystems. 2024 Oct 22;9(10):e0092924. doi: 10.1128/msystems.00929-24. Epub 2024 Sep 17. PMID: 39287373; PMCID: PMC11494892.

https://pubmed.ncbi.nlm.nih.gov/39287373/

22] Dell'Anna G, Fanizzi F, Zilli A, Furfaro F, Solitano V, Parigi TL, Ciliberto A, Fanizza J, Mandarino FV, Fuccio L, Facciorusso A, Donatelli G, Allocca M, Massironi S, Annese V, Peyrin-Biroulet L, Danese S, D'Amico F. *The Role of Vitamin D in Inflammatory Bowel Diseases: From Deficiency to Targeted Therapeutics and Precise*

Nutrition Strategies. Nutrients. 2025 Jun 29;17(13):2167. doi: 10.3390/nu17132167. PMID: 40647273; PMCID: PMC12252289.

https://pubmed.ncbi.nlm.nih.gov/40647273/

23] Grant WB, Al Anouti F, Boucher BJ, Dursun E, Gezen-Ak D, Jude EB, Karonova T, Pludowski P. *A Narrative Review of the Evidence for Variations in Serum 25-Hydroxyvitamin D Concentration Thresholds for Optimal Health.* Nutrients. 2022 Feb 2;14(3):639. doi: 10.3390/nu14030639. PMID: 35276999; PMCID: PMC8838864.

https://pubmed.ncbi.nlm.nih.gov/35276999/

24] Baek GH, Yoo KM, Kim SY, Lee DH, Chung H, Jung SC, Park SK, Kim JS. *Collagen Peptide Exerts an Anti-Obesity Effect by Influencing the Firmicutes/Bacteroidetes Ratio in the Gut.* Nutrients. 2023 Jun 2;15(11):2610. doi: 10.3390/nu15112610. PMID: 37299573; PMCID: PMC10255498.

https://pubmed.ncbi.nlm.nih.gov/37299573/

25] Chen Q, Chen O, Martins IM, Hou H, Zhao X, Blumberg JB, Li B. *Collagen peptides ameliorate intestinal epithelial barrier dysfunction in immunostimulatory Caco-2 cell monolayers via enhancing tight junctions.* Food Funct. 2017 Mar 22;8(3):1144-1151. doi: 10.1039/c6fo01347c. PMID: 28174772.

https://pubmed.ncbi.nlm.nih.gov/28174772/

26] Feng J, Li Z, Ma H, Yue Y, Hao K, Li J, Xiang Y, Min Y. *Quercetin alleviates intestinal inflammation and improves intestinal functions via modulating gut microbiota composition in LPS-challenged laying hens.* Poult Sci. 2023 Mar;102(3):102433. doi: 10.1016/j.psj.2022.102433. Epub 2022 Dec 16. PMID: 36587451; PMCID: PMC9816806.

https://pmc.ncbi.nlm.nih.gov/articles/PMC9816806/

27] Lamichhane G, Godsey TJ, Liu J, Franks R, Zhang G, Emerson SR, Kim Y. *Twelve-Week Curcumin Supplementation Improves Glucose Homeostasis and Gut Health in Prediabetic Older Adults: A Pilot, Double-Blind, Placebo-Controlled Trial.* Nutrients. 2025 Jun 29;17(13):2164. doi: 10.3390/nu17132164. PMID: 40647269; PMCID: PMC12251931.

https://pubmed.ncbi.nlm.nih.gov/40647269/

28] Ge J, Li M, Yao J, Guo J, Li X, Li G, Han X, Li Z, Liu M, Zhao J. *The potential of EGCG in modulating the oral-gut axis microbiota for treating inflammatory bowel disease.* Phytomedicine. 2024 Jul 25;130:155643. doi: 10.1016/j.phymed.2024.155643. Epub 2024 Apr 14. PMID: 38820660.

https://pubmed.ncbi.nlm.nih.gov/38820660/

29] Costantini L, Molinari R, Farinon B, Merendino N. *Impact of Omega-3 Fatty Acids on the Gut Microbiota.* Int J Mol Sci. 2017 Dec 7;18(12):2645. doi: 10.3390/ijms18122645. PMID: 29215589; PMCID: PMC5751248.

https://pubmed.ncbi.nlm.nih.gov/29215589

30] Jankowski WM, Fichna J, Tarasiuk-Zawadzka A. *The interplay between diet and the enteric nervous system in the pathophysiology of colorectal cancer.* Folia Med Cracov. 2024 Sep 15;64(2):5-16. doi: 10.24425/fmc.2024.150147. PMID: 39324673.

https://pubmed.ncbi.nlm.nih.gov/39324673/

31] Yang Y, Fu Y, Wu C. *Gut microbe-derived pentadecanoic acid could represent a novel health-promoter via multiple pathways.* Food Funct. 2025 Jun 16;16(12):4636-4653. doi: 10.1039/d5fo01278c. PMID: 40439551.

https://pubmed.ncbi.nlm.nih.gov/40439551/

32] Singh D, Mehghini P, Rodriguez-Palacios A, Di Martino L, Cominelli F, Basson AR. *Anti-Inflammatory Effect of Dietary Pentade-canoic Fatty Acid Supplementation on Inflammatory Bowel Disease in SAMP1/YitFc Mice.* Nutrients. 2024 Sep 8;16(17):3031. doi: 10.3390/nu16173031. PMID: 39275347; PMCID: PMC11397537.

https://pubmed.ncbi.nlm.nih.gov/39275347/

33] Pihelgas S, Ehala-Aleksejev K, Kutti ML, Kuldjärv R, Kazantseva J. *Impact of fresh and fermented vegetable consumption on gut microbiota and body composition: insights from diverse data analysis approaches.* Front Nutr. 2025 Jul 15;12:1623710. doi: 10.3389/fnut.2025.1623710. PMID: 40735240; PMCID: PMC12306187.

https://pubmed.ncbi.nlm.nih.gov/40735240/

34] Bui G, Marco ML. *Impact of Fermented Dairy on Gastrointestinal Health and Associated Biomarkers.* Nutr Rev. 2025 Jul 24:nuaf114.

doi: 10.1093/nutrit/nuaf114. Epub ahead of print. PMID: 40706019.

https://pubmed.ncbi.nlm.nih.gov/40706019

Chapter 14 – Promoting Health to Prevent Chronic Disease

1] Jones, D. W., Ferdinand, K. C., Taler, S. J., Johnson, H. M., Shimbo, D., Abdalla, M., Altieri, M. M., Bansal, N., Bello, N. A., Bress, A. P., Carter, J., Cohen, J. B., Collins, K. J., Commodore-Mensah, Y., Davis, L. L., Egan, B., Khan, S. S., Lloyd-Jones, D. M., Melnyk, B. M., ... Whelton, P. K. (2025). 2025 AHA/ACC/AANP/AAPA/ABC/ACCP/ACPM/AGS/AMA/ASPC/NMA/PCNA/SGIM *guideline for the prevention, detection, evaluation and management of high blood pressure in adults: A report of the American College of Cardiology/American Heart Association Joint Committee on Clinical Practice Guidelines.* Hypertension, 0(0). https://doi.org/10.1161/HYP.0000000000000249

https://pubmed.ncbi.nlm.nih.gov/40811516/

2] Rock, C. L., Thomson, C., Gansler, T., Gapstur, S. M., McCullough, M. L., Patel, A. V., Andrews, K. S., Bandera, E. V., Spees, C. K., Robien, K., Hartman, S., Sullivan, K., Grant, B. L., Hamilton, K. K., Kushi, L. H., Caan, B. J., Kibbe, D., Black, J. D., Wiedt, T. L., ... Doyle, C. (2020). *American Cancer Society guideline for diet and physical activity for cancer prevention.* CA: A Cancer Journal for Clinicians, 70(4), 245–271. https://doi.org/10.3322/caac.21591

https://experts.arizona.edu/en/publications/american-cancer-society-guideline-for-diet-and-physical-activity-/

3] Knowler WC, Barrett-Connor E, Fowler SE, Hamman RF, Lachin JM, Walker EA, Nathan DM; Diabetes Prevention Program Research Group. Reduction in the incidence of type 2 diabetes with lifestyle intervention or metformin. N Engl J Med. 2002 Feb 7;346(6):393-403. doi: 10.1056/NEJMoa012512. PMID: 11832527; PMCID: PMC1370926. Knowler WC, Barrett-Connor E, Fowler SE, Hamman RF, Lachin JM, Walker EA, Nathan DM; *Diabetes Prevention Program Research Group. Reduction in the incidence of type 2 diabetes with lifestyle intervention or metformin.* N Engl J Med. 2002 Feb 7;346(6):393-403. doi: 10.1056/NEJMoa012512. PMID: 11832527; PMCID: PMC1370926.

https://pubmed.ncbi.nlm.nih.gov/11832527/

4] Lindström J, Ilanne-Parikka P, Peltonen M, Aunola S, Eriksson JG, Hemiö K, Hämäläinen H, Härkönen P, Keinänen-Kiukaanniemi S, Laakso M, Louheranta A, Mannelin M, Paturi M, Sundvall J, Valle TT, Uusitupa M, Tuomilehto J; Finnish Diabetes Prevention Study Group. *Sustained reduction in the incidence of type 2 diabetes by lifestyle intervention: follow-up of the Finnish Diabetes Prevention* Study. Lancet. 2006 Nov 11;368(9548):1673-9. doi: 10.1016/S0140-6736(06)69701-8. PMID: 17098085.

https://pubmed.ncbi.nlm.nih.gov/17098085/

5] American Diabetes Association Professional Practice Committee. (2025). 3. *Prevention or delay of diabetes and associated comorbidities: Standards of care in diabetes—2025.* Diabetes Care, 48(Suppl. 1), S50–S58. https://doi.org/10.2337/dc25-S003

https://diabetesjournals.org/care/article/48/Supplement_1/S50/157550/3-Prevention-or-Delay-of-Diabetes-and-Associated

6] Goldstein, L. B., Adams, R., Alberts, M. J., Appel, L. J., Brass, L. M., Bushnell, C. D., Culebras, A., ... Sacco, R. L. (2006*). Primary prevention of ischemic stroke: A guideline from the American Heart Association/American Stroke Association Stroke Council*: Cosponsored by the Atherosclerotic Peripheral Vascular Disease Interdisciplinary Working Group; Cardiovascular Nursing Council; Clinical Cardiology Council; Nutrition, Physical Activity, and Metabolism Council; and the Quality of Care and Outcomes Research Interdisciplinary Working Group. Stroke, 37(6), 1583–1633. https://doi.org/10.1161/01.STR.0000223048.70103.F1

https://pubmed.ncbi.nlm.nih.gov/16675728/

7] National Heart, Lung, and Blood Institute. (n.d.). *DASH eating plan.*

https://www.nhlbi.nih.gov/education/dash-eating-plan

8] Litke R, Garcharna LC, Jiwani S, Neugroschl J. *Modifiable Risk Factors in Alzheimer Disease and Related Dementias: A Review.* Clin Ther. 2021 Jun;43(6):953-965. doi: 10.1016/j.clinthera.2021.05.006. Epub 2021 Jun 6. PMID: 34108080; PMCID: PMC8440362.

https://pmc.ncbi.nlm.nih.gov/articles/PMC8440362/

9] Lennon MJ, Lam BCP, Lipnicki DM, Crawford JD, Peters R, Schutte AE, Brodaty H, Thalamuthu A, Rydberg-Sterner T, Najar J, Skoog I, Riedel-Heller SG, Röhr S, Pabst A, Lobo A, De-la-Cámara C, Lobo E, Bello T, Gureje O, Ojagbemi A, Lipton RB, Katz MJ, Derby CA, Kim KW, Han JW, Oh DJ, Rolandi E, Davin A, Rossi M, Scarmeas N, Yannakoulia M, Dardiotis T, Hendrie HC, Gao S, Carrière I, Ritchie K, Anstey KJ, Cherbuin N, Xiao S, Yue L, Li W, Guerchet MM, Preux PM, Aboyans V, Haan MN, Aiello AE, Ng TP, Nyunt MSZ, Gao Q, Scazufca M, Sachdev PSS. *Use of Antihypertensives, Blood Pressure, and Estimated Risk of Dementia in Late Life: An Individual Participant Data Meta-Analysis*. JAMA Netw Open. 2023 Sep 5;6(9):e2333353. doi: 10.1001/jamanetworkopen.2023.33353. PMID: 37698858; PMCID: PMC10498335.

https://pubmed.ncbi.nlm.nih.gov/37698858/

10] Zeng J, Hu K, Wang Z, Huang YC, Zhang Y, Peng H, Ma S. *Cognitive Dysfunction and Dementia in Type 2 Diabetes Mellitus: Insights into Mechanisms, Models, and Therapeutics*. ACS Pharmacol Transl Sci. 2025 Jul 7;8(8):2337-2352. doi: 10.1021/acsptsci.5c00086. PMID: 40810170; PMCID: PMC12340629.

https://pubmed.ncbi.nlm.nih.gov/40810170/

11] Liu Y, Fowler H, Wang DD, Barnes LL, Cornelis MC. *Mediterranean-DASH Intervention for Neurodegenerative Delay (MIND) Trial: Genetic Resource for Precision Nutrition*. Nutrients. 2025 Aug 4;17(15):2548. doi: 10.3390/nu17152548. PMID: 40806132; PMCID: PMC12348084.

https://pubmed.ncbi.nlm.nih.gov/40806132/

12] Chen H, Dhana K, Huang Y, Huang L, Tao Y, Liu X, Melo van Lent D, Zheng Y, Ascherio A, Willett W, Yuan C. *Association of the Mediterranean Dietary Approaches to Stop Hypertension Intervention for Neurodegenerative Delay (MIND) Diet With the Risk of Dementia*. JAMA Psychiatry. 2023 Jun 1;80(6):630-638. doi: 10.1001/jamapsychiatry.2023.0800. PMID: 37133875; PMCID: PMC10157510.

https://pubmed.ncbi.nlm.nih.gov/37133875/

13] Xu L, Gu H, Cai X, Zhang Y, Hou X, Yu J, Sun T. *The Effects of Exercise for Cognitive Function in Older Adults: A Systematic Review and Meta-Analysis of Randomized Controlled Trials*. Int J Environ

Res Public Health. 2023 Jan 7;20(2):1088. doi: 10.3390/ijerph20021088. PMID: 36673844; PMCID: PMC9858649.

https://pubmed.ncbi.nlm.nih.gov/36673844/

14] Ernst M, Folkerts AK, Gollan R, Lieker E, Caro-Valenzuela J, Adams A, Cryns N, Monsef I, Dresen A, Roheger M, Eggers C, Skoetz N, Kalbe E. *Physical exercise for people with Parkinson's disease: a systematic review and network meta-analysis.* Cochrane Database Syst Rev. 2024 Apr 8;4(4):CD013856. doi: 10.1002/14651858.CD013856.pub3. PMID: 38588457; PMCID: PMC11001292.

https://pubmed.ncbi.nlm.nih.gov/38588457/

15] Guay-Gagnon M, Vat S, Forget MF, Tremblay-Gravel M, Ducharme S, Nguyen QD, Desmarais P. *Sleep apnea and the risk of dementia: A systematic review and meta-analysis.* J Sleep Res. 2022 Oct;31(5):e13589. doi: 10.1111/jsr.13589. Epub 2022 Apr 2. PMID: 35366021.

https://pubmed.ncbi.nlm.nih.gov/35366021/

16] Li L, Zhang Q, Yang D, Yang S, Zhao Y, Jiang M, Wang X, Zhao L, Liu Q, Lu Z, Zhou X, Gan Y, Wu C. *Tooth loss and the risk of cognitive decline and dementia: A meta-analysis of cohort studies.* Front Neurol. 2023 Apr 17;14:1103052. doi: 10.3389/fneur.2023.1103052. PMID: 37139053; PMCID: PMC10150074.

https://pubmed.ncbi.nlm.nih.gov/37139053/

17] Park JC, Chang L, Kwon HK, Im SH. *Beyond the gut: decoding the gut-immune-brain axis in health and disease.* Cell Mol Immunol. 2025 Aug 14. doi: 10.1038/s41423-025-01333-3. Epub ahead of print. PMID: 40804450.

https://pubmed.ncbi.nlm.nih.gov/40804450/

18] Ugwu OP, Okon MB, Alum EU, Ugwu CN, Anyanwu EG, Mariam B, Ogenyi FC, Eze VHU, Anyanwu CN, Ezeonwumelu JOC, Egba SI, Uti DE, Onohuean H, Aja PM, Ugwu MN. *Unveiling the therapeutic potential of the gut microbiota-brain axis: Novel insights and clinical applications in neurological disorders.* Medicine (Baltimore). 2025 Jul 25;104(30):e43542. doi: 10.1097/MD.0000000000043542. PMID: 40725913; PMCID: PMC12303509.

https://pubmed.ncbi.nlm.nih.gov/40725913/

19] Zhong G, Wang Y, Zhang Y, Guo JJ, Zhao Y. *Smoking is associated with an increased risk of dementia: a meta-analysis of prospective cohort studies with investigation of potential effect modifiers.* PLoS One. 2015 Mar 12;10(3):e0118333. doi: 10.1371/journal.pone.0118333. Erratum in: PLoS One. 2015 Apr 13;10(4):e0126169. doi: 10.1371/journal.pone.0126169. PMID: 25763939; PMCID: PMC4357455.

https://pubmed.ncbi.nlm.nih.gov/25763939/

20] Cuperfain AB, Black SE, Fostoc M, Freedman M, Ma C, Rajji T, Strother S, Tang-Wai DF, Tartaglia MC, Kumar S, Research TC. *Delineating the Effects of Alcohol Use on Cognition in Individuals With Neurocognitive Disorders.* J Clin Psychiatry. 2025 Aug 6;86(3):24m15738. doi: 10.4088/JCP.24m15738. PMID: 40767839.

https://pubmed.ncbi.nlm.nih.gov/40767839/

21] Yu X, Wang J, Qin S, Du E, Yin Y, Shan E, Li X. *Dementia friendly communities: A concept analysis.* Arch Psychiatr Nurs. 2025 Aug;57:151895. doi: 10.1016/j.apnu.2025.151895. Epub 2025 May 28. PMID: 40816800.

https://pubmed.ncbi.nlm.nih.gov/40816800/

22] Centers for Disease Control and Prevention. (n.d.). *Preventing chronic diseases: What you can do now.*

https://www.cdc.gov/chronic-disease/prevention/index.html

23] Cleveland Clinic. (2024). *Mediterranean diet.*

https://my.clevelandclinic.org/health/articles/16037-mediterranean-diet

24] Estruch R, Ros E, Salas-Salvadó J, Covas MI, Corella D, Arós F, Gómez-Gracia E, Ruiz-Gutiérrez V, Fiol M, Lapetra J, Lamuela-Raventos RM, Serra-Majem L, Pintó X, Basora J, Muñoz MA, Sorlí JV, Martínez JA, Fitó M, Gea A, Hernán MA, Martínez-González MA; PREDIMED Study Investigators. *Primary Prevention of Cardiovascular Disease with a Mediterranean Diet Supplemented with Extra-Virgin Olive Oil or Nuts.* N Engl J Med. 2018 Jun 21;378(25):e34. doi: 10.1056/NEJMoa1800389. Epub 2018 Jun 13. PMID: 29897866.

https://pubmed.ncbi.nlm.nih.gov/29897866/

25] Gharby S, Asbbane A, Nid Ahmed M, Gagour J, Hallouch O, Oubannin S, Bijla L, Goh KW, Bouyahya A, Ibourki M. *Vegetable oil oxidation: Mechanisms, impacts on quality, and approaches to enhance shelf life.* Food Chem X. 2025 May 10;28:102541. doi: 10.1016/j.fochx.2025.102541. PMID: 40491699; PMCID: PMC12146556.

https://pubmed.ncbi.nlm.nih.gov/40491699/

26] Winstone JK, Pathak KV, Winslow W, Piras IS, White J, Sharma R, Huentelman MJ, Pirrotte P, Velazquez R. *Glyphosate infiltrates the brain and increases pro-inflammatory cytokine TNFa: implications for neurodegenerative disorders.* J Neuroinflammation. 2022 Jul 28;19(1):193. doi: 10.1186/s12974-022-02544-5. Erratum in: J Neuroinflammation. 2024 Jan 17;21(1):20. doi: 10.1186/s12974-023-02990-9. PMID: 35897073; PMCID: PMC9331154.

https://pubmed.ncbi.nlm.nih.gov/35897073/

27] Ma W, Zhao L, Zhou W. *Risk factors for multiple myeloma and its precursor diseases.* Zhong Nan Da Xue Xue Bao Yi Xue Ban. 2025 Apr 28;50(4):560-572. English, Chinese. doi: 10.11817/j.issn.1672-7347.2025.240594. PMID: 40785671; PMCID: PMC12329731.

https://pubmed.ncbi.nlm.nih.gov/40785671/

28] Boretti A. *Comprehensive risk-benefit assessment of chemicals: A case study on glyphosate.* Toxicol Rep. 2024 Nov 7;13:101803. doi: 10.1016/j.toxrep.2024.101803. PMID: 39606775; PMCID: PMC11600065.

https://pubmed.ncbi.nlm.nih.gov/39606775/

29] Environmental Working Group. (n.d.). EWG's 2025 *Clean Fifteen & Dirty Dozen lists.*

https://www.ewg.org

30] Martineau AR, Jolliffe DA, Hooper RL, Greenberg L, Aloia JF, Bergman P, Dubnov-Raz G, Esposito S, Ganmaa D, Ginde AA, Goodall EC, Grant CC, Griffiths CJ, Janssens W, Laaksi I, Manaseki-Holland S, Mauger D, Murdoch DR, Neale R, Rees JR, Simpson S Jr, Stelmach I, Kumar GT, Urashima M, Camargo CA Jr. *Vitamin D supplementation to prevent acute respiratory tract infections:*

systematic review and meta-analysis of indi-vidual participant data. BMJ. 2017 Feb 15;356:i6583. doi: 10.1136/bmj.i6583. PMID: 28202713; PMCID: PMC5310969.

https://pubmed.ncbi.nlm.nih.gov/28202713/

31] Al-Khalidi B, Kimball SM, Rotondi MA, Ardern CI. *Standardized serum 25-hydroxyvitamin D concentrations are inversely associated with cardiometabolic disease in U.S. adults: a cross-sectional analysis of NHANES, 2001-2010.* Nutr J. 2017 Feb 28;16(1):16. doi: 10.1186/s12937-017-0237-6. Erratum in: Nutr J. 2017 May 22;16(1):32. doi: 10.1186/s12937-017-0251-8. PMID: 28241878; PMCID: PMC5329954.

https://pubmed.ncbi.nlm.nih.gov/28241878/

32] Zeb F, Osaili T, Hashim M, Alkalbani N, Papandreou D, Cheikh Ismail L, Naja F, Radwan H, Hasan H, Obaid RS, Savvaidis I, AlBlooshi S, Alam I. *Effect of Vitamin D Supplementation on Human Gut Microbiota: A Systematic Review of Randomized Controlled Trials.* Nutr Rev. 2025 Jul 17:nuaf120. doi: 10.1093/nutrit/nuaf120. Epub ahead of print. PMID: 40673989.

https://pubmed.ncbi.nlm.nih.gov/40673989/

33] Yan Y, Guo Y, Li Y, Jiang Q, Yuan C, Zhao L, Mao S. *Vitamin D, Gut Microbiota, and Cancer Immunotherapy-A Potentially Effective Crosstalk.* Int J Mol Sci. 2025 Jul 22;26(15):7052. doi: 10.3390/ijms26157052. PMID: 40806182; PMCID: PMC12346249.

https://pubmed.ncbi.nlm.nih.gov/40806182/

34] Grant WB, Al Anouti F, Boucher BJ, Dursun E, Gezen-Ak D, Jude EB, Karonova T, Pludowski P. *A Narrative Review of the Evidence for Variations in Serum 25-Hydroxyvitamin D Concentration Thresholds for Optimal Health.* Nutrients. 2022 Feb 2;14(3):639. doi: 10.3390/nu14030639. PMID: 35276999; PMCID: PMC8838864.

https://pubmed.ncbi.nlm.nih.gov/35276999/

35] Office of Dietary Supplements. (n.d.). *Vitamin D: Fact sheet for health professionals.* National Institutes of Health.

https://ods.od.nih.gov/factsheets/VitaminD-HealthProfessional/

36] van Ballegooijen AJ, Pilz S, Tomaschitz A, Grübler MR, Verheyen N. *The Synergistic Interplay between Vitamins D and K for*

Bone and Cardiovascular Health: A Narrative Review. Int J Endocrinol. 2017;2017:7454376. doi: 10.1155/2017/7454376. Epub 2017 Sep 12. PMID: 29138634; PMCID: PMC5613455.

https://pmc.ncbi.nlm.nih.gov/articles/PMC5613455/

37] Rusu ME, Bigman G, Ryan AS, Popa DS. *Investigating the Effects and Mechanisms of Combined Vitamin D and K Supplementation in Postmenopausal Women: An Up-to-Date Comprehensive Review of Clinical Studies.* Nutrients. 2024 Jul 20;16(14):2356. doi: 10.3390/nu16142356. PMID: 39064799; PMCID: PMC11279569.

https://pubmed.ncbi.nlm.nih.gov/39064799/

38] Liu T, Wang J, Ren C, Yu R, Fu C. *Association between magnesium depletion score and atherosclerotic cardiovascular disease: Findings from NHANES 2005 to 2018.* Medicine (Baltimore). 2025 Aug 15;104(33):e43914. doi: 10.1097/MD.0000000000043914. PMID: 40826784; PMCID: PMC12367052.

https://pubmed.ncbi.nlm.nih.gov/40826784/

39] Wang X, Zeng Z, Wang X, Zhao P, Xiong L, Liao T, Yuan R, Yang S, Kang L, Liang Z. *Magnesium Depletion Score and Metabolic Syndrome in US Adults: Analysis of NHANES 2003 to 2018.* J Clin Endocrinol Metab. 2024 Nov 18;109(12):e2324-e2333. doi: 10.1210/clinem/dgae075. PMID: 38366015; PMCID: PMC11570370.

https://pubmed.ncbi.nlm.nih.gov/38366015/

40] Chen M, Xue R, Zhang M, Zhang J, Zheng J, Ye D, Sun J. *Magnesium Depletion Score as a Novel Predictor of Cognitive Impairment: A Population-Based Cross-Sectional Study From NHANES.* J Am Med Dir Assoc. 2025 Jul 25;26(9):105776. doi: 10.1016/j.jamda.2025.105776. Epub ahead of print. PMID: 40659052.

https://pubmed.ncbi.nlm.nih.gov/40659052/

41] Zhao T, Li C, Wang H, Li J, Wang C, Gao Z, Du J, Teng W, Shan Z. *Effects of Maternal Iodine Deficiency in Women with Mild Thyroid Dysfunction During Early Pregnancy on Mental and Motor Growth of Their Offspring During Levothyroxine Treatment.* Biol Trace Elem Res. 2025 Sep 4. doi: 10.1007/s12011-025-04810-y. Epub ahead of print. PMID: 40903653.

https://pubmed.ncbi.nlm.nih.gov/40903653/

Chapter 15 – Living Your Healthiest Life

1] Garmany A, Terzic A. *Global Healthspan-Lifespan Gaps Among 183 World Health Organization Member States.* JAMA Netw Open. 2024;7(12):e2450241. doi:10.1001/jamanetworkopen.2024.50241

https://jamanetwork.com/journals/jamanetworkopen/fullarticle/2827753

2] Grgic J, Garofolini A, Orazem J, Sabol F, Schoenfeld BJ, Pedisic Z. *Effects of Resistance Training on Muscle Size and Strength in Very Elderly Adults: A Sys-tematic Review and Meta-Analysis of Random-ized Controlled Trials.* Sports Med. 2020 Nov;50(11):1983-1999. doi: 10.1007/s40279-020-01331-7. PMID: 32740889.

https://pubmed.ncbi.nlm.nih.gov/32740889/

3] Nose D, Shiga Y, Takahashi RU, Yamamoto Y, Suematsu Y, Ku-wano T, Sugihara M, Kanda M, Tahara H, Miura SI. *Association Be-tween Telomere G-Tail Length and Coronary Artery Disease or Statin Treatment in Patients With Cardiovascular Risks - A Cross-Sectional Study.* Circ Rep. 2023 Jul 11;5(8):338-347. doi: 10.1253/circrep.CR-23-0038. PMID: 37564879; PMCID: PMC10411992.

https://pubmed.ncbi.nlm.nih.gov/37564879/

4] Luealai P, Pongcharoen T, On-Nom N, Suttisansanee U, Temviri-yanukul P, Kriengsinyos W, Khemthong C, Chupeerach C. *Shorten-ing Leukocyte Telomere Length Associated With Elevated Blood Dia-betes-Related Cardiovascular Risk Factor in Thai Adolescents.* Food Sci Nutr. 2025 Aug 5;13(8):e70546. doi: 10.1002/fsn3.70546. PMID: 40772020; PMCID: PMC12325094.

https://pubmed.ncbi.nlm.nih.gov/40772020/

5] Verma AK, Singh P, Al-Saeed FA, Ahmed AE, Kumar S, Kumar A, Dev K, Dohare R. *Unravelling the role of telomere shortening with ageing and their potential association with diabetes, cancer, and re-lated lifestyle factors.* Tissue Cell. 2022 Dec;79:101925. doi: 10.1016/j.tice.2022.101925. Epub 2022 Sep 12. PMID: 36137363.

https://pubmed.ncbi.nlm.nih.gov/36137363/

6] Rodríguez-Fernández B, González-Escalante A, Genius P, E Ev-ans T, Ortiz-Romero P, Minguillón C, Kollmorgen G, Ashton NJ,

Zetterberg H, Blennow K, Gispert JD, Navarro A, Suárez-Calvet M, Sala-Vila A, Crous-Bou M, Vilor-Tejedor N; ALFA Study. *Longitudinal association of shorter leukocyte telomere length with CSF biomarker dynamics across early Alzheimer's disease stages in at-risk individuals.* EBioMedicine. 2025 Aug 19;119:105886. doi: 10.1016/j.ebiom.2025.105886. Epub ahead of print. PMID: 40834628; PMCID: PMC12395440.

https://pubmed.ncbi.nlm.nih.gov/40834628/

7] Polom J, Boccardi V. Employing Nutrition to Delay Aging*: A Plant-Based Telomere-Friendly Dietary Revolution.* Nutrients. 2025 Jun 14;17(12):2004. doi: 10.3390/nu17122004. PMID: 40573115; PMCID: PMC12196515.

https://pubmed.ncbi.nlm.nih.gov/40573115/

8] Sun L, Zhang T, Luo L, Yang Y, Wang C, Luo J. *Exercise delays aging: evidence from telomeres and telomerase -a systematic review and meta-analysis of randomized controlled trials.* Front Physiol. 2025 Jun 26;16:1627292. doi: 10.3389/fphys.2025.1627292. PMID: 40642293; PMCID: PMC12241061.

https://pubmed.ncbi.nlm.nih.gov/40642293/

9] Huang X, Lv J, Zhu D, Peng H, Yu T. *Effectiveness of mindfulness-based interventions on inflammaging: a systematic review and meta-analysis.* Biogerontology. 2025 Jul 18;26(4):145. doi: 10.1007/s10522-025-10287-y. PMID: 40679650.

https://pubmed.ncbi.nlm.nih.gov/40679650/

10] Rönne-Petersén L, Niemi M, Walach H, Lavebratt C, Yang LL, Gerdle B, Ghafouri B, Falkenberg T. *Exploring emotional well-being, spiritual, religious and personal beliefs and telomere length in chronic pain patients-A pilot study with cross-sectional design.* PLoS One. 2024 Sep 4;19(9):e0308924. doi: 10.1371/journal.pone.0308924. PMID: 39231146; PMCID: PMC11373805.

https://pubmed.ncbi.nlm.nih.gov/39231146/

11] Eşel G, Olguner Eker Ö, Amraliyev A, Asdemir A, Biçer EÖ, Badur Mermer D, Dündar M, Eşel E, İsmailoğulları S. *Telomere length in sleep disorders.* Exp Gerontol. 2025 Oct 1;209:112851. doi: 10.1016/j.exger.2025.112851. Epub 2025 Jul 31. PMID: 40752890.

https://pubmed.ncbi.nlm.nih.gov/40752890/

12] Chen D, Tam WWS, Zhang J, Lu J, Wu VX. *Association between the inflammageing biomarkers and clinical outcomes amongst the community-dwelling middle-aged and older adults: A systematic review and meta-analysis.* Ageing Res Rev. 2025 Aug;110:102811. doi: 10.1016/j.arr.2025.102811. Epub 2025 Jun 23. PMID: 40562315.

https://pubmed.ncbi.nlm.nih.gov/40562315/

13] Franceschi C, Olivieri F, Moskalev A, Ivanchenko M, Santoro A. *Toward precision interventions and metrics of inflammaging.* Nat Aging. 2025 Aug;5(8):1441-1454. doi: 10.1038/s43587-025-00938-7. Epub 2025 Aug 14. PMID: 40813813.

https://pubmed.ncbi.nlm.nih.gov/40813813/

14] Gaziev AI, Abdullaev S, Podlutsky A. *Mitochondrial function and mitochondrial DNA maintenance with advancing age.* Biogerontology. 2014;15(5):417-38. doi: 10.1007/s10522-014-9515-2. Epub 2014 Jul 12. PMID: 25015781.

https://pubmed.ncbi.nlm.nih.gov/25015781/

15] Pinto M, Moraes CT. *Mechanisms linking mtDNA damage and aging.* Free Radic Biol Med. 2015 Aug;85:250-8. doi: 10.1016/j.freeradbiomed.2015.05.005. Epub 2015 May 13. PMID: 25979659; PMCID: PMC4508218.

https://pubmed.ncbi.nlm.nih.gov/25979659/

16] Valero T. *Mitochondrial biogenesis: pharmacological approaches.* Curr Pharm Des. 2014;20(35):5507-9. doi: 10.2174/138161282035140911142118. PMID: 24606795.

https://pubmed.ncbi.nlm.nih.gov/24606795/

17] Kakara R, Bergen G, Burns E, Stevens M. *Nonfatal and Fatal Falls Among Adults Aged ≥65 Years* - United States, 2020-2021. MMWR Morb Mortal Wkly Rep. 2023 Sep 1;72(35):938-943. doi: 10.15585/mmwr.mm7235a1. PMID: 37651272.

https://pubmed.ncbi.nlm.nih.gov/37651272/

18] Hoyt, J. (n.d.). *Nursing home costs in 2025.* SeniorLiving.org. https://www.seniorliving.org/nursing-homes/costs/

Chapter 16 – Patient Empowerment

1] Parmar J, L'Heureux T, Anderson S, Lobchuk M, Charles L, Pollard C, Powell L, Chaudhuri ER, Fawcett-Arsenault J, Mosaico S, Sim C, Walker P, Shapkin K, Weir C, Sproule L, Strickfaden M, Tarnowski G, Lee J, Cameron C. *Bridging the Care Gap: Integrating Family Caregiver Partnerships into Healthcare Provider Education. Healthcare (Basel).* 2025 Aug 4;13(15):1899. doi: 10.3390/healthcare13151899. PMID: 40805932; PMCID: PMC12346123.

https://pubmed.ncbi.nlm.nih.gov/40805932/

2] Keehan SP, Fiore JA, Poisal JA, et al. *National Health Expenditure Projections, 2024–33: Spending Growth Outpaces Economic Growth.* Health Affairs. 2024;43(8):1099-1108. doi:10.1377/hlthaff.2024.00428

https://pubmed.ncbi.nlm.nih.gov/40561359/

Chapter 17 – The HOPE Blueprint For Success

1] ARA, Integrative and Functional Medicine, ya Shah Kapoon, MD. *A Closer Look at the 5R Protocol for Improved Gut Health, and How It Can Benefit You.* No author or date. Collected 31st Oct. 2025.

https://www.araintegrative.com/blog/a-closer-look-at-the-5r-protocol-for-improved-gut-health-and-how-it-can-benefit-you

2] The Institute for Functional Medicine, *Gut & Microbiome Health,* no author or date. Collected 31st October 2025.

https://www.ifm.org/gut-microbiome-health

www.ingramcontent.com/pod-product-compliance
Lightning Source LLC
Chambersburg PA
CBHW071918150726
47999CB00001B/31